The *AIDS* Pandemic

STUDIES IN SOCIAL MEDICINE

ALLAN M. BRANDT AND LARRY R. CHURCHILL, EDITORS

The *AIDS*

Pandemic

Complacency, Injustice, and
Unfulfilled Expectations

Lawrence O. Gostin

Foreword by Michael Kirby

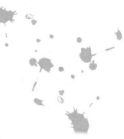

The University of North Carolina Press
Chapel Hill and London

Designed by April Leidig-Higgins
Set in Monotype Garamond by Copperline Book Services, Inc.
Manufactured in the United States of America

This book was published with the assistance of the William Rand Kenan Jr. Fund of the University of North Carolina Press.

The paper in this book meets the guidelines for permanence and durability of the Committee on Production Guidelines for Book Longevity of the Council on Library Resources.

Library of Congress Cataloging-in-Publication Data
Gostin, Larry O. (Larry Ogalthorpe)
The AIDS pandemic: complacency, injustice, and unfulfilled expectations / Lawrence O. Gostin; foreword by Michael Kirby.
   p. cm.— (Studies in social medicine)
Includes bibliographical references and index.
ISBN 0-8078-2830-0 (cloth: alk. paper)
1. AIDS (Disease)—Social aspects. 2. AIDS (Disease)—
Government policy.
   [DNLM: 1. Acquired Immunodeficiency Syndrome.
2. HIV Infections. 3. Disease Outbreaks—history.
4. Jurisprudence. 5. Public Policy. WC 503 G682a 2003]
I. Title. II. Series.
RA643.8.G675 2003
362.1'969792—dc22   2003016078

08 07 06 05 04 5 4 3 2 1

Contents

Part 3. Policy, Politics, and Ethics

Part 4. Special Populations

Part 5. AIDS in the World

Illustrations

Figures, Tables, and Maps

Figures

Tables

Maps

Foreword

Something New

It is only twenty years since HIV/AIDS burst upon the world. Hard now for us to imagine a world free of it. It crept up on us. Soon its awful reality was everywhere.

I first heard about it in a gay newspaper in Sydney early in the 1980s. Stories began to appear about a strange new condition among gay men in the United States, especially San Francisco. The weird symptoms seemed exotic and therefore not too troubling. Early comments from the Centers for Disease Control and Prevention suggested that the phenomenon might be linked with the use of the recreational drug amyl nitrite.

From such small beginnings and tiny news stories the problem soon expanded. By 1982, the acronym AIDS had been adopted. By 1984, Luc Montagnier and Robert Gallo had isolated the virus. By 1985, a test was available to determine the presence of the virus in human blood. Soon friends began to manifest the symptoms. The quiet confidence that had been carried along by the post-Kinsey sexual revolution, the belief that with knowledge of social facts would come acceptance of sexual reality and law reform, began to fade. Then came the funerals.

For a time, at least in gay circles in countries such as Australia and the United States, scarcely a month went by but another friend acknowledged that he was living with HIV. One by one friends were taken to the hospital. Sitting with them, by their bedside, it was impossible not to feel empathy. One knew that there, but for the grace of God or luck, was oneself. Brave assertions that we would overcome, optimistic assurance that a cure was just around the corner, naive faith in the power of will over the virus crumbled in the face of the realities. The dreadful truth was that friends were dying. Most of them should have been in the bloom of youth.

The funerals were highly charged. Typically, the participants were divided. On one side sat the grieving biological family, holding an image of their lost member as they knew him. On the other side was another family of more recent friends who knew a different image. They knew, and possibly shared, the underground of sexual truth or drug use through which the virus had been acquired. Sometimes the two sides reached out to each other to understand what was happening. Often they did not. Through fear, ignorance, and occasional hate, they went their separate ways, each keeping in mind a different memory of their friends.

It is essential to say such personal things at the opening of this book. It is about an extraordinary epidemic. But HIV/AIDS is not just another medical condition—like malaria, influenza, or tuberculosis. It is a force more powerful than all the nuclear blasts. It brings together the dynamics of life-threatening illnesses, sex and drugs topped off too often with death. Fear has propelled many of those with the power to respond into cowardly silence, hypocritical condemnation, or banal words not followed by action.

It is important to speak the personal things about the human side of HIV/AIDS for two further reasons. This epidemic has led to terrible suffering, now in every corner of the world. It continues to eat away at human beings everywhere. The infected are children and brothers, aunts and teachers, judges and garbage collectors, farmers and street children. Their suffering is human suffering. It afflicts them and burdens their families, their communities, and the world. It is all too easy to be dispassionate about a pandemic of millions. We have seen evidence of similar indifference in earlier reactions to genocide and to human hunger, homelessness, and political oppression. It is when HIV/AIDS is translated into human terms and one comes to know friends living in the epicenter of the epidemic that feelings are aroused.

This is what happened to me. By the early 1980s, I began to involve myself in Australian responses to HIV/AIDS I went to conferences. I described the good and the bad that was happening in other lands, especially the United States. I supported the brave decisions of the Australian government, spurred on by AIDS organizations, to tackle the epidemic imaginatively. I began to attend international meetings. I encountered many of those who, like the author of this book, took a leadership role in developing the global response to HIV/AIDS. I met Jonathan Mann, and he appointed me to the Global Commission on AIDS.

To know and to have experienced suffering should cause any moral being to want to do something, however inadequate, to relieve the pain and prevent its extension. So this is another reason why it is vital to read every page of this book remembering that it is a page about individuals and their families. It is not just about statistics and political theories, legal and medical problems. It is about human beings. Whenever we forget this we lose our sense of perspective. We also risk losing the dynamic that will propel us to defeat HIV/AIDS through social and eventually medical means.

The AIDS Paradox

Jonathan Mann is properly celebrated in these pages. What might have been a quiet, but interesting life as an epidemiologist in Central Africa was converted, by a series of chances, into a remarkable force for seeing connections essential to the struggle to contain HIV/AIDS and to relieve its manifestations.

A chance meeting between Jonathan Mann and the then director general of the World Health Organization (WHO), Halfden Mahler, in the Congo during a thunderstorm led to Mann's appointment as the first director of the Global Programme on AIDS. As this book tells it, he started duties with nothing but a tiny office and a Swiss secretary. But under his dynamic leadership the response to HIV/AIDS soon became the biggest program in WHO's history.

It was Jonathan Mann who taught the connections between public health and human rights. In the past (and in many places still) there is a sharp antithesis between these forces. In the name of public health, individual human rights are often subordinated. Yet, spurred on by other members of the Global Commission on AIDS, most notably June Osborn, then of the Michigan School of Public Health, Mann identified the AIDS paradox. Paradoxically, the most effective way to tackle the HIV/AIDS pandemic, given the limited medical tools, was to protect the human rights of the people most at risk of receiving and spreading the virus. It was a paradox because it defied the normal assumptions about public health. It was a brilliant insight because, at the start, behavior modification, ineffective without such rights protection, was just about all we had to tackle the spread of HIV. Stigmatization that came with diagnosis added grievously to the burdens of those living with HIV/AIDS. Responding in a rights-respecting way was something new, untried.

WHO endorsed Jonathan Mann's paradox. It began the difficult task of promoting these insights around the world. In most countries, as this book discloses, the leaders and their officials fell into embarrassed silence. Many and varied were the excuses for inaction. Every day, including in the United States, large numbers became infected and large numbers who were infected (or were at risk) suffered stigma and avoidable disadvantages.

Australia was one of the few countries that, from the start, embraced and boldly acted on the message that Mann was teaching. Words were translated into ideas. Honesty replaced silence. Education reached all sections of the community. Sex education was introduced in schools. Condom distribution was stepped up. Free needle exchange was promoted. Law reforms were passed to proscribe HIV discrimination. Laws on homosexual offenses, drugs, and commercial sex work were changed. The picture was by no means perfect. But compared to the reactions elsewhere, described in this book, Australia's response was admirable.

In January 2003 I joined in the first meeting of a Global Panel on Human Rights convened by the Joint United Nations Programme on AIDS (UNAIDS) in Geneva. This initiative has been taken by Peter Piot, the director of UNAIDS, who has assumed the mantle and extended the work of Jonathan Mann following Mann's tragic death in 1998. One of the participants in the panel, from a developing country, asked how we could be sure that the AIDS paradox really worked. How could we demonstrate to skeptical countries, whose social, religious, and cultural values were so different, that taking strong protective measures as urged by WHO/UNAIDS would have an impact on the spread of HIV and cut the frightening growth of the figures that threaten 100 million infections by 2006.

I answered this question with a simple graph (see Figure F-1). It illustrates more vividly than words the number of HIV infections in Australia before and after the radical initiatives were adopted in 1984. Although there may have been other relevant factors, the diagram represents a vivid illustration of the truth of the AIDS paradox.

As in other countries, the Australian graph after 2000 rises a little. This demonstrates the constant need to reinforce the messages of information and persuasion. Failures are inevitable in any attempt to influence human behavior in matters so intimate and important to identity as sexual, psychological,

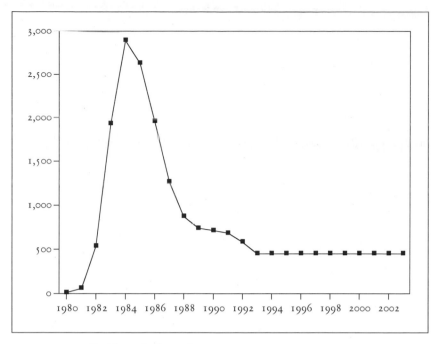

FIGURE F-1. HIV Incidence in Australia

and recreational conduct. But if, allowing for different social factors, a partly similar impact could be achieved in Sub-Saharan Africa, in India, and in China, we could turn the tide of this epidemic. We could save an immeasurable toll of suffering, stigma, and death.

Call to Action

Once it is appreciated that social and legal policies, together with education, can have a big impact on the HIV/AIDS pandemic, there is suddenly an appreciation that lawyers, politicians, and social scientists have things to teach. For once, they can play a constructive role in a global matter of public health. This is where this book may have its largest impact. It describes the contours of the pandemic, the stages into which its course can be divided, and the problems that it presents, particularly to developing countries with limited budgets for public health and many obstacles to speaking and acting resolutely and honestly in matters connected with sex and drugs.

The book describes the way in which cases involving HIV/AIDS have come before courts in the United States. Most developed, and many developing, countries have had their own such decisions. I have participated in them myself. The solutions offered by the courts vary in quality depending, in part, on the extent to which the judges are familiar with the realities of the pandemic and the truth of the AIDS paradox. The legal responses, in and out of the courts, bear out Professor Gostin's descriptions of the clashes we have witnessed over the directions that should be taken in resolving the interface of public health and individual rights.

However, court cases represent only the tip of the iceberg of a nation's law and policy. Most issues of that character never get near a courtroom. They are dealt with in the community. Yet, until now, that is where there has been much ignorance, fear, and misinformation. As the author points out, the basic policies for preventing the spread of HIV and AIDS are already clear and effective. So are the policies for reducing stigma and discrimination. All too often, what is lacking is the political will and commitment to safeguarding public health and human rights at home and abroad.

American readers (like those of other lands) may find it puzzling to discover some of the steps taken in their name by their government—for example:

1. The indecision over needle exchange, for which former president Bill Clinton has recently apologized.
2. The continued hypocrisy over "don't ask don't tell" in the military.
3. The lone resistance of the United States to the exclusion of generic drugs, essential for public health in developing countries, from international regimes on intellectual property.
4. The continued objection to condom promotion in the developing world as one of the strategies for safer sex.

President George W. Bush, in his State of the Union address in January 2003, promised new initiatives to tackle the HIV/AIDS epidemic in Sub-Saharan Africa. Whether these words will be translated into action remains to be seen. Whether the action will be informed by the AIDS paradox, and will target effectively the people and behaviors at special risk, only the future will tell.

Professor Gostin suggests that we are now in a third phase of the pandemic. He calls it a period of complacency, injustice, and unfulfilled expectations. This is a sobering assessment. Yet in these pages there is plenty of evidence for his assertion. The early optimism about a "magic bullet" cure or an effective vaccine within a couple of years has been dashed. In terms of medicine, we remain travelers on a hard and long road. Even the therapies that we have are expensive. They are not readily available in most epicenters of the pandemic. Even if generic equivalents could be freely available, there are countless problemoi problems of supply, monitoring, and adjustment in countries with few health care workers and overwhelming obstacles to effective treatment.

Yet it is impossible, even in the current phase, to put this book down without a sense of optimism. After all, there will be a fourth phase. Freed from other distractions, the world will turn its attention once again to HIV/AIDS. Better therapies will be discovered. Safe and powerful vaccines will be developed. Their advent will trigger a new determination voiced in this book by James Wolfensohn, president of the World Bank, in the epigraph to Chapter 1. We will win and stop the spread of AIDS. One day, a future generation will see a world free of the scourge of AIDS. But in the meantime there is work to be done.

In terms of history, twenty years is no more than the blinking of an eye. In Peter Piot's words, we are only at the beginning of this epidemic and at the earliest stages of humanity's fight against it. Many more human lives have been, and will be, lost through HIV/AIDS than through terrorism or weapons of mass destruction. If only something of the same resolution, commitment, and resources could be devoted to tackling HIV/AIDS, we would save lives, prevent suffering, and win this struggle more quickly.

It is proper to dream. It is part of our nature to have ideals. Today, many human ideals rest on the principles of the United Nations and the treaties of global human rights that have been built these past fifty years. But HIV/AIDS will not be tamed by dreams and ideals alone. The lesson of this book is that strong action is needed. Inevitably, that action must begin in earnest in the United States. It is in the United States that much of the effort for a cure and a vaccine will be centered. It is in the United States that the resources will be found to mobilize initiatives more effectively. Only in the United States is there the economic and political power that can breathe new life into such an international effort. Yet in the United States, as all too often among the developing countries, one finds the same impediments to tried and trusted strategies. Perhaps, in its own peculiar way, the United States of America is a second AIDS paradox.

Completing this book, not a few readers will feel discouraged. Yet objectively humanity has learned much in the past twenty years. It has learned not only about HIV/AIDS but also about epidemics more generally; about public health and human rights; about the role of politics, law, and social policy in changing human behavior quickly in the face of an unusual epidemic. We will win. But we will need insights and strategies, courage and imagination, resources and global leadership. Those who care will find these precious lessons in this important book. That is why it is so timely. In these pages we are called upon to choose between resolute action and frozen inaction, between life and death. Lawrence Gostin explains why, for the sake of humanity, there is no real choice.

The Honorable Justice Michael Kirby, AC, CMG
Justice of the High Court of Australia
One-time member of the WHO Global Commission on AIDS
Member of the UNAIDS Global Panel on Human Rights
Laureate of the UNESCO Prize for Human Rights Education

Canberra
March 2003

We live in a world threatened by unlimited destructive force, yet we share a vision of creative potential. .... AIDS shows us once again that silence, exclusion, and isolation of individuals, groups, or nations, creates a danger for us all. —**Jonathan M. Mann,** former director, WHO Global Programme on AIDS (1988)

Preface

The HIV/AIDS pandemic is probably the defining historical event of the late twentieth century and threatens to further define our future (see Figure P-1). The first cases of gay men with pneumocystis pneumonia, an unusual opportunistic infection, were reported in the United States in June 1981.[1] By 1982 the Centers for Disease Control and Prevention (CDC) established the term "Acquired Immune Deficiency Syndrome" (AIDS),[2] and within two years Luc Montagnier and Robert Gallo isolated the human retrovirus that causes AIDS;[3] the retrovirus would later be named the Human Immunodeficiency Virus (HIV). The following year the Food and Drug Administration (FDA) licensed the first test to identify antibodies to HIV, and blood banks began screening the nation's blood supply.[4]

In the United States, more than 800,000 cases of AIDS have been reported since the beginning of the epidemic and a half a million people have died of AIDS.[5] AIDS consistently has been one of the leading causes of death for persons aged twenty-five to forty-four. An estimated 900,000 Americans are living with HIV/AIDS,[6] and one-fourth of these people do not know they are in-

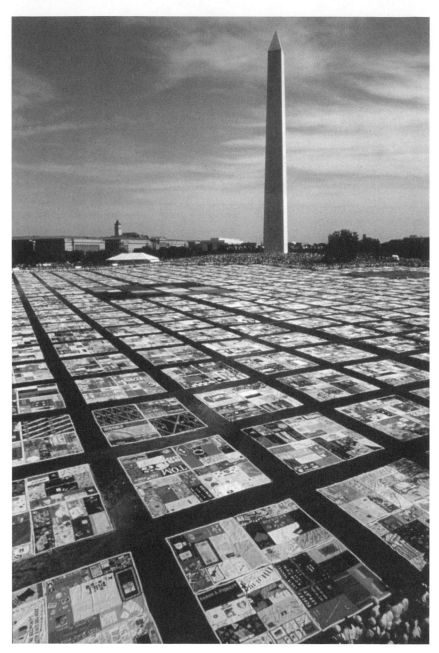

The AIDS Memorial Quilt allows friends and families to commemorate those they have lost to the AIDS epidemic. This image shows the quilt spread across the Mall in Washington, D.C., in 1992. The Memorial Quilt began in 1986 and now has more than 44,000 panels. Over 14 million people have visited the quilt at displays worldwide. (© 1992 The NAMES Project Foundation/The AIDS Memorial Quilt; photograph by Mark Thiessen)

fected.[7] Although public health officials predicted a reduction, HIV incidence rose between 1999 and 2001, especially among vulnerable populations.[8]

Globally, the picture is even more grim. Three-quarters of all countries report HIV/AIDS as their most significant demographic issue.[9] More than 20 million people have already died from AIDS and an estimated 42 million people are currently infected with HIV.[10] HIV/AIDS has been reported in all regions of the world, but the vast majority of people (95 percent) live in resource-poor countries, particularly within Sub-Saharan Africa. In less than ten years, many countries in southern Africa will see life expectancies fall to near thirty years of age, levels not experienced since the end of the nineteenth century.[11] Without AIDS, life expectancy in Botswana would be seventy-four years in 2010; with AIDS, it is projected to be twenty-seven.[12] Worldwide, nine out of ten persons living with HIV are unaware that they are infected.[13] AIDS is the leading cause of death in Africa and the fourth leading cause of death globally. Half of all adults living with HIV/AIDS worldwide are women,[14] who are more vulnerable to infection due to poverty, inadequate access to health care, and discrimination. Over 13 million children have lost their mothers or both parents to AIDS.[15] The media has vividly portrayed the tragic images of people living with HIV/AIDS, once young and vibrant, then weakened, desperately ill, and wasting away.

The epidemic not only causes illness and death, but also influences social norms. AIDS exposes the social fault lines of fear, hate, and discrimination. New phrases entered the English language such as "gay-related immune deficiency" (GRID) or "gay cancer" and "AIDS phobia," closely related to "homophobia."[16] AIDS fueled animus not only against persons living with the disease, but also against groups disproportionately affected—gays, injection drug users, and sex workers.

At the same time, the epidemic has inspired pride and a sense of purpose. Never before had the gay community come together so openly and with such determination to expose the evils of stigma, discrimination, and underfunded research. Never before had vulnerable communities been so politically active and service oriented. As early as 1982, the San Francisco AIDS Foundation and the Shanti Project developed a model of care emphasizing home- and community-based services. In 1983 the first AIDS Candlelight Memorial was held. Within two decades, four hundred cities and towns worldwide would hold similar memorials. In 1986 the first panel of the AIDS Memorial Quilt was created. New advocacy (e.g., ACT UP, AIDS Action Council, National Association of People with AIDS, National Minority AIDS Council), service (e.g., Gay Men's Health Crisis, San Francisco AIDS Foundation, AIDS Project Los Angeles, Whitman Walker Clinic District of Columbia), and funding (e.g., American Foundation

1981 CDC reports first cases of the illness that will be known as AIDS.

1982 National Institute of Health rejects proposed study to determine whether women get AIDS.

1983 First congressional hearings held on HIV/AIDS.

1984 Dr. Luc Montagnier in France and Dr. Robert Gallo in the United States isolate a new retrovirus, later known as Human Immunodeficiency Virus (HIV).

1985 HIV antibody test is licensed; First International Conference on AIDS; AIDS reported in every continent of the world.

1986 Clinical trials begin for antiretroviral drug AZT; first panel of the AIDS Memorial Quilt created; President Reagan first mentions the word AIDS in public.

1987 AIDS Clinical Trials Group (ACTG) formed; Presidential Commission on AIDS formed; AIDS Drug Assistance Program (ADAP) initiated to ensure the availability of medications; United States prohibits immigration of persons infected with HIV (PWAS).

1988 Women named the fastest-growing group of PWAS; FDA speeds up approval process for experimental drugs; first annual World AIDS Day commemorated; National Civil Rights Commission holds hearing on the "right" to discriminate against PWAS.

1989 Congress creates the National Commission on AIDS.

1990 Americans with Disabilities Act (ADA) enacted; first national Women and HIV Conference; CDC calls for end to U.S. restrictions on HIV-infected immigrants; Ryan White Comprehensive AIDS Resource Emergency (CARE) Act passes; 8 to 10 million HIV cases worldwide.

1991 CDC recommends restrictions on the practice of HIV-infected health care workers (HCWS), and Congress enacts law requiring states to take similar action; Congress enacts Housing Opportunities for People with AIDS (HOPWA) Act.

1992 President Clinton promises full funding of the Ryan White CARE Act and appointment of a national AIDS "czar."

1993 President Clinton establishes the White House Office of National AIDS Policy (ONAP); Clinton signs HIV immigration exclusion policy into law; CDC revises AIDS definition to include CD4 cell counts below 200 and cervical cancer.

1994 AIDS declared the leading cause of death for Americans ages 25 to 44; FDA approves oral HIV test; researchers find that perinatal HIV transmission dramatically reduced with treatment.

1995 First White House Conference on AIDS; Clinton establishes Presidential Advisory Council on HIV/AIDS.

1996 Congress approves higher spending on AIDS programs; viral load testing begins; Clinton signs a welfare reform bill that deprives countless numbers of PWAS of public benefits.

1997   CDC reports a 42 percent decrease in deaths due to AIDS.

1998   In *Bragdon v. Abbott*, the U.S. Supreme Court rules that ADA covers persons with asymptomatic HIV infection; Congress enacts the Ricky Ray Hemophilia Relief Fund Act; African Americans account for 49 percent of AIDS deaths; first large-scale human trials (Phase III) for an HIV vaccine.

1999   U.S. stops opposing South Africa's attempts to produce and/or purchase generic drugs, as long as South Africa adheres to existing world trade rules; IOM urges screening of all pregnant women.

2000   Ryan White CARE Act reauthorized; Congress enacts the Global AIDS and Tuberculosis Relief Act of 2000; UNAIDS estimates 40 million people are living with HIV/AIDS worldwide.

2001   Approximately 17 percent of Americans with HIV are in correctional facilities; generic drug manufacturers offer to produce discounted, generic forms of HIV/AIDS drugs.

2002   Secretary of State Colin L. Powell advocates the use of condoms to prevent the spread of HIV; USAID reports that the life expectancy in Botswana fell from 72 to 39 years due to AIDS.

2003   President George W. Bush announces $15 billion pledge for the global fight against HIV/AIDS; CDC recommends routine HIV screening in health care settings; the first Phase III AIDS vaccine fails to show evidence of efficacy.

Source: Adapted from timelines prepared by the Kaiser Family Foundation, Gay Men's Health Crisis, and New York State AIDS Institute.

for AIDS Research [AMFAR]) organizations emerged, while others experienced a resurgence (e.g., Lambda Legal Defense and Education Fund).

Vast social changes that took place in the late twentieth century led inexorably to legal changes. Legislators at the federal, state, and local levels enacted a spate of new laws. Some laws reflected society's worst instincts such as exclusion of HIV-infected immigrants, segregation of prisoners, and criminal sanctions against persons who knowingly transmit HIV infection. Other laws were protective, such as those requiring informed consent, privacy, and nondiscrimination. At the same time, the epidemic provoked litigation on almost every conceivable issue, including constitutional rights, social institutions, and personal and professional obligations.[17]

The AIDS epidemic has reached deeply into the political sphere. At times, politicians signaled their ignorance and antipathy through silence. The persistent refusal to speak about AIDS from the highest levels of government was soul-destroying for those fighting the disease. Other politicians displayed their irrational fears and biases through calls for shame and punishment of persons living with HIV/AIDS. A few lawmakers exemplified political strength by passing statutes such as the Ryan White CARE Act in 1990 (most recently reauthorized in 2000) to ensure an HIV/AIDS care infrastructure.

The AIDS epidemic also has had a detrimental effect on the economy. Many industries have lost workers in their most skilled and productive years of life. As the number of persons with the disease rose and the available treatment options expanded, the costs of treatment escalated. The nation had to devote resources to research and development, counseling, education, treatment, and services.

Perhaps most importantly, the United States has had to grapple with its role in the world as a political, military, and economic leader. Questions of humanitarian aid, patents for AIDS medications, international trade, and research ethics have become salient. In 2000 the U.S. government declared AIDS a national security threat.[18] However, it has failed to devote sufficient resources to poor countries, encourage the pharmaceutical sector to make drugs accessible, or work cooperatively with international agencies and nongovernmental organizations to reduce the global burden of the pandemic. For example, at a United Nations population conference in Bangkok in December 2002, the American delegation tried to block an endorsement of condom use to prevent HIV/AIDS. The consequences of this behavior in the international arena go beyond resentment and ridicule. Girls and young women often contract HIV because they are pressured into sex by older men. To deny them access to condoms and counseling about how to negotiate safe sex is a deadly strategy.[19]

In January 2003, in his State of the Union address, President George W. Bush announced $15 billion over the next five years to fight AIDS in twelve countries in Africa as well as Haiti and Guyana.[20] The declaration was met with elation, hope, and, given the administration's past policies, skepticism.[21] Time will tell if the promised funding is spent wisely in ways that will make a true impact on this global tragedy.

Three Phases of the HIV/AIDS Epidemic

The history of the AIDS epidemic in the United States can be roughly divided into three phases: Denial, Blame, and Punishment, 1981–87; Engagement and Mobilization, 1987–97; and Complacency, Injustice, and Unfulfilled Expectations (1997–present).

tively simple interventions to prevent HIV transmission such as health education and condom use have not been implemented in many poor countries. Pregnant women and infants often do not receive treatment that would dramatically reduce the risk of perinatal transmission. Less than 1 percent of persons living with HIV/AIDS in developing countries receive antiretroviral therapy.[51] More than ever, the AIDS pandemic has created two worlds—one with relatively low burdens of disease and sophisticated treatments and the other with staggering burdens and paltry health care resources. It was not until 2000 that the first international AIDS conference was held in a developing country. The Thirteenth International AIDS Conference in Durban, South Africa, took place under the slogan "Break the Silence."

In response to overwhelming global health problems, the United Nations in January 2002 established a Global Fund to Fight AIDS, Tuberculosis, and Malaria.[52] Yet pledges from industrial nations were far below United Nations expectations or Third World needs. President George Bush unveiled an International Mother and Child HIV Prevention Initiative in June 2002 but had actually cut bipartisan anti-AIDS funding provided by Congress.[53] President Bush's promise of $15 billion for global AIDS funding in 2003 could signal American willingness to finally make a difference. However, critics remain skeptical about the way the funds will be spent and the strings that may be attached.[54] It remains to be seen whether in the third decade of the HIV/AIDS pandemic, the world will respond or continue to tolerate injustice.

Organization of the Book

This book examines the social, legal, political, and ethical controversies surrounding AIDS in the early twenty-first century. I originally set out to provide a collection of essays about AIDS written over the span of two decades. These essays were originally published in legal, medical, and policy journals, as well as in books and reports on the subject. However, AIDS is so complex and dynamic that essays written years ago could not convey the modern dilemmas in politics, policy, and law. Consequently, I have rewritten and updated the chapters, providing a detailed descriptive and analytic account of the field in the early twenty-first century.

The book is divided into five parts: I. AIDS in the Courtroom; II. Rights and Dignity; III. Policy, Politics, and Ethics; IV. Special Populations; and V. AIDS in the World.

Part I. AIDS in the Courtroom

Part I gives an overview of AIDS policy, politics, and law and presents data from the AIDS Litigation Project (ALP). Chapter 1 places the AIDS epidemic in historical perspective, examines the positions of the major players, assesses contemporary policies, and predicts future directions. Chapters 2 and 3 describe the findings of the ALP, which tracked all significant court cases involving HIV/AIDS from the beginning of the epidemic through the 1990s. Chapter 2 considers the social impact of AIDS—the effect of litigation on social institutions, constitutional law, and interpersonal relationships. Chapter 3 discusses the role of litigation relating to personal privacy and discrimination. Taken together, the latter two chapters reveal the deep controversies surrounding HIV/AIDS that have played out in the nation's courtrooms.

Part II. Rights and Dignity

Part II begins a more in-depth examination of the use of law to safeguard the rights of persons living with HIV/AIDS. Chapter 4 looks at the role of international human rights in the AIDS pandemic, including civil, political, social, and economic rights. Chapter 5 considers health information privacy; it explores the conflict between confidentiality and privacy on the one hand and the right to know and the duty to warn on the other. In examining discrimination against persons living with HIV/AIDS, Chapter 6 reviews modern legislation and case law, notably the salient role of the Americans with Disabilities Act and HIV-specific antidiscrimination law at the state and local levels.

Part III. Policy, Politics, and Ethics

Part III covers the most contentious debates of the HIV/AIDS epidemic in the United States. This part seeks to use legal and ethical analyses to understand the politics and controversies that have permeated AIDS discourse. Chapter 7 examines proposals and policies for HIV testing and screening. It provides an analytic framework for evaluating testing and screening that pays close attention to science and public health, as well as ethics and human rights. Chapter 8 considers the thorny issue of HIV reporting. Reporting cases of CDC-defined AIDS to state health departments is routine and widely accepted, but reporting cases of HIV infection by name is politically charged. This chapter explains the importance of HIV surveillance and examines alternatives to named reporting, including the use of unique identifiers (UIS).

Chapter 9 discusses the many variations of partner notification, including classic governmental contact tracing programs, the duty of health care professionals to warn persons at risk, and the responsibility of persons infected with HIV to inform their partners. Chapter 10 deals with civil and criminal confinement. Given the fact that HIV cannot be transmitted casually, one might expect that civil and criminal confinement would not be seriously discussed. Yet politicians and the media often have argued for isolation or quarantine, and legislatures have enacted HIV-specific criminal laws. This chapter offers a critique of civil and criminal confinement of persons living with HIV/AIDS.

Part IV. Special Populations

Part IV covers the rights and obligations of groups at heightened risk or identified as having special responsibilities. Chapter 11 looks at the emotive issue of perpetrators and survivors of sexual assault. Survivors of sexual assault frequently fear contracting HIV infection. Although the risk is usually low, testing the accused as well as counseling and prophylaxis for the victim have become important and highly charged subjects. Chapter 12 is concerned with the rights and duties of HIV-infected health care workers (HCWs). In 1990 Kimberly Bergalis contracted HIV infection from her dentist, sparking major public debate. I was actively involved with the CDC at that time, and the ensuing CDC guidelines resulted in the exclusion of many HIV-infected HCWs from practicing exposure-prone procedures. More recent data have now shown the risk of HCW-to-patient transmission to be exceedingly low. This chapter presents my new position that HIV-infected HCWs should be permitted to practice as long as they can do so competently and safely.

Chapter 13 turns to perinatal transmission of HIV. Since the results of ACTG 076 were published in 1994, there has been extensive debate over the screening and treatment of pregnant women and newborns. This chapter examines this debate in light of Institute of Medicine (IOM) and CDC recommendations to reduce the risk of mother-to-infant transmission. Chapter 14 focuses on the interconnected epidemics of HIV/AIDS and drug dependency. Sharing drug-injection equipment poses a serious risk of HIV infection, leading many public health professionals to propose increased access to sterile needles and syringes. At the same time, many politicians have argued that needle exchanges and repeal of laws that criminalize possession of needles encourage drug use. This chapter shows why harm-reduction policies significantly reduce the risk of HIV/AIDS and do not increase drug use.

Part V reviews the global devastation of the HIV/AIDS pandemic. Chapter 15 discusses the U.S. policy of screening and exclusion of travelers and immigrants, one that activists have vigorously opposed to the point of boycotting AIDS conferences held in the United States. The chapter demonstrates why this American policy is ill-conceived from a public health and human rights perspective. Chapter 16, on the global HIV/AIDS pandemic, shows the enormous scope and unfair distribution of disease around the world. It also examines the central issues of HIV/AIDS in the world: the absence of political leadership, an international trade system that militates against access to affordable treatment in poor countries, and the ethics of international collaborative research. Finally, Chapter 17 offers reflections on the AIDS pandemic past, present, and future, focusing on AIDS law, policy, and politics in the United States and beyond.

The AIDS pandemic has reached deeply into all major spheres of modern life—public health, medicine, law, economics, and politics. The pandemic has transformed society and restructured ethical values. This book provides an account of the major themes of the pandemic during the last two decades and analyzes contemporary and future policy.

Working on AIDS with Friends and Partners: Acknowledging the Leaders

Having spent more than a decade in the United Kingdom as the head of the British Civil Liberties Union (National Council of Civil Liberties), as legal director of the National Association for Mental Health, and as a Fellow at Oxford University, I returned to the United States in the mid-1980s to work with William J. Curran at the Harvard School of Public Health. The late Professor Curran, who wrote an acclaimed series of columns on legal medicine for the *New England Journal of Medicine*, was a mentor.

During those early years, Harvard University was already gearing up to study the HIV/AIDS epidemic in America and globally. Harvey Fineberg, then dean of the School of Public Health, encouraged the faculty to work cooperatively on AIDS; Max Essex, an internationally renowned laboratory researcher, helped form the Harvard AIDS Institute (as of this writing directed by Richard Marlink); and prominent clinicians such as Jerry Groopman, Martin Hirsch, and Kenneth H. Mayer devoted their careers to serving persons living with HIV/AIDS. I had the privilege of working closely with young scholars and valued friends such as Allan Brandt and Paul Cleary at Harvard and Ronald Bayer at

Columbia, all of whom were beginning their brilliant careers in AIDS and public policy. Influenced by these and many other scholars, I began a period of sustained engagement in the world of AIDS.

When I arrived at Harvard in 1985, Secretary of Health and Human Services Margaret Heckler asked William Curran, Mary Clark, and me to write a report on AIDS law and policy in the United States.[55] That report predicted an explosion in legal activity that would unfold during the next decade, beginning with the first AIDS discrimination law enacted in Los Angeles. A study of global AIDS legislation for the World Health Organization (WHO) in 1990 revealed a similar pattern of legal and regulatory policy on AIDS in most regions of the world.[56] By 1992, Lane Porter and I had edited a volume on international law and AIDS for the American Bar Association (ABA).[57]

Work in the area of global AIDS policies required travel to populous countries where HIV/AIDS was newly emerging. In 1996 a delegation of experts visited Beijing, China, at the invitation of the minister of justice. The following year the prime minister and chief justice of India hosted a global AIDS conference in Delhi. During these visits we witnessed the poverty and lack of education that would lead to an explosive growth of the pandemic in Asia. In India, a working group led by Michael Kirby (the admired Australian High Court justice and global leader on AIDS) drafted the "Delhi Declaration" on the rights of persons living with HIV/AIDS.

The year after I arrived at Harvard, I visited my close friend Sev Fluss, then head of health legislation at the WHO in Geneva. He told me that a young American, Jonathan Mann, had just been appointed to run WHO's Global Programme on AIDS (GPA). When I met Dr. Mann in the summer of 1986, GPA was comprised of only him and a Swiss secretary. The Global Programme on AIDS eventually turned into the largest program in WHO's history.

During the rise of the GPA, Mann's strategy for curtailing the AIDS pandemic transformed. At first, he applied conventional ideas of education, screening, and partner notification. Later, he felt that persons at risk of HIV should have the means to protect themselves by possession of condoms and sterile injection equipment. Finally, he recognized that public health and human rights were inseparable ideas. People could not avoid risk without civil, political, social, and economic rights. Mann often illustrated this point by explaining that vulnerable women could not remain healthy if they were economically dependent on, or in fear of, their sex or needle-sharing partners.

In 1990, after a bitter dispute with then director general of WHO, Dr. Hiroshi Nakajima, Jonathan left the GPA to join the faculty at the Harvard School of Public Health. In 1993 he became the founding chair of Harvard's François-

Xavier Bagnoud Center for Health and Human Rights, where he established himself as one of the great figures in health and human rights in the twentieth century. I had the great fortune to teach the first class on health and human rights at Harvard with Dr. Mann and to collaborate with him on early papers on the intersection of these two great fields.[58] On September 2, 1998, after leaving Harvard, he and his wife, prominent AIDS researcher Mary Lou Clements-Mann, died in the Swiss Air 111 disaster on their way to Geneva. Jonathan was survived by his mother, Ida Mann, his first wife Marie-Paule, and his children Naomi, Lydia, and Aaron. In September 2001 Scott Burris, Zita Lazzarini, and I chaired an international conference on health and human rights in Philadelphia dedicated to the memory of Jonathan Mann.

The Harvard AIDS Institute provided an outlet for collaboration within the university. William Curran and I drafted the Harvard Model AIDS Legislation Project from 1988 to 1990.[59] That project proposed legal reforms on privacy and discrimination. Harvard legal scholars Martha Field and Kathleen Sullivan (as of this writing dean of Stanford Law School) joined in the model law project. I also chaired the track on social science, policy, and law for the Eighth International Conference on AIDS, held in Amsterdam in 1992, which was the first international AIDS conference to focus on social science and law.

From 1990 to 1996 I worked on the AIDS Litigation Project with Kathleen Flaherty, Zita Lazzarini, Lane Porter, and Hazel Sandomire. This project was originally funded by the National AIDS Program Office, of the Department of Health and Human Services (HHS),[60] led by James Allen, and then by the Henry J. Kaiser Family Foundation,[61] led by Drew E. Altman. The ALP summarized the case law, offered an analysis, and forecast the trends in AIDS law and policy.[62] The ALP revealed the fundamental misunderstandings of judges and legislators about HIV, its methods of transmission, and the most effective and humane policies. As a result, colleagues and I engaged in a series of workshops to train leaders in the judicial and legislative branches. This training was done in collaboration with the National Judicial College, the State Justice Institute, and the Agency for Healthcare Research and Quality.

The training mission expanded to include AIDS and human rights, and audiences grew to comprise WHO, CDC, and the U.S. Agency for International Development (USAID).[63] The human rights training at USAID became a model. This training began in 1997 with Jonathan Mann and continued in 2000 with Stephen Marks and Sofia Gruskin of the François-Xavier Bagnoud Center for Health and Human Rights. Clif Cortez and Rebecca Cook from the University of Toronto also participated in the USAID training.

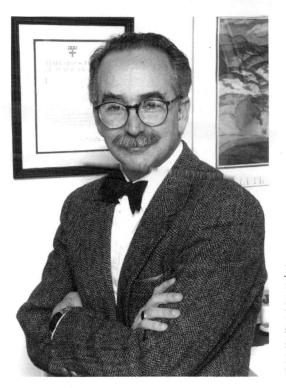

Jonathan Mann (1947–98), founding director, World Health Organization's Global Programme on AIDS (1986) and François-Xavier Bagnoud Center for Health and Human Rights at Harvard University (1993).

I have been fortunate to work with the major public health agencies in the United States and globally. These organizations frequently hold consultations and advisory meetings to develop AIDS policies. I served in several capacities for the CDC under able directors such as William Roper, David Satcher, Jeffrey P. Koplan, David Fleming, and Julie Gerberding. I served as a member of the CDC National Advisory Committee on HIV and STD (Sexually Transmitted Disease) Prevention, chaired at various times by Kristine Gebbie, Mark Maggenheim, and Robert E. Fullilove. I engaged in numerous policy-making projects with the CDC, particularly the National Center for HIV, STD, and TB (Tuberculosis) Prevention, with leading public health professionals such as James Curran, Helene Gayle, Kevin DeCock, and Ronald O. Valdiserri. I had the opportunity to work on stimulating projects including research ethics (James Buehler, Marjorie Spears, and Dixie Snyder), the Model State Public Health Privacy Act (Patricia Fleming, David R. Holtgrave, and John W. Ward),[64] partner notification (Gary R. West),[65] HIV-infected health care workers (David Bell and Robert Janssen), and injection drug users (T. Stephen Jones).[66] Perhaps most of all, I worked closely with the Office of the General Counsel (Gene Matthews and Verla Neslund) and the public health law program (Edward L. Baker, Richard A. Goodman, Martha Katz, and Anthony Moulton). Several experts at CDC reviewed this book, including Patricia Fleming, Mary Glenn Fowler, Ida Onorato, and Thomas Peterman. I prepared several policy reviews for NIH, including a report on law and ethics for international collaborative HIV research.[67] I currently serve on the Office of AIDS Research Advisory Council of NIH. I am particularly grateful for the opportunity to work for many years with the indefatigable head of the National Institute of Allergy and Infectious Diseases, Anthony S. Fauci.

I have been privileged to serve on several boards and advisory committees for the Joint United Nations Programme on AIDS (previously WHO's Global Programme on AIDS), working with Peter Piot, Daniel Tarantola, Susan Timberlake, and Helen Wachirs. In 1997 an expert committee drafted the United Nations Guidelines on HIV/AIDS and Human Rights (E/CN.4/1997/37) (amended in 2002 by UNAIDS/02.49E).

Through the years, I have had the pleasure of working with some of the great advocates and innovators in the field of HIV/AIDS such as A. Cornelius Baker, Scott Burris, Chai Feldblum, Jeffrey Levi, William Rubenstein, David Schulman, and David W. Webber. Sadly, many valiants have lost their battle with AIDS such as Terry Beirn (who worked on Senator Edward Kennedy's staff) and Tom Stoddard (who worked on a Hastings Center AIDS project). I am particularly grateful to David Schulman for his careful prepublication review of this book.

I received generous funding for my work on HIV/AIDS from UNAIDS and the WHO, Department of Health and Human Services, Centers for Disease Control and Prevention, National Institutes of Health, AMFAR, and Henry J. Kaiser Family Foundation.

My colleague, James G. Hodge Jr., ably led a team of bright and energetic Fellows, students, and staff at Georgetown University Law Center, including Stephen Barbour, Dan Cooper, Gabe Eber, Lance Gable, Megan Gunther, Kevin Haeberle, Laura Kidd, Jane Kim, Katherine Kirking, Jennifer Leonard, Marguerite Middaugh, and Anna Selden. I want to single out Lesley Stone, Lauren Marks, and Kathryn Watson for their outstanding work in efficiently coordinating the research and editing of the book. I want to thank Professor Denis Galligan for giving me the opportunity to work on this book during my year at the Centre for Socio-Legal Studies at Oxford University.

The editors for this book series, Allan M. Brandt and Larry R. Churchill, originally approached me with the idea for this volume. Sian Hunter, my editor at the University of North Carolina Press, offered advice and encouragement throughout the process. I am most grateful to each of them.

My wife Jean and children, Bryn and Kieran, have been by my side throughout I love them and thank them for all of their love and support.

Lawrence O. Gostin, J.D., LL.D. (Hon.)
Professor and Director, Center for Law and the Public's
Health at Georgetown and Johns Hopkins Universities

Washington, D.C.
March 2003

Abbreviations

ABA	American Bar Association
ACLU	American Civil Liberties Union
ACTG	AIDS Clinical Trials Group
ADA	Americans with Disabilities Act
ADEA	Age Discrimination and Employment Act
AIDS	Acquired Immune Deficiency Syndrome
ALP	AIDS Litigation Project
AZT	azidothymidine or zidovudine
BCIS	Bureau of Citizenship and Immigration Services (formerly the INS), Department of Homeland Security
CARE	Ryan White Comprehensive AIDS Resources Emergency Act of 1990
CDC	Centers for Disease Control and Prevention
CESCR	United Nations Committee on Economic, Social, and Cultural Rights
CIOMS	Council of International Organisations of Medical Sciences
DOD	Department of Defense
DOS	Department of State

EEOC	Equal Employment Opportunity Commission
EIA	enzyme immuno-assay
ERISA	Employee Retirement Income Security Act
ESAP	Expanded Syringe Access Demonstration Program
FDA	Food and Drug Administration
GATT	General Agreement on Tariffs and Trade
GPA	Global Programme on AIDS
GRID	"gay-related immune deficiency"
HAART	highly active antiretroviral therapy
HBV	hepatitis B virus
HCV	hepatitis C virus
HCW	health care worker
HHS	U.S. Department of Health and Human Services
HIPAA	Health Insurance Portability and Accountability Act of 1996
HIV	human immunodeficiency virus
HOPE	Health Omnibus Programs Extension
HOPWA	Housing Opportunities for People with AIDS
ICCPR	International Covenant on Civil and Political Rights
ICESCR	International Covenant on Economic, Social, and Cultural Rights
IDU	injection drug user
IND	Treatment Investigational New Drug
INS	Immigration and Naturalization Service, U.S. Department of Justice
IOM	Institute of Medicine, National Academy of Sciences
IRB	Institutional Review Board
LAV	Lymphadenopathy-associated virus
MDPA	Model Drug Paraphernalia Act
MSM	men who have sex with men
NIH	National Institutes of Health
OAR	Office of AIDS Research
OHCHR	Office of the High Commissioner for Human Rights, United Nations
OSHA	Occupational Safety and Health Administration
PCT	placebo-controlled trial
PTSD	post-traumatic stress disorder
SEP	syringe exchange program
SNA	Social Network Analysis
SSA	Social Security Administration
STD	sexually transmitted disease

TAC	Treatment Action Campaign
TB	tuberculosis
TRIPS	Agreement on Trade-Related Aspects of Intellectual Property Rights
UAC	Uganda AIDS Commission
UDHR	Universal Declaration of Human Rights
UI	unique identifier
UNAIDS	Joint United Nations Programme on AIDS
USAID	U.S. Agency for International Development
USPHS	U.S. Public Health Service
WHO	World Health Organization
WTO	World Trade Organization

Part 1 AIDS in the Courtroom

We can win. We can stop the spread of AIDS. We can prevent new infections. We can [better] treat those who suffer. In time, we can hope to find a cure. I propose to confidently hold up the prospect of a world free of AIDS.—**James D. Wolfensohn,** president, World Bank (2001)

Chapter 1

AIDS Policy, Politics, and Law in Context

This introductory chapter places the principal themes of the book in context. It frames the major AIDS policy debates retrospectively and outlines their current and ongoing implications. This discussion will put the AIDS epidemic in historical perspective, examine the positions of the major players, assess contemporary policies, and predict future directions. AIDS policies are covered in greater depth, and with more detailed support, in the following series of essays. This chapter follows the book's five-part organization: AIDS in the Courtroom; Rights and Dignity; Policy, Politics, and Ethics; Special Populations; and AIDS in the World.

AIDS in the Courtroom

The first essay (Chapter 2) examines AIDS in the courtroom and presents data from the U.S. AIDS Litigation Project (ALP). The ALP is a historically important

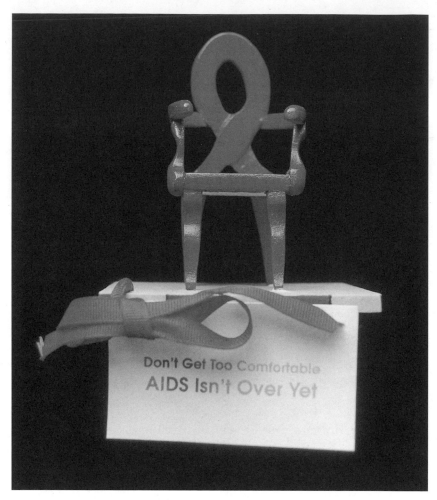

Originating from the United States, the red ribbon has become an international symbol for the fight against AIDS. In 2000 Michael Ransom carved the AIDS Ribbon Chair as a symbol of support in this indiscriminate pandemic.

event because it systematically tracked all significant court cases involving HIV/AIDS for more than a decade. Twentieth-century America is well known for being a highly litigious society. Even so, there had never been a disease that provoked as much litigation as HIV/AIDS. The ALP tracked several thousand court and human rights cases on almost every imaginable topic. Just to give a few illustrations, civil litigation was brought in the fields of torts, family law, and constitutional law. Litigation penetrated most social institutions, ranging from prisons to the blood supply system. Even judges found themselves as defendants. The fact patterns in these cases vividly illustrate the social upheaval wrought by this modern pandemic.

Torts

Contracting an infectious disease used to be perceived as a matter of chance or inadvertent misfortune. But in the first decade of the HIV/AIDS epidemic, it was not uncommon for an exposed person to search for fault and, with it, liability. Claims of lack of due care, even bad faith, by those who were exposed to HIV found their way to the courtroom. The depth of mistrust spanned many relationships: patients against physicians, health care professionals against hospitals, and sex partners against their lovers. Tort litigation was instigated, for example, concerning false diagnoses of HIV infection, failure to diagnose, and fear of exposure. The judiciary wrestled with the issue of whether to provide a remedy for those who were not actually harmed but exhibited fear and anxiety resulting from a perceived exposure to infection. For the most part, the courts required some actual harm before awarding damages to ensure that the plaintiff's case was genuine.[1]

Family Law

The potential for HIV/AIDS to stir conflict within the family is apparent. Infection can be transmitted sexually and perinatally, affecting the spouse and future offspring. The attachment of blame to persons living with HIV/AIDS can be used as a weapon in divorce, custody, and visitation disputes. Finally, the person's health, including his or her mental health, can be used to imply incapacity to care for, or supervise, a child. Cases on all of these issues, and more, found their way to the courts. AIDS cases did not have a significant effect on the development of family law. However, the fact patterns demonstrate that HIV, because it could be transmitted sexually and perinatally, caused serious upheaval in many marriages and families.

Constitutional Law

The HIV/AIDS epidemic forced the courts to grapple with some of the most fascinating constitutional issues in the field of public health. The judiciary issued important rulings in relation to cherished freedoms—association, expression, and liberty. Bitter disputes over the freedom to associate occurred when public health authorities closed bathhouses in the mid-1980s. Gay men claimed the right to select their sex partners and to have privacy in places of their own choosing. Public health officials, however, felt that bathhouses posed unacceptably high risks of HIV transmission because they provided a venue for anonymous sexual encounters. From a public health perspective, the issue was not easy. Bathhouses were high-risk settings, but if they were closed, health officials might lose the opportunity to provide education and distribute condoms to patrons. The courts, for the most part, upheld the discretion of public health officials.[2]

The issue of free expression was raised when politicians regulated adult book stores and cinemas, arguing that they endangered the public's health. Although many restrictions on video shops or bookstores did promote the state's moral agenda, it is doubtful whether they promoted the public's health. At most, state restrictions prevented masturbation and other activities that pose no risk of HIV transmission. Yet the federal courts upheld local ordinances that required viewing booths to be open and visible to the public.[3]

Litigation within the Nation's Major Institutions

AIDS-related litigation penetrated the nation's major institutions such as blood suppliers, prisons, and the judiciary. Court cases substantially affected how these institutions operate and the rights afforded to those who interact with the system.

Prior to wide-scale screening, the transfusion of blood or blood products constituted one of the principal modes of HIV transmission.[4] A large number of cases seeking compensation on behalf of HIV-infected individuals, their sex partners, and their family members ensued. These cases raised a number of interesting policy issues. Many courts found that the identity of blood donors could be forcibly disclosed during the course of a trial. In this context, the judiciary appeared more concerned with the smooth administration of justice than the privacy of blood donors.[5] The courts also generally limited the liability of blood suppliers when HIV was contracted during a transfusion. The courts usually required a showing of negligence (rather than strict liability), which was consistent with legislative policy. Since many suppliers followed the industry standard for HIV screening procedures, courts were reluctant to impose liability. Most controversial of all was the fact that the industry transfused HIV-contaminated blood-clotting agents to persons with hemophilia. This led not only to litigation, but also to political investigations into the safety of the system and the veracity of industry leaders.[6]

Litigation against federal and state prison officials was rife in the early years of the epidemic. Prisoners, and organizations representing their interests, were angry at what they saw as repressive policies. Many prisoners were compulsorily tested, and if they were HIV positive they could be segregated and excluded from many activities.[7] At the same time, prisoners often complained that they did not receive adequate medical treatment.[8] In most of these cases, the courts upheld the discretion of prison officials, often without a searching inquiry about whether such policies were necessary for the public's health.[9] In a small number of cases, however, the courts vindicated the rights of inmates living with HIV/AIDS, particularly the right to privacy.[10]

The prejudicial treatment of persons living with HIV/AIDS in the early years of the epidemic extended even to courts—the branch of government designed to promote justice. Consider the 1988 New York State judicial guidelines suggesting that judges could press defendants to waive their right to appear in court; surgical gloves, masks, and plastic shields could be kept on hand but out of sight; and "court officers may guard an afflicted person . . . from a distance of up to 10 feet."[11] These kinds of policies, born of irrational fear and prejudice, were reflected in cases across the country in which HIV-infected defendants claimed that they were denied a fair trial because court officers wore rubber gloves or face masks.[12]

The quantity of litigation surrounding HIV/AIDS is smaller now than it was during the early years of the epidemic. Many interpersonal and societal struggles have been diffused. Although HIV/AIDS still evokes trepidation and intolerance among some individuals, many people see the human side. There is less of a tendency to attribute blame and more to facilitate access to services. Citizens will continue to resort to the courts, but it is hoped that most of the disputes will be settled through scientific inquiry and ethical discourse. That may be an overly optimistic assessment, but history shows that epidemics often start with social turmoil and then become assimilated into the culture. As families and communities begin to see AIDS in their own members, they will perceive it less as being a plague of "the other" and more as a part of the human condition.

Rights and Dignity

In retrospect, it should not be surprising that the social construction of HIV/AIDS would be so similar to, and yet so different from, diseases that preceded it. The similarities to other epidemics are unmistakable. Like bubonic plague, cholera, and smallpox in the nineteenth century and tuberculosis (TB), polio, and syphilis in the twentieth century, HIV/AIDS instilled dread.[13] Fears led to animus, prejudice, and separation. Persons living with HIV/AIDS, particularly those associated with disfavored groups, such as gays and injection drug users (IDUS), were blamed for their disease—in contrast to "innocent" AIDS babies and hemophiliacs. This is reminiscent of venereal insontium (venereal disease of the innocent) in the early twentieth century.[14] Popular indignation was evident in proposals for punitive measures, such as branding with a tatoo, isolation, and establishing special institutions. AIDS earned its own sobriquet (AIDS phobia, often associated with homophobia), just as TB did in the early twentieth century (phthisiophobia, or fear of TB).[15]

But AIDS is also quite different from diseases of the past. AIDS was the first major epidemic to emerge after the civil rights movement of the 1960s.[16] This was an era of "rights rhetoric," with the discourse of entitlement voiced on the streets as well as in the courts. The social protests over injustice toward African Americans and women carried over to include gay men and sex workers. It was in this context that persons living with HIV/AIDS had rights—"negative" rights to be free from discrimination, restraint, or punishment and "positive" rights to benefits, services, and expedited access to life-prolonging treatments.

Around the same time as the civil rights era, there emerged a parallel discourse expressed as "human rights." Certainly, international human rights law could be traced back to the Universal Declaration of Human Rights (UDHR) signed on December 10, 1948. Yet the International Covenant on Civil and Political Rights (ICCPR) and the International Covenant on Economic, Social, and Cultural Rights (ICESCR) were not adopted until 1966 and did not enter into force until 1976. The United States ratified the ICCPR in 1992 but has still not ratified the ICESCR. The language of human rights came naturally to those advocating for respect and dignity of persons living with HIV/AIDS.[17] International human rights offered a particularly incisive tool for dealing with the devastating epidemic in resource-poor countries.[18] Human rights principles required sharing the benefits of scientific advances, protecting the right to education, and ultimately safeguarding the right to health.

Two "rights" issues were especially important in the civil rights and human rights movements: privacy and antidiscrimination. Privacy and antidiscrimination are at the core of the "rights" agenda. They represent society's respect for the dignity of the person and willingness to ensure justice for all people.[19]

Because persons living with HIV/AIDS experienced stigma and ostracism, they strove to keep their health status private. Unauthorized disclosures not only revealed the person's health status, but also generated speculation as to his or her sexual orientation or use of injection drugs. Invasions of privacy could have serious and enduring consequences—alienation from family or friends, loss of care or support, and discrimination in employment, housing, and public accommodations.

Public health professionals frequently joined persons living with HIV/AIDS in their struggle for privacy. Those in public health realized that individuals would not come forward for testing, counseling, and treatment without assurance of privacy. The lay public and politicians, on the other hand, often could not understand why persons with a potentially lethal infectious disease could keep it secret. Some sex and needle-sharing partners sought a "right to know" the person's HIV status; others went further, calling for dissemination of HIV information to teachers and health care or emergency workers exposed to infection.[20]

These battles between privacy and disclosure were often contentious, but the coalition of consumers and public health professionals, for the most part, prevailed. Most states enacted AIDS-specific privacy laws,[21] and most recently the federal government promulgated national privacy regulations.[22] HIV-specific privacy laws often have permitted a number of disclosures, particularly to health care and emergency workers, as well as sex and needle-sharing partners. But the principle of privacy has been largely accepted.

Notably, the CDC urged states to enact strong privacy and security safeguards. In the late 1990s the CDC and the Council of State and Territorial Epidemiologists asked legal scholars at Georgetown University to draft a model public health information privacy act. This began a two-year process of seeking consensus on legal safeguards for privacy that, at the same time, would allow public health officials to use data for the public good. Despite acrimonious debate (and even threatened litigation by the American Civil Liberties Union [ACLU] against the secretary of health and human services), AIDS activists and civil libertarians joined with public health professionals to endorse the model act.[23] The CDC recommended that states consider adopting the safeguards in the Model State Public Health Privacy Act.[24] In 2002 the CDC initiated a process to develop guidelines for states on the "legitimate uses" of public health information. This is expected to result in recommendations to be published in *Morbidity and Mortality Weekly Reports* in 2004.

All human beings deserve fair treatment. People understand when they are passed over because they are unqualified, incapable, or pose a risk to others. But there is nothing as hurtful as being denied an opportunity because of a personal characteristic that is irrelevant to individual abilities. There has perhaps been no fight as important to the AIDS community as the struggle for equity and justice.

Persons living with HIV/AIDS have experienced discrimination in many spheres of life, including health care, employment, housing, and insurance. Much of the discrimination has been based purely on their HIV status or association with groups at risk. For instance, there have been reports of people being denied basic medical or dental treatment.[25] Despite their obvious need for services, persons living with HIV/AIDS were turned away by those professionals who had an ethical duty to provide care.[26]

Struggles over discriminatory treatment in other contexts have not been so clear-cut. Many employers have claimed that persons living with HIV/AIDS cannot perform the functions of the job because they are too ill, need time off from work, or pose a risk to others. Although this may be true in some cases, many persons living with HIV/AIDS are able to work effectively, particularly if they are given reasonable accommodations such as flexible work schedules. Too often, employers' claims of justifiable termination from employment are simply a subterfuge for discrimination.

Life and health insurance companies have also claimed that persons living with HIV/AIDS are uninsurable, pointing to their substantial health care costs and shortened life expectancies. Certainly, HIV/AIDS is an expensive disease to treat and often leads to premature death. Yet the key question is how insurers deal with people suffering from other chronic, costly illnesses such as cancer or cardiovascular disease. Too often, insurance companies have adversely treated persons living with HIV/AIDS even though, from an actuarial perspective, the economic burdens have been comparable to other health conditions.

The Americans with Disabilities Act (ADA) was a remarkable achievement in the fight against discrimination. The AIDS community joined a coalition of disability rights organizations to campaign for the ADA's passage in 1990.[27] Many disputes over discriminatory treatment should have been resolved by the ADA and HIV-specific antidiscrimination laws at the state and local levels. The Supreme Court's 1998 decision in *Bragdon v. Abbott*,[28] that asymptomatic HIV infection is covered under the ADA, clearly was promising. Since *Abbott*, however, the Rehnquist Court has narrowed the scope of the ADA and seriously eroded its protection.[29] In approximately 87 percent of ADA cases from 1992 to 2009, for example, federal appellate courts favored employers, usually on grounds that individuals failed to meet the statutory definition of disability.[30]

The Supreme Court has held that to receive protection under the ADA, an individual must actually suffer from a *substantial* impairment of a *major* life activity.[31] The disability must restrict the ability to perform tasks of central importance to daily life, not just those associated with the job.[32] Moreover, corrective and mitigating measures must be considered in determining whether an individual is disabled.[33] This reasoning could have a profound impact on the rights of persons living with HIV/AIDS as medications become more effective in controlling symptoms. Finally, the Court has held that employers can refuse to hire persons with disabilities whose performance on the job would present a threat to their *own* health.[34] This decision could embolden employers to exclude persons living with HIV/AIDS from the workforce on the grounds that employment could affect the health and safety of the employee.

The new conservative mood in the courts does not bode well for protecting the rights of persons living with HIV/AIDS and other disabilities. As the Supreme Court emphasized in 2002, the ADA's language requires a "demanding standard for qualifying as disabled."[35]

Policy, Politics, and Ethics

Like most epidemics in the past, HIV/AIDS poses sharp conflicts between civil liberties and public health.[36] According to this view, some restraint on individual freedom is necessary to achieve common goods. Conversely, some diminution in public health may be necessary to ensure a free and open society. Politicians and commentators often have lamented "AIDS exceptionalism"—the idea that persons living with HIV/AIDS are afforded rights and freedoms that are denied to others with infectious diseases.[37] Under this conception, persons living with HIV/AIDS should be subject to restraints and loss of privacy when necessary to protect the public's health.

Those who complain about AIDS exceptionalism sometimes fail to appreciate the significant differences between AIDS and other infectious diseases. HIV infection is not contagious through the air but usually requires conscious behavior for transmission. In this way, HIV is different from, say, tuberculosis or smallpox where persons may need to be separated during periods of contagiousness. Some diseases do have similar patterns of transmission such as syphilis, gonorrhea, chlamydia, and hepatitis B virus (HBV). But even here there are differences. The risk of HIV transmission often is considerably lower than for other sexually transmitted infections. For example, the likelihood of transmission of the HBV from a single exposure is significantly greater than for HIV. Moreover, a discrete, unintrusive form of treatment often can eliminate infectiousness for sexually transmitted diseases (STDS) (e.g., an antibiotic to treat syphilis).

Although treatment probably does reduce infectiousness for HIV, taking antiviral medication is an arduous and lifelong task. Thus, even though the focus on civil liberties of persons living with HIV/AIDS may seem counterintuitive, there are sound reasons for avoiding coercion whenever possible. The public's perception of AIDS is still unduly influenced by fear. After all, during the early years of the epidemic, AIDS was seen as untreatable and invariably fatal. Today, AIDS is much more like a chronic disease, and, with counseling and education, the epidemic can be contained without resorting to compulsion in almost all cases.[38]

Criteria for Testing and Screening

The perceived conflict between public health and civil liberties has been intensely debated in various policy forums. In the early years of the HIV epidemic, testing and screening policy was at the center of these debates. Persons living with HIV/AIDS were suspicious of government proposals for testing and screening due to their fear of violation of privacy and discrimination. At that time, the clinical benefits of treatment were unclear, leading people in the AIDS community to question the need for testing. Public health authorities, on the other hand, sought to make testing routine, especially among persons at increased risk. They reasoned that people would change their behavior only if they knew their serological status. Screening would also benefit the public's health by providing much needed data for surveillance and partner notification programs.

The sharp disagreements over testing and screening have dissipated considerably in recent years, due mainly to the clinical benefits of early diagnosis and treatment. The AIDS community has argued correctly that testing should be linked to access to care. Provided that individuals give informed consent and gain access to modern treatments, HIV testing should move into the mainstream of diagnostic services for the general population. There remain, however, bitter disagreements over screening that is used for separation, exclusion, or punishment of persons living with HIV/AIDS.

It is crucial to develop objective standards to guide screening policy in the United States. Too often, it is assumed that knowing the serological status of individuals and populations is an inherent good.[39] Yet screening requires rigorous justification based on science and human rights. Chapter 7 proposes screening criteria that include (1) technical excellence in testing procedures, (2) a sound public health objective, (3) minimal burdens on individual rights (e.g., counseling and informed consent), (4) the least restrictive alternative, and (5) public acceptability.

These principles have not always been put into practice. There remain intractable disagreements between government officials and the AIDS community on a number of controversial screening policies. Decisions to screen criminal defendants, prisoners, military personnel, and immigrants, for example, are fiercely resisted by advocates. Despite this vocal opposition, government shows little indication that it will change these policies.

Many of the most interesting future issues involve the development and use of innovative testing technologies. There is strong support for rapid testing because it enables patients to receive their results quickly, often without the need for a second visit to the clinic. In 2002 the FDA approved a rapid HIV diagnostic test that returns results in less than twenty minutes and is 99.6 percent accurate.[40] There is also support for tests that evaluate different bodily fluids (e.g., oral fluid and urine). Although there remain questions about the accuracy of such tests, they do allow less invasive and more acceptable forms of testing.[41] Thus, rapid and less intrusive testing technologies should expand the number of people who know their HIV status. Capitalizing on these new technologies, the CDC recommended in April 2003 that HIV testing should become a routine part of medical care.[42]

Perhaps the most controversial testing option is the home collection kit. Initially, there were genuine concerns with this technology because individuals who did not go to a clinic for blood collection would not have ready access to counseling and support services. Many people in the community now think that restricting access to home collection kits is paternalistic. They argue that people have a right to be tested in the privacy of their homes. This should increase knowledge about HIV and ultimately expedite treatment. Although the Food and Drug Administration (FDA) has approved home collection kits, it has not approved home-use test kits that allow consumers to interpret their own HIV test results.[43] Many public health officials are deeply concerned with this technology because it is not as accurate as laboratory tests and because home testing makes it even more difficult to ensure access to services.

The Politically Charged Issue of Named HIV Reporting

The idea that government would collect the names of persons living with HIV seemed unacceptable from a civil liberties perspective. Advocates feared that the health department might disclose the names to people outside the agency, for example, if compelled to do so by the legislature. Moreover, advocates had evidence of compelled disclosure in the past such as the Illinois decision (never implemented) to match AIDS data with health care worker (HCW) records. Public health officials, on the other hand, were determined to move from AIDS reporting to a national system of HIV surveillance. They reasoned that surveillance of late-stage disease was ineffective. Public health agencies could track the epidemic and predict trends only if a national surveillance system could monitor individuals from the earliest stages of infection.

Over the years, the CDC held numerous consultations with experts and advocates, designed in part to secure the AIDS community's approval for named HIV reporting. That approval, however, was never forthcoming. Instead, advocates were prepared to accept a non-named system of HIV reporting based on unique identifiers (UIs). They argued that such a system would achieve public health goals while still maintaining confidentiality.

The CDC moved ahead without the community's support (which was unusual for an agency that generally sought the cooperation of AIDS advocates). It issued guidance to states encouraging them to move to a system of named HIV reporting.[44] Most states have now complied with CDC guidance, although a minority have implemented a UI system.

Research has yet to demonstrate whether unique identifiers are sufficiently reliable and cost-effective to meet surveillance needs. The CDC argues that UI systems create duplicate records and make it difficult to track cases. There also remains considerable disagreement as to whether UI systems actually afford better protection of privacy. Public health officials argue that they can be trusted with the names of persons living with HIV. Under a UI system, however, private health care providers may keep lists of names that match each patient's code, thus creating greater risks to privacy. The AIDS community believes that UI systems can work if they are well designed and adequately funded. The future of HIV reporting will depend on whether the CDC or advocates' view of unique identifiers is supported by research studies.

Partner Notification and the "Right to Know"

Because AIDS advocates often distrust government involvement in the lives of persons living with HIV/AIDS, it is not surprising that they often have resisted partner notification programs.[45] In classic partner notification, public health officials help patients trace their past and current sex and needle-sharing partners. The partners are then notified of their exposure and offered testing, counseling, and treatment.

Although partner notification is intended to be anonymous, many partners know who disclosed their names to public health officials. These partners may feel embarrassed, even betrayed, by the disclosure. Not only do AIDS advocates regard partner notification as a potential invasion of privacy, but they also express concern about the safety of people involved in partner notification. Studies have documented that persons whose HIV status has been disclosed often suffer from physical or emotional abuse.[46]

Public health officials focus on the benefits of partner notification, which has long been used to curtail the spread of sexually transmitted diseases. HIV/AIDS may not be identical to other STDs, but there are enough similarities to include HIV within partner notification programs. Partner notification, health officials argue, is voluntary, anonymous, and effective. It informs individuals that they may have been exposed to infection and gives them the opportunity to access prevention and clinical services. Perhaps more importantly, sex or needle-sharing partners claim a "right to know" whether they have been exposed to a serious infectious disease. Failure to inform them, according to some ethicists, may be morally unacceptable.[47]

At present, the CDC recommends partner notification for HIV/AIDS and most states have programs in place.[48] It will be important to conduct additional research on evidence of the effectiveness and harms of partner notification. Although public health professionals often claim that partner notification is cost-effective in preventing STDs, the data are mixed.[49] At the same time, there is relatively little information about how frequently, and to what extent, partner notification actually infringes on the right to autonomy and privacy. More research is also needed to determine how frequently these programs expose partners to physical and emotional abuse.

The first two decades of the AIDS epidemic have produced clashes over policies that have been staples of public health practice in the past: testing and screening, reporting, and partner notification. Some of the disputes simply represent entrenched positions—advocates struggle for personal rights and health officials for the common good. Other disagreements can be settled through additional research. How effective is the intervention? How great a burden does it impose? Are there measures that can achieve the public health objective better and less intrusively? Public health agencies increasingly are judged on their objective performance,[50] and they will continue to come under strict scrutiny from the body politic and interest groups in the coming years.

Special Populations

Many AIDS policies apply specifically to designated populations. Since these policies often burden vulnerable communities, they require special justifications. The essays in this part of the book examine policies relating to three populations: HIV-infected health care workers, pregnant women and infants, and injection drug users.

Rights and Duties of HIV-infected Health Care Professionals

There have been acrimonious disagreements over policies relating to HIV-infected HCWs ever since Dr. David Acer infected six patients in his Florida dental office in 1990.[51] One of his patients, Kimberly Bergalis, went on to become a visible political symbol. The CDC, under intense pressure from Congress and the White House, urgently commenced a consultative process to formulate guidelines. Several contentious meetings were held in Atlanta in 1990–91 with representatives of medical organizations, advocates, and scholars in ethics and law. Advocacy groups and medical organizations formed an alliance, urging few, if any, restrictions on professional practice.[52]

The CDC guidelines published in 1991 were far more restrictive than either medical organizations or the AIDS community wanted. The CDC recommended that HCWs infected with HIV or hepatitis B (HbeAg positive) should be reviewed by an expert panel and should inform patients of their serologic status before engaging in exposure-prone procedures.[53] The guidance did not recommend mandatory testing but urged HCWs at risk to discover their serologic status.

What is historically interesting about that recommendation is that the CDC had concluded from its deliberations that HCWs should not invariably have to inform their patients of their HIV status. The White House, however, overruled the CDC on this issue, and guidance was ultimately published recommending that patients give informed consent in all cases. (Indeed, I understand that the initial print runs of the CDC guidance did not require informed consent of patients in all cases; these copies of the recommendations had to be destroyed after the White House intervened.) Later in 1991, Congress enacted the Kimberly Bergalis Act, which required states to adopt CDC guidelines or their equivalent.[54] This statute was passed after highly emotive testimony in Congress, particularly by Ms. Bergalis.

I was involved in the CDC's deliberative process and supported the idea of an expert review panel but did not accept that informed consent was an appropriate safeguard. I advocated for the expert review because the data on the nature and probability of risk to patients were, at the time, inconclusive. It was better, I thought, to err on the side of patient safety. I opposed patient notification because it would be a significant violation of the HCW's privacy and would effectively ruin his or her professional career.[55]

It is important to emphasize that the CDC sought an independent review only for those HCWs engaged in "exposure-prone" procedures. At the time, the agency requested that specialized medical organizations devise guidance on these procedures, but medical organizations declined. (They probably felt that the task was too complex and did not want to be seen as contributing to a system that would exclude some of their members from professional practice.) This failure to sufficiently define exposure-prone procedures and to narrow the scope of the policy to those engaged in truly high-risk practices would be telling. Many HCWs have been excluded from practice even though they were not engaging in exposure-prone procedures as originally contemplated by the CDC.

In the years since the CDC guidance, many HIV-infected HCWs have been prevented from pursuing their livelihoods. Hospitals, fearing liability and adverse publicity, have been quick to test HCWs perceived to be at risk and exclude those who test HIV positive. The courts, more often than not, have upheld restrictive hospital practices.[56] These restraints have been placed not only on surgeons engaged in seriously invasive procedures, but also on internists, nurses, dentists, and others.

It is now more than a decade since the initial cluster of cases contracted from a HCW in Florida, and the risks to patients are well understood. It is clear that the probability of transmission to patients is exceedingly low. Given the new data, I have changed my mind and support broad reform of the CDC's policy. Current national policy offers no discernible risk reduction for patients— few, if any, new blood-borne infections are prevented. At the same time, the policy imposes human rights burdens, undermines efforts to retain experienced professionals, and poses liability risks. Consequently, new national policy should focus on structural changes to make the health care workplace safer for both patients and HCWs (e.g., universally required infection control techniques) rather than on identification and management of HIV-infected HCWs.[57] Certainly, patient safety remains the most important part of any national policy, but it ought to be possible to ensure patient safety while not undermining the HCW's interests in autonomy, privacy, and livelihood.

Many senior CDC officials concur in this analysis, which led the agency to conduct consultations for changing the guidance in the late 1990s. I was present at those meetings, and there appeared to be clear, almost unanimous, agreement in favor of policy reform. Nevertheless, there was no follow-up to these consultations, and the committee of experts was not informed of the reasons why the agency did not pursue needed reforms. Most probably, reform of the policy for HIV-infected HCWs would have rekindled the political and public conflicts that had occurred a decade earlier in the Florida dental cases. That was a battle that the agency was not prepared to wage, and, given its political vulnerability in Washington D.C., the CDC is unlikely to seek reform in the near future.

Perinatal Transmission of HIV: Screening and Treatment of Women and Infants

In 1994 AIDS policy was transformed with the scientific discovery (Protocol ACTG 076) that perinatal (mother-to-infant) HIV transmission could be dramatically reduced with treatment.[58] This research set in motion fierce debates about HIV screening and treatment. Public health agencies and legislatures acted quickly to identify infected mothers and babies. The CDC issued guidelines for the treatment of pregnant women in 1994,[59] for counseling and screening in 1995,[60] and for antiretroviral drug treatment in 2002.[61] In 1996 Congress required the secretary of health and human services to determine by 1998 whether HIV screening of infants was "routine practice."[62] In January 2000 the secretary determined that infant screening had not become routine practice.[63] Only New York and Connecticut required mandatory HIV testing of all newborns whose mothers had not undergone prenatal HIV testing, and only New York had fully implemented this requirement. The sponsor of the New York mandatory screening statute, Assemblywoman Nettie Mayersohn, reasoned that it was "criminal" to allow the suffering of "innocent and helpless victims."[64] However, mere evidence of the HIV status of infants does not reduce perinatal transmission.

Public health authorities recognized that reductions in perinatal transmission can be achieved only by screening pregnant women and treating those who are HIV positive.[65] In response, the Institute of Medicine (IOM) issued a bold report in 1999 urging universal screening of all pregnant women.[66] The panel concluded that existing requirements for pretest counseling and specific informed consent posed a barrier to prenatal HIV screening. The report flew in the face of traditional AIDS dogmas in two respects. First, the proposal would target all pregnant women, not just those at high risk. This meant that low-prevalence populations would be screened even though it might not be cost-effective. The IOM made this proposal believing that screening targeted to high-risk women would inevitably be unjust; it would disproportionately affect poor women and women of color, adding to their stigma. Second, the IOM recommended routine screening without routine pretest counseling. This would mean that some women might be tested without their full knowledge and consent. In 2001 the U.S. Public Health Service issued revised recommendations for HIV screening of pregnant women.[67] The 2001 guidelines follow the IOM structure except in one crucial respect; they recommend counseling and informed consent in advance of testing. By emphasizing the importance of counseling and consent, the agency sought to ensure that women's autonomy and liberty would be protected during the screening process. By 2003, the CDC amended its recommendations to conform more closely with the IOM.[68] The agency eliminated the requirement of formal pretest counseling to make it easier to do testing in private doctors' offices.

The practice of universal screening and treatment of pregnant women has substantially reduced perinatal transmission in the United States. It is too early, however, to understand the effects of pretest counseling. This is one of the profound dilemmas that marks the field of AIDS policy. Should public health officials take the path of maximum cost-effectiveness in reducing the burden of disease, or should they take special care to respect the rights and dignity of individuals and groups? That is the perennial question for public health law and ethics.

The Interconnected Epidemics of AIDS and Drug Dependency

The interconnected epidemics of HIV/AIDS and drug dependency pose a profound health threat. Injection drug use is the second most frequently reported risk factor for AIDS in the United States,[69] where nearly 10,000 IDUs are infected with HIV annually.[70] Moreover, since drug users have sex and reproduce, the needle-borne HIV epidemic has spread rapidly to partners and children. This is a major reason for the disproportionate burden of HIV/AIDS among racial minorities,[71] women, and the poor.

HIV and other blood-borne infections (e.g., HBV and HCV) are caused by multi-person use of injection equipment. The sharing of drug-injection equipment is a highly complicated behavior. It involves direct sharing of needles and syringes between friends or lovers, anonymous sharing of pooled injection equipment in shooting galleries, and indirect sharing when drug paraphernalia are used communally by the group when preparing drugs for injection. Sharing behavior was originally reported as part of the subculture and routines of the drug world; it represented an initiation into drug use and a social bonding mechanism.[72] However, sharing is not merely part of drug subcultures but is principally caused by an artificially induced scarcity of injection equipment.[73] This scarcity can deny IDUs a realistic opportunity to engage in safer behavior.

The limited supply of sterile injection equipment is the result of a conscious policy choice by government within its drug control strategy. Several interrelated legislative and regulatory provisions have the effect of systematically restricting the availability of syringes: drug paraphernalia laws, syringe prescription laws, and pharmacy regulations.

Drug paraphernalia statutes, enacted in forty-nine states, ban the manufacture, distribution, or possession of a wide range of devices if knowledge exists that they may be used to introduce illicit substances into the body. Since these laws have an element of intent, pharmacists are permitted to sell hypodermic syringes and needles over the counter if they have no knowledge that the equipment will be used for drug injection.

Syringe prescription laws, enacted in twelve states, proscribe the dispensing or possession of a syringe without a valid medical prescription. Since syringe prescription laws do not have an element of intent, pharmacists cannot lawfully dispense injection equipment without a prescription. In this sense, prescription laws potentially encompass many more transactions than paraphernalia laws.

A majority of states have regulations or guidelines that significantly affect pharmacy practices. These rules or guidelines may prevent pharmacists from dispensing syringes to drug users, restrict the display of syringes in retail establishments, and require pharmacists to keep detailed written records of sales. Thus, even if drug paraphernalia or syringe prescription laws are not an issue in some states, pharmacy regulations and guidelines may significantly restrict the purchase and sale of sterile injection equipment.

This pervasive network of laws, regulations, and guidelines presents formidable obstacles to disease prevention. They render it much more difficult for pharmacists to sell syringes over the counter, pose a chilling effect on IDUs seeking to comply with public health advice, and hinder the operation of syringe exchange programs. Providing the means for safer injection is an effective prevention strategy that can significantly reduce needle-borne infections among drug users.[74] The tragedy is that the government itself may be exacerbating the HIV/AIDS epidemic among the poorest and most vulnerable populations in society. For example, despite concluding that sterile injection equipment reduced HIV transmission and did not discourage drug use, the Clinton administration refused to reinstate federal funding for needle exchanges.[75] Indeed, I understand that on the very day Secretary Donna Shalala was going to announce the resumption of federal funding, the White House overturned the decision.

AIDS in the World

The public health and AIDS communities in developed countries can take comfort in the fact that they have time to deliberate over "nice" questions of law and ethics. In addition to considering these questions, developing countries have to confront an overwhelming burden of HIV with meager public health and health care resources. The final part of this book tackles problems in resource-poor countries. It also deals with the obligations of developed countries to provide economic and scientific assistance to reduce the global burden of HIV/AIDS. Before examining the profound problems of HIV/AIDS in resource-poor countries, it will be helpful to see why the U.S. policy of screening travelers and immigrants has enraged AIDS activists worldwide.

Screening and Exclusion of Travelers and Immigrants

Global strategies to control infectious disease have historically included the erection of barriers to international travel and immigration.[76] Keeping people with infectious diseases outside national borders reemerged as a controversial public health policy in the HIV/AIDS pandemic. Sixty countries have introduced border restrictions on foreigners infected with HIV, usually those planning an extended stay in the country, such as students, workers, or seamen.[77]

Although many countries impose immigration and travel restrictions on persons living with HIV/AIDS, the United States has one of the most comprehensive systems. In fact, similar restrictions were rejected in Canada in 2001.[78] National[79] and international[80] organizations have sharply criticized the U.S. policy as being contrary to public health goals and human rights principles. The Eighth International Conference on AIDS, scheduled to be held at Harvard University in July 1992, was moved to Amsterdam in protest of the American immigration policy. Some AIDS and human rights organizations still boycott international meetings held in the United States.

The U.S. Immigration and Nationality Act makes any applicant who has a communicable disease of public health significance ineligible for admission or a visa.[81] In 1987, in response to congressional direction in the Helms Amendment,[82] the Public Health Service added HIV infection to the list of communicable diseases of public health significance;[83] HIV infection still remains on the list.

The complex rules under the Immigration and Nationality Act, examined in Chapter 15, have pernicious effects for international travelers and immigrants living with HIV/AIDS. Travelers are not routinely tested for HIV, although they must declare their serologic status when applying for a visa. An immigration officer may require a test if there is "suspicion" that the person is infected.[84] Immigrants must undergo a medical examination that includes an HIV test.[85] Those who test positive must be denied permanent residence unless they can meet the stringent requirements for an exclusion waiver.

The Bureau of Citizenship and Immigration Services (BCIS; formerly the INS) is conducting one of the largest HIV screening programs in the world, yet the program has never been evaluated for its effectiveness. From a global perspective, the testing and exclusion of international travelers is a specious public health policy.[86] Restricting travel is unlikely to reduce the reservoir of infection in the world. More importantly, the absence of provisions for education and counseling suggests that the program is not intended to reduce the global burden of HIV/AIDS. Furthermore, there is no attempt to identify and educate HIV-infected citizens who leave the United States to travel abroad. The only potential global effect of restrictions on international travel, then, might be to shift the geographic distribution of infection marginally.

U.S. policy restricting travel violates international law and global health guidelines. The *International Health Regulations* provide that the only document that can be required in international traffic is a valid certificate of vaccination against yellow fever.[87] The World Health Organization has stated that "no country bound by the Regulations may refuse entry into its territory to a person who fails to provide a medical certificate stating that he or she is not carrying the AIDS virus."[88]

A just and efficacious travel and immigration policy would not exclude people because of their serologic status unless they posed a danger to the community. It is inequitable to use cost as a reason to exclude people infected with HIV, for there are no similar exclusionary policies for those with other costly chronic diseases. Rather than arbitrarily restrict the movement of a subgroup of infected people, we should dedicate ourselves to the principles of justice, scientific cooperation, and a global response to the HIV pandemic.

HIV/AIDS truly is a global pandemic, imposing a burden on all countries and regions and leaving no one immune from its devastating impact. As of December 2002, 42 million people were living with HIV/AIDS, with the highest infection rates concentrated in countries that can least afford the sickness, death, and loss of productivity. The vast majority (95 percent) of people living with HIV/AIDS reside in developing countries, particularly Sub-Saharan Africa.[89] If the current trend continues, there will be 100 million people infected by 2006.

Given the undeniable global effects of HIV/AIDS, one might expect the international community to unite in an effort to reach the common goal of preventing and treating HIV/AIDS. Yet the response by governments has been fragmented. There is often an absence of political will, an unwillingness to share strategies and resources, and wide philosophical and pragmatic differences, principally between countries in the North/West and those in the South/East. This unwillingness to cooperate often is caused by insular attitudes to world health, economics, and politics. Narrow self-interest seems to prevent many countries from engaging in truly global cooperative approaches.

Three salient questions must be asked: Why have many political leaders turned a blind eye to AIDS or, worse still, actively resisted necessary reforms? Why have highly developed countries used the international trade and patent systems to keep the price of HIV/AIDS drugs inordinately high, placing them out of the reach of resource-poor countries? Finally, why is there such rancor over the ethics of international collaborative AIDS research designed to promote the health of people in the poorest countries?

With notable exceptions, such as in Uganda and Senegal, many politicians have thwarted AIDS prevention, treatment, and research by imposing societal prohibitions. Some have prevented the use of graphic educational materials targeted to groups at risk; others have refused to recognize AIDS and the prevalence of risk behaviors in their country. Still others have actively resisted the AIDS community's efforts to make treatments available to children, pregnant women, and the rest of the infected population. South African president Thabo Mbeki, for example, made it difficult for pregnant women and infants to obtain antiretroviral medication. In 2002 the South African Constitutional Court ruled that this political resistance was a violation of the human right to health.[90]

Pharmaceutical companies, supported by advanced industrialized countries, often seek to maintain a high price for HIV medications. These largely northern-based transnational companies claim that a market price is necessary to recoup the substantial costs of research and development. That is one reality. But another, more poignant reality is that without access to treatments, large parts of the world will experience devastating illness and death. Resource-poor countries have no hope of affording the high market price of HIV treatments, and they receive few reciprocal benefits from the international patent system. The United States has been particularly obstructive in attempts to craft a compromise. In December 2002, for instance, 143 of the World Trade Organization's 144 members agreed on a solution that would allow the import and export of drugs in a public health crisis. The lone holdout, the United States, blocked the deal but has now reconsidered.[91]

Perhaps the most important use for antiretroviral treatments is to reduce perinatal HIV transmission. The problem, of course, is that the ACTG 076 regimen is expensive and difficult to implement in resource-poor countries. In the mid-to-late 1990s, international collaborative research was undertaken in African, Asian, and Caribbean countries on the effectiveness of short-course antiretroviral treatment. The intention was to develop more affordable and practical interventions for developing countries.

These trials touched off a storm of protest because they used a placebo-controlled model. Such trials would be unethical in the United States and Western Europe since human subjects must have access to known, effective treatments. The question arose, should ethical standards prevalent in the First World be transplanted to the Third World? On the face of it, the answer is yes. Why should investigators not protect the rights and interests of all human subjects, irrespective of the research venue?

On deeper reflection, however, it was essential to have an understanding of whether less expensive, more affordable therapies are effective in resource-poor countries. The standard of care is not the same everywhere, and in parts of Africa, Asia, and the Caribbean, persons living with HIV/AIDS would not have access to state-of-the-art therapies. Policymakers had to make treatment allocation decisions under conditions of poverty, scarcity, and urgent need. The research subjects were informed, consented, and not exposed to risk; the study was designed to benefit host countries, which desired the research and ethically approved the protocol; and the results may vastly improve the lives of the world's poorest and most disadvantaged mothers and children. Given the social and economic context, it may have been unethical not to conduct the most rigorous and efficient international studies to prevent perinatal transmission in the least developed countries.

Conclusion

HIV is a virus with potentially lethal effects on human populations. But the effects of this pathogen go well beyond the physical. HIV/AIDS deeply affects families and communities—partners die alone, children live without parents, and ordinary people lose friends and neighbors. HIV/AIDS also has powerful social and economic effects that penetrate into all spheres of life from the household to the workplace and from health care to insurance.

Once the virus gains a foothold in a population it can spread rapidly, fueled by sex and injection drug use. The only vaccine is education. There is no cure, but only a complex therapeutic regimen that is burdensome and often causes debilitating adverse effects. For most people in the world, there is neither adequate education on how to avoid infection nor medical treatment. The epidemic has taken a dreadful toll in Sub-Saharan Africa, and it will do so in other great population centers such as Russia, India, and China if prevention does not become the first priority.

Governments know how to dramatically reduce the burden of disease. But the resources and political courage needed are often tragically absent. When that occurs, it is up to the people to speak out against the apathy, and sometimes antipathy, so evident in the evolving HIV/AIDS pandemic.

Wherever it takes hold, the AIDS epidemic feeds on existing economic and social problems. Ultimately, the test of our leadership will be how decisively we address the enduring poverty, inequality and inadequate infrastructures that are the enablers of this terrible disease. It is only by doing so that we can empower individuals, communities and countries to play their full part as leaders in the fight against HIV/AIDS.—**Kofi A. Annan,** secretary general, United Nations (2001)

Chapter 2

The AIDS Litigation Project

The Social Impact of AIDS

Throughout the 1990s my colleagues and I conducted a systematic national review of court and human rights commission decisions relating to the AIDS epidemic. This study, known as the AIDS Litigation Project (ALP), revealed a vast terrain of judicial policy-making. This chapter and the next provide a representative sample of the most important cases, updating the ALP to December 1, 2002. (For a comprehensive list of cases, see the original ALP reports).[1] This chapter discusses the social impact of AIDS, and the next chapter covers the rights of persons living with HIV/AIDS, primarily the rights to privacy and to be free from discrimination. These themes—social response and civil rights— reverberate throughout this book.

No other infectious disease in recent history compares with AIDS in the ways that it affects our relationships with each other and with our social institutions. Sharp differences in perception of public health, ethics, and civil liberties have

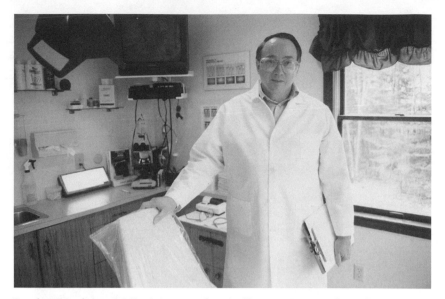

Randon Bragdon, DMD. During a 1994 dental office visit, Dr. Bragdon refused to provide routine care to patient Sidney Abbott, who had disclosed on her patient information form that she was HIV positive. In *Bragdon v. Abbott* (1998), the U.S. Supreme Court held that persons living with asymptomatic HIV infection are protected from discrimination under the Americans with Disabilities Act (ADA) of 1990. However, the Supreme Court recently has been narrowing the protections afforded by the ADA.

created the largest body of legal cases attributable to a single disease in the history of American jurisprudence.

Litigation related to AIDS has had powerful impacts on the major social institutions of our nation—schools, health care, the blood supply, the judiciary, prisons, and the military.[2] The litigation has had an equal effect on cherished constitutional principles of privacy, freedom of speech and association, and liberty. The AIDS epidemic reaches into intimate personal relationships, sparking litigation against sex partners and family members. Courts and human rights commissions operate as a lens magnifying public policy and social tensions. The factual patterns of cases provide intriguing insights into the history of the AIDS epidemic.

This chapter considers findings of the AIDS litigation project in the social arena:

   1. *AIDS education and health promotion.* One would have thought that the need for education is obvious, but the content (e.g., sex and drug use) and targets (e.g., gay men and sex workers) of AIDS education are highly controversial.

   2. *The blood supply system.* In the early years of the epidemic many individuals

contracted HIV from the transfusion of blood or blood products, resulting in a flood of litigation.

3. *Public health surveillance.* Public health and civil liberties advocates challenged compulsory testing in various populations such as military recruits, immigrants, and inmates. The courts, however, often upheld many of these HIV screening programs.

4. *State regulation of public places such as bathhouses and adult bookstores.* These cases raised important questions about the freedom of association and the best way to achieve the public health goals of reducing unsafe sex.

5. *Tort litigation in the HIV/AIDS epidemic.* This involves a wide range of fascinating issues such as the false diagnosis of HIV, failure to diagnose HIV, and fear of exposure.

6. *Occupational safety and health,* including federal regulations and employee claims of risk of HIV infection.

7. *The administration of justice in the nation's courtrooms.* Although judges should be the last group to discriminate, many early judicial practices were highly prejudicial, notably allowing court staff to wear gloves when dealing with persons living with HIV/AIDS.

8. *Family law,* including issues involving divorce and child custody.

AIDS Education: Health Promotion

From the earliest moments of the AIDS epidemic, educational messages were influenced not only by public health, but also by morality, law, and politics.[3] In 1988 Congress prohibited federal funds from being used to provide AIDS prevention materials that "promote or encourage, directly, homosexual or heterosexual sexual activity" and required that the educational content of AIDS prevention materials must not be "judged by a reasonable person to be offensive to most educated adults."[4] Consequently, community-based organizations in receipt of federal funds were limited in their ability to disseminate frank, well-targeted messages to people in the gay community. Because public health messages had to reflect mainstream moral positions, Congress impeded the most effective health promotion campaigns.

Similarly, efforts to educate in California were obstructed by that state's AIDS Material Review Committee, created in 1985. The committee restricted the use of slang or "street language" in AIDS educational material, stating that it was "preferable to use clinical or descriptive terms describing sexual contact or behavior."[5]

In addition, efforts by Surgeon General C. Everett Koop in 1988 to institute AIDS education "at the lowest grade possible" met vehement opposition from within the Reagan administration and from members of Congress.[6] Eventually, Koop issued a statement that emphasized abstinence as the best method of avoiding AIDS and abandoned the plan for safer sex education.[7]

The government's power to restrict public health messages, of course, is bounded by the First Amendment. AIDS education by health care professionals and community organizations are forms of expression protected under the U.S. Constitution, and the courts have prohibited government-imposed censorship. For example, in striking down congressional regulation of indecent communications to minors on the Internet, the Supreme Court noted the First Amendment's protection of safer sex information.[8] Similarly, a federal court struck down Centers for Disease Control and Prevention (CDC) guidelines that prohibited federal funding for nonobscene, but "offensive" or "indecent," HIV educational materials.[9] Generally, because of the social and educational value of sexually explicit AIDS educational materials, they are not catagorized as obscene.

Courts have also upheld the free speech rights of individuals and organizations to distribute HIV-related information on college campuses and in other public places.[10] For example, the First Circuit Court of Appeals held unconstitutional a ban on AIDS educational activities on public transportation vehicles in Boston.[11]

Programs to educate school children about sex and sexually transmitted diseases have long been a source of controversy.[12] The First Circuit Court of Appeals upheld a state requirement that high school students participate in a sexually explicit AIDS awareness assembly without prior parental approval. The court concluded that parents possess no "broad-based right to restrict the flow of information in public schools" and found no violation of the parents' constitutional right to direct their children's upbringing.[13] Similarly, courts have upheld school-based programs to distribute condoms without parental consent.[14]

Protection of the Blood Supply

Liability of Blood Suppliers and Hospitals

Reported cases of *Pneumocystis carinii* pneumonia among persons with hemophilia[15] and blood transfusion recipients[16] in late 1982 first brought into question the safety of the national blood supply.[17] By March 1983 the CDC had recommended self-deferral of donors who had engaged in high-risk behavior.[18] A test to detect antibody resistance to HIV was not commercially available until early 1985. Prior to wide-scale screening, the transfusion of blood or blood products constituted one of the principal modes of HIV transmission; more than half of the 168,000 hemophiliacs and over 12,000 blood transfusion recipients became infected with HIV during that period.[19] A large number of cases seeking compensation on behalf of HIV-infected individuals, their sex partners, and family members ensued.[20]

For policy reasons, state legislatures have deemed blood and blood products a "service" (subject to liability on a negligence or fault basis), rather than a "product" (subject to strict liability without evidence of fault or negligence). Legislatures and courts reason that imposition of strict liability would defeat the important state goal of ensuring a voluntary and inexpensive blood supply.[21] Blood suppliers, therefore, are judged not under a strict liability standard, but instead under a negligence standard (e.g., the ordinary level of prudence used by blood suppliers in the same or similar circumstances).[22]

What constitutes proper evidence of negligence in the blood-collection industry has been frequently disputed. Generally, if exposure occurred prior to the standard practice of screening donated blood in early 1985, the supplier is not negligent, simply because there was no accepted means to detect HIV and prevent contamination.[23] Some courts, however, have imposed liability for the failure of blood suppliers to more stringently select donors. Other courts have imposed liability for the failure of blood suppliers to offer the option of autologous or directed donation, in which the patient (autologous) or a friend or family member (directed) donates blood prior to elective surgery. Failure of hospitals or blood-collection agencies to identify HIV-infected blood donors and to inform the recipients of the transfusion after the fact ("look-back" notification) has also been asserted as a basis for liability.[24]

Discovery of the Donor's Identity

In attempting to prove that contaminated blood was collected negligently, plaintiffs' attorneys often seek information directly from the donor regarding the actual collection practices. Blood suppliers generally oppose disclosing identifying information regarding donors, citing the need to maintain confidentiality. In resolving these disputes, judges balance the plaintiff's need for the information and the state's interest in the administration of justice against the donor's privacy, the blood bank's guarantees of confidentiality, and maintenance of a voluntary blood supply. Many courts find the balance to favor disclosure,[25] particularly when the donor is deceased.[26] Commonly, courts allow limited discovery of the donor's testimony but prohibit revealing the identity of the donor.[27] In some cases, state HIV confidentiality laws prohibit disclosure.[28]

Hemophilia, Clotting Factors, and AIDS

Numerous persons with hemophilia have filed suits against the manufacturers of clotting factors.[29] These cases raise fascinating legal questions because the plaintiff cannot know with certainty which organization supplied the contaminated blood. Some plaintiffs have used imaginative legal theories such as "market-share liability." Under this theory, plaintiffs sue all potential blood suppliers and collect from each according to its proportion of the market.[30] Other plaintiffs have used the "learned intermediary" argument, which places responsibility on the hematologist rather than the blood supplier.[31] In perhaps the most significant ruling, the Seventh Circuit Court of Appeals refused to certify as a class action a lawsuit brought by plaintiffs claiming to have been exposed to contaminated clotting factors;[32] as a result, claimants sought a negotiated settlement with the manufacturers or compensation approved by Congress.[33]

Public Health Powers and Epidemiologic Surveillance

Since the beginning of the HIV epidemic, a debate has ensued about compulsory versus voluntary public health approaches.[34] Although the dividing lines have not always been clear, community-based organizations and public health officials have often supported voluntarism, whereas some medical organizations have espoused selective use of compulsion. Such was the context when the New York State Medical Society sued to compel the health commissioner to include HIV in the official list of sexually transmitted diseases (STDs). By failing to classify HIV as an STD, the commissioner declined to trigger his powers for compulsory testing, reporting, and contact tracing. New York's highest court held that the classification of diseases was within the commissioner's discretion and affirmed the reasonableness of his belief that mandatory powers would not serve an important public health purpose.[35]

Testing and Screening

Throughout the epidemic many policymakers have called for a "tougher" approach to fighting HIV/AIDS. This tougher approach has included compulsory testing and screening of persons who engage in high-risk behavior or who are members of a group perceived to engage in high risk behavior. The federal government and/or the states have required testing for certain populations such as firefighters and paramedics,[36] military personnel,[37] overseas employees in the State Department,[38] immigrants,[39] and sex offenders.[40] In each of these cases, the courts have upheld the screening (see Chapter 7).

Government screening programs must comply with the Fourth Amendment's standards of reasonable search and seizure.[41] The Supreme Court has held that when the state has "special needs beyond the normal need for law enforcement," the warrant and probable or reasonable cause requirements of the Fourth Amendment may not be applicable.[42] Most HIV screening programs are not conducted for law enforcement purposes, thus falling within the "special needs" doctrine; for example, even mandated HIV screening for persons accused or convicted of sexual assaults are considered special needs because the results are not used as evidence in a criminal trial (see Chapter 11). The Supreme Court, however, has held that drug testing of pregnant women in hospitals does not fit within the special needs doctrine when test results are shared with police.[43] Thus, any HIV screening policy devised or implemented in conjunction with law enforcement authorities is likely to be judged under a stricter Fourth Amendment standard.

If screening is for public health—rather than criminal justice—purposes, the courts balance governmental and privacy interests to determine the reasonableness of the search. On one side of the balance is the government's interest in public health; on the other side is the individual's expectations of privacy. The courts have weighed the state's interest in public health and safety quite heavily but have perceived individual interests as nominal: "Society's judgement [is] that blood tests do not constitute an unduly extensive imposition on an individual's privacy and bodily integrity."[44] As a result, most courts have assumed a permissive posture when reviewing government screening programs.[45]

Many state statutes require informed consent for HIV testing and allow only specified, limited exceptions. An Alabama statute permitted testing without consent if (1) the patient was at "high risk" for infection, (2) knowledge of the patient's serologic status was necessary for medical care, or (3) knowledge of the patient's serologic status was necessary for the protection of health care personnel. A federal district court found the "high risk" classification to be unconstitutional because a patient could be arbitrarily classified but upheld the other two classifications.[46]

Most states have "alternative" test sites where individuals can receive anonymous testing. Against the advice of the CDC, North Carolina closed all of its anonymous HIV test sites. The state's purpose was to require universal, named

HIV reporting. The North Carolina courts upheld the closure as a valid exercise of the state's public health powers.[47]

State Regulation of Public Places: Bathhouses and Adult Bookstores

Government action to impede the spread of HIV has included the closure or regulation of public places such as bathhouses,[48] adult cinemas or video shops,[49] and bookstores.[50] Several municipal public health agencies have closed bath-houses in response to the HIV epidemic, believing that these establishments create opportunities for anonymous sex. In response, the gay community has argued that closure infringes upon the freedom of association, whereas positive measures, such as education and condom distribution, would help prevent high-risk sexual behavior.[51] The judiciary has consistently sided with public health authorities in such debates.[52] The courts have regarded places that fa-cilitate unsafe sexual activity as public nuisances, and they have granted public health agency requests to abate these nuisances.

Less clear is the impact of adult video shops or bookstores in contributing to the spread of HIV. When the state controls the sale of literature or movies, it may affect not only the right to privacy and association, but also the right to free expression guaranteed under the First Amendment. The federal courts have found local ordinances that require viewing booths to be open and visible to the public constitutional.[53] The ostensible goal is to prevent sexual activity, including masturbation.[54] These ordinances have been upheld because they are content neutral (i.e., they do not favor certain messages over other messages), serve a public health purpose, and do not interfere with the right to view films.[55] Although many restrictions on video shops or bookstores may promote a state's moral agenda, it is doubtful whether they promote the public's health. Masturbation, for example, does not pose a health risk and may even benefit the public by providing a safe outlet for sexual expression.

Tort Law

Contracting an infectious disease used to be perceived as a matter of chance or inadvertent misfortune. Today, it is not unusual for an exposed person to search for fault and, with it, liability. Claims of lack of due care, even bad faith or betrayal, by those who have been exposed to HIV have found their way to the courtroom. The depth of mistrust spans many relationships: patients against physicians or hospitals, health care professionals against the facility that employs them, one health care professional against another, and sex partners against their lovers. (Tort actions among sex partners are discussed in Chapter 3).

False Diagnosis of HIV Infection

A number of patients who have been incorrectly informed that they are infected with HIV have filed suit against their health care providers for negligent infliction of emotional distress.[56] Some of these plaintiffs have argued that an HIV-positive diagnosis is a "death sentence" that inflicts extreme psychological harm. Courts have been divided in their approach to these cases. Some courts have refused to allow the plaintiff to recover damages unless the mental distress arose from or led to a physical injury. For example, courts have held that increased blood pressure is not an adequate injury, but that harmful side effects of AIDS treatments or a patient's attempt at suicide would suffice to justify liability.[57] A few courts have not imposed a physical injury requirement at all.[58]

Failure to Diagnose HIV/AIDS

Since the advent of effective antiretroviral therapy, patients have had a strong interest in early diagnosis. The courts, therefore, sometimes have held physicians liable for negligently failing to diagnose HIV infection. In one case, a jury awarded more than $1 million because an earlier diagnosis would likely have delayed by one year the onset of symptoms, disability, and death.[59] A physician may also be liable for unnecessary delay in notifying a patient of exposure to HIV,[60] as well as the patient's sex partner who is subsequently infected.[61] However, physicians have not been held liable for failure to diagnose and effectively treat HIV unless the plaintiff has shown a causal connection between their failure and the injury suffered.[62]

Early diagnosis of HIV infection is particularly important for pregnant women.[63] The Institute of Medicine[64] and the CDC[65] both recommend routine HIV screening of pregnant women. Federal law incorporates the CDC recommendations for HIV counseling and voluntary testing for pregnant women as the standard of care.[66] Since early diagnosis is the standard of care, physicians who fail to offer testing to pregnant women (especially if they are at increased risk of HIV) may face tort liability for wrongful life or wrongful birth.[67]

Fear of exposure to HIV has created a burgeoning area of litigation. In these cases, the plaintiffs express fear that they were put at risk for HIV transmission, but typically they are not infected. Such plaintiffs seek compensation for their mental distress and anguish. Fear of HIV infection has even been asserted as a basis for refusing venipuncture for a blood alcohol test.[68]

Recognizing the litigious nature of American society, courts usually limit fear of HIV claims by requiring proof that the plaintiff's mental distress is a result of circumstances posing a meaningful exposure to infection. Most courts require that, for a plaintiff's fear to be reasonable, the virus must be present and the method of contact between the infected material and the plaintiff must be a "scientifically accepted channel for transmission of the disease." This requirement is needed to avoid an "explosion of frivolous litigation" regarding AIDS phobia claims.[69] Plaintiffs who fear an objectively nonexistent or unprovable risk usually are not compensated.[70] This requirement has been used in cases filed by patients of HIV-infected health care professionals (see Chapter 12), a surgeon who unknowingly operated on an HIV-positive patient,[71] a mortician embalming an HIV-infected corpse,[72] health care workers and others who have sustained needlestick injuries,[73] and sex partners of persons at risk for HIV.[74] If risk of exposure is proven, as in the case of a security officer whose skin was broken when he was bitten by an HIV-infected patient, damages are awarded.[75] If there is no evidence that the source patient was HIV-infected, the claim is denied.[76] Furthermore, many courts limit compensation to distress occurring during the "window of anxiety," the period between learning of possible exposure and obtaining a reliable HIV-negative test result.[77]

Fear of AIDS also has been used to justify the basis for court orders requiring HIV testing, for example, in cases in which the defendant has assaulted and bitten the plaintiff. In one such case, the Wisconsin Supreme Court, despite the lack of legislative authorization, upheld court-ordered testing even though the bite had occurred five years previously; thus, testing the defendant could not have determined whether HIV transmission had occurred as a result of that bite.[78] In a similar case, an inmate was ordered to undergo HIV testing so that the results would be available to a correctional officer who had been bitten three and one-half years earlier.[79]

Duty to Protect Workers

Employers, including health care and correctional facilities, have a duty to provide a reasonably safe workplace.[80] The Occupational Safety and Health Administration (OSHA) has issued a major blood-borne pathogen safety standard.[81] This standard requires, among other things, universal precautions against blood-borne transmission of infection. The OSHA regulations have been challenged as overly broad and excessively expensive,[82] but they remain the primary safety standard. OSHA permits health care professionals to refuse to work if the health care facility maintains inadequate infection control practices. The courts have held, however, that the worker's fear must be objective, meaning that the fear must be based on reliable evidence.[83]

Employee claims involving occupational transmission (or fear of occupational transmission) are generally covered by worker compensation statutes that provide exclusive remedies for work-related claims against employers.[84]

Administration of Justice

The prejudicial treatment of persons living with HIV/AIDS in the early years of the epidemic extended even to courts—the branch of government designed to promote justice. In 1988 New York State judicial guidelines suggested that judges may press defendants to waive their right to appear in court; surgical gloves, masks, and plastic shields may be kept on hand but out of sight; and "court officers may guard an afflicted person . . . from a distance of up to 10 feet."[85]

These kinds of policies, born of irrational fear and prejudice, were reflected in cases across the country when defendants living with HIV/AIDS claimed that they were denied a fair trial because court officers wore rubber gloves[86] or face masks,[87] sheriffs refused to transport the defendant to trial,[88] or the judge required that pleas be made by telephone, from behind glass, or by closed circuit television.[89]

Disclosure of HIV Infection: Prejudice versus Relevance

The Supreme Judicial Court of Massachusetts observed that "widespread ignorance about the nature of this disease and the accompanying prejudice against persons suffering from it . . . pose dangers to the accuracy and fairness of the legal process in many ways."[90] During the early era of the epidemic, appellate courts let stand decisions where the defendant's serologic status or high-risk behavior were needlessly disclosed to the judge or jury.[91] Specific cases included jurors being asked detailed questions about their attitudes toward homosexuality[92] or toward sitting with a defendant living with HIV/AIDS.[93] In virtually all of these cases, information about HIV was extraneous to the defendant's innocence or guilt, undermining the fairness of the fact-finding process. The modern legal standard for disclosure of HIV is whether the disclosure is inevitable and the evidence is relevant to the case.[94] If HIV information is irrelevant[95] or prejudicial,[96] it should be excluded.

HIV/AIDS is a health status that often results in social stigma and unfair treatment. The nation's judicial system should not be a place that tolerates injustice.

Expedited Trial

Plaintiffs living with HIV/AIDS have sought expedited litigation of their claims. Without such accommodation, illness or death may frustrate the prosecution of their claims. Particularly before the advent of effective treatment, courts sometimes granted trial preference to plaintiffs infected with HIV, finding it judicially indistinguishable from AIDS.[97]

Disclosure and Identity: Use of Pseudonyms

Many litigants living with HIV/AIDS fear that disclosure of their health status in the public forum of litigation may result in discrimination. Speaking in the context of an employment lawsuit by a plaintiff living with HIV/AIDS infection, a New Jersey superior court stated that a "plaintiff should not be compelled to turn himself or herself into a social outcast or forego what may be a valid claim for wrongful termination."[98] Generally, courts permit litigants to use pseudonyms (most commonly "Doe")[99] and otherwise accommodate their privacy interests, including by sealing court records from public access.[100] In some cases, however, courts have prohibited the use of a pseudonym where the plaintiff's identity had already been revealed in earlier proceedings.[101]

Family Law

The potential for HIV/AIDS to stir conflict within the family is apparent. Infection can be transmitted sexually and perinatally, affecting the spouse and future offspring. The attachment of blame to persons living with HIV/AIDS has been used as a weapon in divorce, custody, and visitation disputes. Finally, the infected person's health, including his or her mental health, can be used to imply incapacity to care for or supervise a child.

A spouse who knows he or she has a sexually transmitted infection, lies to his or her spouse, and actually transmits the infection can be held liable.[102] A jury awarded $2.1 million to the ex-wife of a man who died of AIDS. The husband failed to tell his wife that he was HIV-infected.[103] However, if a husband who is committing adultery does not know that he is infected with HIV and has not in fact transmitted the infection to his wife, he may not be held liable. One court refused to open a "Pandora's Box" where "a party who alleged adultery would have a tort action for AIDS phobia because any infidelity might lead to HIV."[104]

Apart from the limited tort of intentionally concealing an STD from a spouse, the courts usually have not found HIV infection to be relevant in deciding family law cases.[105] Most courts also do not mandate an HIV test in this context.[106] The courts reason that even if a person were infected, it would not materially affect his or her ability to be a good parent.

The overriding standard in family law is the child's best interests. The child's welfare is promoted by having loving relationships with both parents. A parent living with HIV/AIDS has as much to give his or her child as any other parent. To divest a parent of the human right to care for his or her child not only devalues the parent, but also deprives the child of the nurturing that the parent can give.[107]

Conclusion: Law, Litigation, and AIDS Policy

AIDS policies, ideally, should be developed by public health authorities using rigorous scientific assessments. Of course, AIDS policies are not created solely by public health officials, but also by the legislature and judiciary. Every state has enacted HIV/AIDS legislation.[108] The judiciary must construe and apply this legislation and adjudicate a bewildering array of disputes generated by the epidemic—ranging from tort, criminal, and constitutional law to family, contract, and insurance law.

Legislators and judges are not always educated about public health approaches to disease epidemics and do not always rely on exacting epidemiological, behavioral, and scientific evidence. Notably absent in many judicial opinions is a careful differentiation between significant and remote risks of transmission. Although courts enunciate a "deference" to scientific opinion, they also may grant "expert" status to testimony that is only loosely grounded in solid science. Accordingly, courts have upheld practice restrictions on health care professionals living with HIV/AIDS (see Chapter 12), found persons civilly or criminally liable for behavior unlikely to transmit the infection (see Chapter 10), approved compulsory testing (see Chapter 7), and undermined HIV education strategies (see discussion earlier in this chapter).

AIDS, perhaps more than any other modern disease, has powerful political and social repercussions. Yet AIDS policy is most effective and humane when illuminated by sound scientific assessments about transmission risks and informed by interventions likely to promote public health and respect individual rights.

The next chapter analyzes a large number of court cases involving the rights of persons living with HIV/AIDS, particularly the rights to privacy and to be free from discrimination.

Ryan White has shown the world that children infected with HIV can carry on normal lives, attend school, skateboard and play with their friends. His battle reminds us of the value of each and every day. It points out how important it is that our federal government commit the necessary money today because tomorrow is too late.—**Elizabeth Glaser,** founder of Pediatric AIDS Foundation (1990)

Chapter 3

The AIDS Litigation Project

Privacy, Discrimination, and Vulnerable Persons

By definition, epidemics alter a population's health; but they also harbor the potential to transform social systems. Epidemics can spur governments to re-allocate resources to promote human health. Epidemics can also illuminate the moral responsibilities of individuals to engage in safer behavior. Chapter 2 on the AIDS Litigation Project focused on government's duties and individuals' responsibilities. This chapter addresses individuals' rights.

Epidemic diseases compel us to consider individuals' rights for a number of reasons. First, public health powers themselves can encroach on personal rights by restricting liberty, autonomy, and privacy through interventions such as iso-lation, compulsory testing, and contact tracing (see, e.g., Chapters 4, 7, 9, and 10). Second, epidemic diseases breed ostracism and stigma. Diseases, particu-larly those involving intimate human behaviors such as sexual intercourse and drug use, are seldom objectively perceived as exclusively biological phenom-

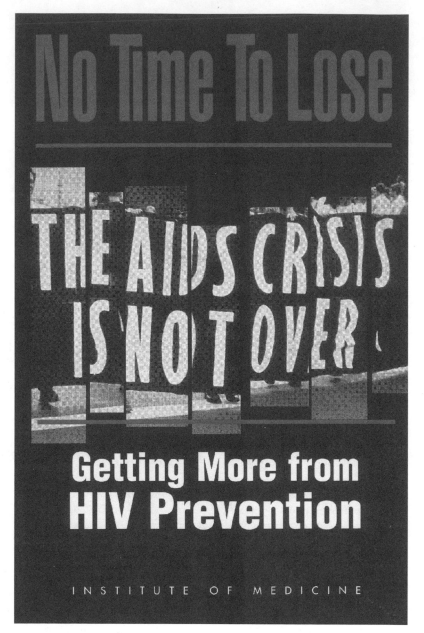

This design appeared on the cover of an influential Institute of Medicine report on HIV prevention published in 1998, when the number of AIDS deaths in the United States had declined by almost two-thirds from the all-time high recorded in 1995. The decline can be attributed to advances in antiretroviral therapies and to HIV prevention. Despite these successes, a growing proportion of HIV/AIDS cases is emerging in women, youth, and communities of color.

ena. Frequently, affected persons are blamed for their illness and viewed primarily as vectors of disease. The public often demands to know how the individual came to be infected and whether the person is likely to infect others. Sex partners, health care professionals, emergency personnel, corrections officers, and others claim a "right to know" whether they have been exposed to HIV.

Finally, epidemics of communicable disease often influence the state as well as private citizens to separate the sick from the healthy. Adverse treatment of individuals because of their health status is the essence of discrimination. When that discrimination invidiously deprives an individual of an important right or privilege—such as employment, housing, services, or insurance—harm and human suffering ensue. For all of these reasons and others, persons living with HIV/AIDS are deeply concerned about the right to privacy and non-discrimination. The CDC, for example, recommended "legal checkups," whereby an attorney counsels newly diagnosed HIV-positive persons to help protect their privacy.[1] Safeguarding privacy in many cases can prevent discrimination.[2]

Privacy and Confidentiality

Privacy, although a highly complex concept, can be defined as the right of individuals to limit access by others to some aspect of their person (see Chapter 5).[3] Informational privacy refers to a person's ability to prevent others from obtaining information about that person.[4] The primary moral justification for privacy is respect for the individual. To respect the privacy of others is to honor their autonomous wish not to be accessed in some way, either through observation or through disclosure of personal information. Privacy also encourages individuals to trust and confide freely. The concept of confidentiality extends a certain level of protection to private information within the context of a special relationship; for example, in the provision of health care, privacy and confidentiality serve to foster and maintain the physician-patient relationship.

The News Media

The First Amendment to the U.S. Constitution grants the media considerable freedom to publish information, even that of a deeply private nature. For instance, a Texas court upheld the right of a television station to air a story identifying a police officer living with HIV/AIDS. The police officer's HIV status became public as a result of his child custody hearing. The court noted that the story was protected by the First Amendment because it involved parental concerns for a child's safety and was therefore of legitimate public interest.[5]

Although many state statutes protect the confidentiality of an individual's HIV status, the courts have allowed the media considerable leeway to share AIDS information with the public. Courts normally balance the public's right to information with the person's privacy interests.[6] In several cases, courts have ruled that, for various reasons, persons living with HIV/AIDS have a reduced privacy interest. For instance, once a defendant's identity has been made public, he or she may no longer be covered by an HIV-specific confidentiality statute.

In another case, a newspaper was permitted to publish the names of three nurses who were assaulted by an HIV-infected patient. The court ruled that the information reported by the newspaper was not private because it was derived from public record police reports.[7] A New York court also permitted a newspaper to use a photograph of an otherwise healthy premature infant to illustrate a story about a hospital's care of infants and mothers suffering from AIDS, rejecting defamation and breach-of-confidentiality claims from the parents.[8]

Publication of a judicial opinion that references a defendant's HIV status is not a violation of his right to privacy.[9] A television station was allowed to broadcast the name of a defendant who was charged for engaging in behavior that led to a risk of transmitting HIV.[10] Publication of false information regarding an individual's HIV status may be considered defamatory.[11] However, if the false information is disclosed in a judicial proceeding, and then is reported as such, there is no liability.[12]

Unauthorized Disclosure

The quintessential aspect of the right to privacy is the ability of a person to control information about herself. Disclosure of HIV information without the person's consent may result in liability. Thus, claims of invasion of privacy or wrongful disclosure of HIV-related information have been brought against hospitals,[13] doctors,[14] pharmacies,[15] schools, education departments,[16] law enforcement agencies,[17] correctional institutions,[18] health departments,[19] social services,[20] coworkers,[21] employers,[22] lawyers,[23] the judicial system,[24] and even human rights commissions.[25]

Guided by the mandates of the physician-patient privilege and state HIV confidentiality laws, health care providers generally are prohibited from revealing a patient's HIV-related information for nontherapeutic purposes. Intentional disclosure is only one way to breach confidentiality. A health care facility's failure to adequately protect a medical record may also violate privacy.[26] However, not all disclosures constitute a breach of privacy. If the health care provider can present a compelling reason to disseminate the information, a court may allow disclosure. The courts balance the need for disclosure against the harm done to both an individual's privacy and the public interest.[27] Using such a test, an Ohio court found a hospital liable for disclosing patients' HIV statuses to a law firm. The law firm wanted to search for potential Supplemental Security Income eligibility for the payment of patients' unpaid medical bills.[28]

The Tenth Circuit Court of Appeals ruled that when a patient brings a malpractice case, the physician can disclose the patient's HIV status if it is relevant to the litigation. The physician-patient privilege is not violated when the doctor's disclosure is offered as part of her defense. Furthermore, by filing the lawsuit, the patient has made her health status a public matter.[29] In another case, a court held that a public health agency was not liable for disclosing confidential information to aid in a criminal prosecution; the criminal activity was deemed a waiver of confidentiality.[30] In contrast, other courts have prohibited law enforcement access to health records.[31]

Some state confidentiality statutes offer no protection outside of the health care or social service setting.[32] In Pennsylvania, for example, a police chief was not liable for posting a memorandum that identified one of his officers as having received a puncture wound from a person living with HIV/AIDS.[33] In another case, monitoring of nonprivileged telephone conversations of prison inmates was held not to violate the state HIV confidentiality statute because there was no compulsion involved.[34] But law enforcement personnel are not immune from liability for disclosing HIV information. The Tenth Circuit Court of Appeals found a police officer liable for informing witnesses, the suspect's family, and the jailer about a suspect's HIV status where there was no risk to these individuals.[35]

Judicially Ordered Disclosure of HIV-Related Information

Occasionally, courts order the disclosure of a person's HIV status. In doing so, the judiciary balances the need for disclosure against the potential harm disclosure presents to private and public interests.[36] For example, a court ordered disclosure in the case of a mental patient who stated that she had AIDS and then bit an attendant. The court reasoned that the patient had effectively waived her privacy rights by announcing her diagnosis.[37]

Courts frequently require that the recipient maintain the confidentiality of judicially disclosed information. One court ordered that patient records of a dentist who died of AIDS be released, provided that the release was limited to public health officials conducting an epidemiological study.[38]

The "Right to Know"

A major tension exists between confidentiality of HIV information and the "right to know." Despite broad privacy protections, many individuals who perceive themselves to be at risk of HIV infection claim the right to be informed of any potential exposure. A New York court characterized the right to know as "the most basic underpinning of a free and open society."[39] This tension has been played out in the nation's courtrooms through cases regarding sexual relationships, HIV-infected health care workers (HCWs), blood transfusions, and postmortem services. (For the HIV-infected HCW's duty to disclose, see Chapter 12).

Duty of Sex Partners to Disclose

Prior to the HIV epidemic, the legal and moral rights and responsibilities of sex partners were rarely articulated. The dominant judicial view holds that persons who know they are infected with HIV have a duty to inform their sex partners.[40] In one case, a woman sued the estate of her deceased boyfriend after he had failed to inform her that he had AIDS. The court ruled that the boyfriend did indeed have a duty to inform his partner.[41] In a case brought against Earvin "Magic" Johnson by a woman who claimed damages for sexual transmission of HIV, the court held that the duty to disclose arises only when a person knows he has HIV, experiences symptoms of HIV, or is aware that a previous sex partner had HIV. Even though, as alleged by the plaintiff, Johnson had numerous sex partners, he had neither been tested for HIV nor exhibited any symptoms at the time the sexual relationship took place and thus was under no duty to disclose.[42]

Duty to Disclose to Blood Transfusion Recipients

Physicians have a duty to inform patients who have been transfused with HIV-contaminated blood. This duty may extend to third parties. A physician in California failed to inform a young woman or her parents that she had been trans-

fused with HIV-contaminated blood. When the woman's sex partner tested
positive for HIV, he successfully sued the woman's physician for failing to inform her.[43] Likewise, in Washington, D.C., the husband of a patient who became infected with HIV from a blood transfusion successfully sued the hospital for negligent failure to warn the patient that she was at risk for contracting
HIV.[44]

Duty to Disclose to Funeral Service Providers

If morticians use universal precautions, the risk of contracting disease from an
infected corpse is negligible. In a West Virginia case, a mortician filed a tort action against a hospital for failing to inform him that a corpse he had handled
had been infected with HIV. The court found no liability in the absence of actual exposure.[45] In a similar case, an Ohio court found that a hospital was not
negligent when it notified the mortician that an HIV test had been performed,
but that no results were yet available.[46] Under the Ryan White CARE Act, states
receiving federal AIDS prevention and treatment funds must comply with federal rules allowing disclosure of HIV information to morticians and emergency
response workers upon their request.[47]

Duty to Disclose HIV Status to Third Parties at Risk

Many state laws allow, but do not require, disclosure by health care professionals to third parties at significant risk of HIV transmission.[48] Some courts have
found that physicians must use reasonable care to protect third parties from
foreseeable exposure to contagious diseases.[49] Consequently, a physician may
disclose a patient's HIV status to the patient's spouse[50] or even to a family member caregiver.[51] A Georgia court found that a doctor had the statutory authority to disclose the HIV status of a dental hygienist because patients had "the
right to make an informed decision about being treated by [the HIV-positive
hygienist]."[52] Other courts have found that health care providers have no duty
to warn third parties.[53] If the risk to the third party is remote, health care professionals may not disclose confidential HIV information.[54] For example, a person cannot claim a right to know his roommate's HIV status.[55]

Occasionally, plaintiffs claim that others are responsible for their exposure
to HIV. However, the Eighth Circuit Court of Appeals held that parole and
probation officers were not liable for failure to warn a parolee's girlfriend that
he was HIV-infected.[56] In an unusual case, a federal court found that an em-

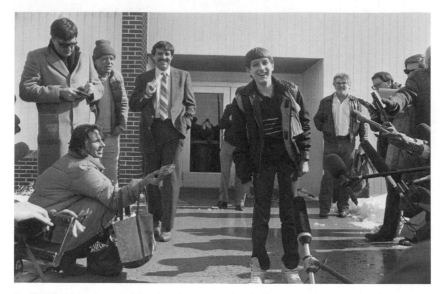

Ryan White (1971–90), who fought to attend public school in Indiana and became a national advocate for the rights and dignity of people living with HIV/AIDS. (© Bettmann/CORBIS)

ployer, an online service provider, was not liable for an employee's actions when the employee had sex without disclosing his HIV infection; the plaintiff had met the employee through a sexual chat room provided by the employer.[57]

Discrimination

Every major governmental,[58] medical,[59] public health,[60] and legal[61] organization to issue a report on the HIV epidemic has condemned discrimination because it violates basic tenets of individual justice and is detrimental to public health (see Chapter 6). Discrimination based on an infectious condition is just as inequitable as discrimination based on race, gender, or disability. People are treated inequitably not because they lack inherent ability, but solely because of a health status. As a result, complex and often pernicious mythologies develop about the nature, cause, and transmission of disease.

Persons living with HIV/AIDS have to endure moral disapproval of their behavior and archaic attitudes that they present a health menace. The public's association of the disease with traditionally disfavored groups—gays, injection drug users, and sex workers—only compounds the bigotry.

Discrimination against persons living with HIV/AIDS is not only unjust; it is also economically and socially detrimental. By rendering talented individuals unemployable or uninsurable, or by impairing their ability to secure housing or receive health care or other services, discrimination tears at the social and economic fabric of the nation. Discrimination also undermines public health. If individuals fear social and economic repercussions, they may forego testing or fail to discuss their health and risk behaviors with counselors or health care professionals and, even more importantly, with their sex or needle-sharing partners.

An array of laws at the federal, state, and local levels prohibits discrimination on the basis of a person's disability or health status.[62] The primary nondiscrimination statute at the federal level is the Americans with Disabilities Act of 1990 (ADA).[63] The ADA prohibits discrimination in employment, government services, public transportation, and public accommodations.[64] The laws of many states and localities specifically prohibit discrimination against individuals with HIV. For more on the ADA and state and local antidiscrimination statutes, see Chapter 6.

Employment

To maintain an employment discrimination suit, a person living with HIV/AIDS must demonstrate that she is qualified to perform the essential functions of the job. Under the ADA, a "qualified" person with a disability is an individual with a disability who, with or without reasonable accommodations, can perform the essential functions of the job.[65] If HIV infection prevents a person from performing the essential aspects of the job, even with reasonable accommodations, the individual is unqualified, and an adverse employment decision is not discriminatory.[66] In the past, several courts found that persons who claimed or received social security disability benefits were per se unqualified, or such benefits were at least evidence of inability to work.[67] However, the Supreme Court has found that an applicant for social security benefits may still be a qualified individual for purposes of the ADA.[68]

Employees can prove discrimination if they meet all of the job requirements but are adversely treated because of their HIV status.[69] Adverse treatment is not limited to hiring and firing decisions but may include promotion decisions and claims of a hostile work environment.[70] The employee must prove that the disability, not some nondiscriminatory reason, was the basis for the employer's actions.[71] Once employers are aware of the employee's disability, they are required to provide "reasonable accommodations" that will make it possible for the employee to perform the job despite the disability.[72]

If an individual poses a significant health risk to others that reasonable accommodations cannot eliminate, the individual is unqualified. For example, an employee with an infectious disease is unqualified if she or he poses a significant risk of transmitting the infection to others.[73] (See Chapter 12 for a discussion of discrimination against HCWs who pose a remote risk of transmitting HIV to patients). In *Chevron U.S.A., Inc. v. Echazabal*, the Supreme Court unanimously held that an individual also is not qualified if she poses a significant risk to her own health.[74] This analysis suggests that individuals infected with HIV could be disqualified if the work environment threatens to worsen their health, such as through exposure to opportunistic infections (even potentially including the common cold). This paternalistic approach to the ADA threatens to limit employment opportunities for persons living with HIV/AIDS.

Federal, state, and local antidiscrimination laws can also protect employees who are associated with persons living with HIV/AIDS.[75] For example, an employee who was fired after taking time off to care for his HIV-infected son successfully sued his employer under the Family Medical Leave Act.[76] A nurse who was terminated for assisting an HIV-infected patient recovered compensatory damages and back pay after the New York State Division of Human Rights found that her employer had engaged in discriminatory conduct against the patient.[77]

Public Accommodations and Commercial Establishments

The ADA provides that no individual "shall be discriminated against on the basis of disability in the full and equal enjoyment of the goods, services, facilities, privileges, advantages, or accommodations of any place of public accommodation."[78] "Places of public accommodation" include private businesses, hotels, restaurants, retail stores, hair salons, funeral parlors, and the professional offices of health care providers.[79] Courts at the federal[80] and state[81] levels have decided numerous cases involving discrimination by health care providers. Notably, New York's highest court has ruled that the offices of private dentists, not operating as clinics, are considered places of public accommodation; but this view is not universally accepted.[82] In other contexts, AIDS discrimination claims have been brought against hotel owners,[83] securities brokerage firms,[84] public transport systems,[85] athletic facilities,[86] day care centers,[87] prisons,[88] and public services.[89]

Health Care

A health care provider cannot lawfully discriminate in treating or caring for a person living with HIV/AIDS. Health care professionals have a duty to dispense equal and appropriate care to all of their patients, irrespective of serological status.[90] Providers must, of course, exercise appropriate clinical judgment. If a professional lacks adequate expertise to competently render care, she may legally refuse to treat the person and may lawfully refer him elsewhere.[91] But a professional cannot simply reject or refer an HIV-infected patient because of his or her HIV status. The Supreme Court has emphasized that professionals must rely on objective, scientific information to determine whether providing services to an HIV-infected patient poses such a substantial risk of transmission that it would be permissible to deny treatment.[92]

The courts have had to decide the difficult question of when health care professionals can treat HIV-infected patients differently from other patients. Although CDC and Occupational Health and Safety Administration (OSHA) standards employ "universal" precautions applicable to all patients without regard to infection status, some courts have upheld the imposition of special precautions for HIV-infected patients.[93] One court, finding that special precautions may be necessary for certain procedures, ruled that a dentist may lawfully refuse to treat a patient who refuses to reveal HIV-related information.[94] But another court found a physician and hospital liable for unlawful discrimination when the physician delayed surgery in order to take precautionary safeguards above and beyond the CDC recommendations.[95]

Housing

Procuring housing for persons living with HIV/AIDS is often problematic. Efforts to establish group homes for persons with HIV frequently encounter roadblocks, such as attempts to use municipal zoning rules or restrictive covenants to exclude such facilities.[96] To combat discrimination, housing providers and persons living with HIV/AIDS have successfully invoked the federal Fair Housing Act[97] or similar state laws.[98]

Such laws require that persons living with HIV/AIDS be treated fairly, not only in the opportunities to rent or buy property, but also in the provision of housing-related services. In one case, a plumbing contractor refused to enter the apartment of an HIV-infected tenant.[99] The court concluded that the landlord was liable for discrimination unless he hired a new contractor or educated the current one about the absence of risk. Landlords who harass tenants based on

HIV status by, for example, posting notices that the tenant is HIV-infected and refusing to accept rent checks have been found liable.[100]

Discrimination in the Military

The U.S. military routinely tests service members for HIV. Although service members living with HIV/AIDS can remain in the military as long as they meet fitness-for-duty standards, recruits living with HIV/AIDS are denied enlistment. The nondiscrimination standards applicable in civilian life, such as the ADA, do not extend to the military. In assessing military policy, courts tend to defer to the judgment of Department of Defense (DOD) officials. For example, the First Circuit Court of Appeals, presuming that the DOD's policy was sound, upheld its discharge of HIV-infected reservists for whom no nondeployable positions were available.[101] On the other hand, the military has not argued that the AIDS epidemic provides a basis for excluding gay service members under the current policy of "Don't Ask, Don't Tell, Don't Pursue, Don't Harass."[102]

Insurance

Many individuals living with HIV/AIDS look to private health and disability insurance to provide access to health care and income in the event of inability to work. However, practices among insurers make maintenance of coverage difficult and obtaining coverage virtually impossible. Health, life, and disability insurance illustrates perhaps the most conspicuous gap in coverage under disability discrimination legislation. Insurers are subject to the public accommodation provisions of the ADA[103] and state nondiscrimination standards.[104] However, the ADA permits insurers, including self-insurers, to engage in the ordinary business of insurance underwriting or risk assessment, but discrimination based on specific disabilities is not permitted.

Most individuals with private insurance obtain coverage as a benefit of employment. Employers may not fire an employee simply because his illness may financially burden the health care benefits plan or cause an increase in premiums.[105] Whether the employer can simply restructure the plan to reduce treatment benefits, however, remains an open question. In a case filed under federal employee benefits law, the Employee Retirement Income Security Act (ERISA), an employer was allowed to reduce coverage for HIV-related treatment from $1 million to $5,000 after an HIV-infected employee began to file claims for health care benefits.[106] The Equal Employment Opportunity Commission (EEOC) has taken the position that the subsequently enacted ADA prohibits such discrimination.[107] Employers may be liable for the discriminatory acts of an insurance company that rejects an employee for coverage based on HIV status.[108]

Since an insured individual's HIV status is relevant to his or her risk of illness or death, insurance companies may legally require an applicant to disclose HIV status, and they may require HIV testing as part of medical underwriting. If an applicant intentionally conceals his or her HIV infection or illness, the insurer may, in some states, rescind the contract.[109] In some states, however, after the expiration of the "contestability" period (typically two years), the contract may not be rescinded, nor can the insurer refuse to pay benefits even if the policy was fraudulently obtained.[110] If the applicant does not perpetrate a fraud and offers the information without the intent to deceive, recision is not allowed.[111] But an insurance applicant who is infected with HIV may, in certain circumstances, be excluded from benefits under preexisting condition clauses.[112] Several courts have held that health insurers may cap benefits to individuals with HIV.[113] In the life insurance context, two courts have held that the ADA prohibits insurance companies from denying policies to applicants who have protected sex with HIV-infected spouses.[114]

An emerging issue is whether services for persons living with HIV are covered. The Eleventh Circuit Court of Appeals held that skilled nursing care was "medically necessary" and should be reimbursed under an employer's self-funded health benefits plan.[115]

The Rights of Vulnerable Persons: Disability, Homelessness, and Indigence

Persons living with HIV/AIDS, who are often among the poorest members of our society, may need to obtain assistance through programs that provide social services, housing, income support, and other related services. Social security regulations setting forth standards for disability benefits have been challenged as discriminating against women and people of color,[116] although subsequently these regulations have been revised.[117] Several cases involved situations where the Social Security Administration (SSA) did not properly evaluate claims of disability presented by individuals with HIV.[118] The SSA in some cases failed to develop evidence and made errors in assessing the evidence.[119] Veterans face other hurdles. To obtain a higher level of veterans' benefits, former service members with HIV must show that their disability is "service-connected" but not the result of misconduct that would be a bar to benefits.[120]

Social service programs, including housing for homeless persons with HIV, have been challenged in several respects. First, homeless persons in New York brought suit contending that services for homeless persons living with HIV/ AIDS were inadequate and posed a health hazard.[121] Second, courts have upheld tuberculosis screening within a congregate living facility because screening was rationally related to reducing the risk of secondary infections.[122] Third, health and social services for persons with AIDS have been challenged as inadequate under the ADA, given the needs of the population.[123] However, one court concluded that states that provide services to one category of disabled individuals need not extend services to all people with disabilities.[124]

The Rights of Prisoners

State's Duty to Protect Inmates

The Eighth Amendment proscribes cruel and unusual punishment.[125] Prison authorities violate the Eighth Amendment if they act with deliberate indifference to prisoner safety or refuse to act when they know, or should know, that an inmate faces a substantial risk of harm.[126] Thus, courts have held that failure to protect an inmate from sexual assault by an HIV-infected inmate may rise to the level of cruel and unusual punishment.[127] Imposing work assignments that might expose inmates to HIV (e.g., cleaning blood spills) has also been held to violate the Constitution.[128]

Inmates have claimed that failure to segregate HIV-infected prisoners from the general population constitutes cruel and unusual punishment, but these claims have been unsuccessful.[129] In one case, the Fourth Circuit Court of Appeals decided that integration was neither unconstitutional nor statutorily mandated; the determination to segregate fell within the prison authorities' discretion.[130] Fear of living with an HIV-infected cellmate is usually based on ignorance. Therefore, to assign an inmate an HIV-infected cellmate is not cruel and unusual punishment.[131] Similarly, courts have held that a prison's failure to test all inmates for HIV and impose segregation does not violate the Eighth Amendment.[132]

Civil Rights of Inmates

Disclosure of Serological Status: Privacy and Confidentiality

To disclose an inmate's HIV status to unauthorized personnel may violate the inmate's right to privacy; not all prison employees are authorized to receive confidential information.[133] In several cases, however, claims of a constitutional violation were rejected on the basis that the privacy right was not clearly established at the time; thus, the violation did not involve deliberate indifference.[134] Generally, dissemination of HIV test results should be limited to prison managers, medical personnel, and others who have a clear need to know. However, a federal district court in New York found that a Spanish-speaking inmate's right to privacy was not violated when the inmate was forced to rely on multiple prison officials and other inmates to communicate with medical personnel treating him for AIDS.[135] In another case, police officers who placed a sign on an arrestee's cell door stating that the arrestee was HIV positive were immune from suit.[136]

Testing: Bodily Autonomy

Prisoners may be denied certain freedoms and privileges if the denial is reasonably related to a legitimate penological objective.[137] Courts have held that mandatory HIV testing is necessary to accomplish a legitimate penological objective.[138] Consequently, although it does not serve an important public health purpose, courts have upheld HIV screening of prisoners. In *Stanley v. Swinson*, an inmate unsuccessfully argued that the mandatory testing of inmates to track the HIV infection rate in prisons violated federal regulations prohibiting human subject research on inmates without informed consent.[139]

Screening and Segregation

Courts have upheld corrections department decisions to exclude HIV-infected inmates from working as food handlers.[140] Prison officials have argued that allowing infected inmates to serve food would provoke unrest and fear among the prison population and might incite violence. This policy, although discriminatory in a nonpenal environment, was allowable because it was reasonably related to security concerns.[141] In another case, however, a prisoner living with HIV/AIDS who was denied yard privileges and forced to wear a face mask outside of his cell brought a successful claim for violation of his Eighth Amendment right to be free from cruel and unusual punishment.[142]

Although integration of inmates living with HIV/AIDS into the general prison population is increasingly common, segregating inmates has been challenged. Courts have upheld this practice on the grounds that it does not violate any clearly established constitutional or statutory rights.[143] For example, the Eleventh Circuit Court of Appeals affirmed a district court holding that a prison could segregate HIV-infected inmates because of the "significant risk" of HIV transmission.[144] The court held that prisons could consider the cost of extra guards needed for integrated programs in deciding whether or not to segregate HIV-infected prisoners.[145] The Federal Bureau of Prisons policy on HIV-infected inmates, which authorizes placement of inmates in controlled housing when "there is reliable evidence indicating that the inmate may engage in conduct posing a health risk to others," has also been upheld against constitutional challenges.[146]

Inadequate Medical Treatment: Cruel and Unusual Punishment

Gross inadequacies in state prison health care systems may rise to the level of a constitutional violation.[147] In New York, inmates living with HIV/AIDS challenged the state's delivery of medical, mental health, educational, and prevention services. The court ordered the state to release records enumerating the inmates, both living and deceased, who had been diagnosed with AIDS or AIDS-related illnesses to help the court determine whether prison authorities deliberately neglected the inmates' health care needs.[148] In another case, inadequate medical care and lack of HIV education services resulted in a court-imposed remedial plan.[149] But when a showing of deliberate indifference is lacking, an Eighth Amendment claim against prison officials will fail.[150]

Immigration and International Travel

One of the most controversial U.S. policies has been the prohibition against entry of HIV-infected visitors and immigrants into the United States.[151] This policy resulted in the confinement of Haitian immigrants with HIV at the U.S. Naval Base at Guantánamo Bay, Cuba, for approximately two years.[152] In considering a challenge on behalf of the Haitians, the court noted that their "imprisonment . . . serves no purpose other than to punish them for being sick."[153] In other immigration cases, fear of persecution based on HIV status has been grounds for a grant of asylum.[154] (For an in-depth discussion of immigration and international travel, see Chapter 15).

Conclusion

For more than two decades, America has fought the HIV/AIDS epidemic on two fronts: through science and medicine to prevent and treat HIV/AIDS and through ethics and law to prevent social injustice. The fields of medicine and public health have confronted HIV/AIDS from the vantage of science. The United States has entered an era of ever more sophisticated advances in the knowledge and treatment of HIV/AIDS.[155] Behavioral approaches—voluntary screening, counseling, and education—have reduced new infections among several populations, but the burden of HIV/AIDS continues to be heavy among communities of color, women, and injection drug users.[156] More recently, infection rates among gay men have also begun to increase.[157]

We like to believe that we have made progress on the social front. Even if science cannot find a vaccine, society surely can learn to treat persons living with HIV/AIDS with dignity and respect. Since HIV is not transmitted through casual contact, it ought to be possible to dispel the fears and prejudices evidenced in public accommodations, employment, and housing. Even in the most challenging contexts (such as the health care and corrections systems), universal precautions virtually eliminate the risk of infection. There is no reason why, in this modern age, fears of contagion should lead to hate and exclusion of persons living with HIV/AIDS.

In addition, society now has a fuller understanding of the potential for stigma and ostracism posed by the disclosure of a person's HIV status. It is well settled that persons living with HIV/AIDS ought to have valid legal and ethical claims to privacy and nondiscrimination.

This review of AIDS litigation shows improvement in the fight against the negative social impact of HIV/AIDS. The Americans with Disabilities Act of 1990 and numerous state statutes that proscribe discrimination or breaches of privacy have spawned a number of successful legal cases. Yet the legislature and judiciary have sometimes failed to protect the rights of persons living with HIV/AIDS. Many challenges still face America in its social and legal response to AIDS: (1) the Supreme Court has significantly narrowed the scope of the ADA, (2) the "significant risk" standard has been bent to permit discrimination in cases where the probabilities of transmission are exceedingly low or where the HIV-infected person's own health is placed at risk, (3) the public's "right to know" has rationalized breaches of privacy, (4) the business interests of insurers have often taken precedence over the health care needs of persons with HIV/AIDS, and (5) the administrative efficiency of the corrections system has justified infringements on the privacy and autonomy of inmates.

As science strives to overcome the formidable biological challenges of the HIV/AIDS epidemic, so too must the law seek to abate the intractable social burdens. AIDS litigation is one key way to strive for individual rights and social justice. In the next part, this book turns to human rights and two of the most important aspects of personal dignity—privacy and fair treatment.

Part 2 Rights and Dignity

It is not necessary to recount the numerous charters and declarations on HIV/AIDS and human rights to understand human rights in the context of HIV/AIDS. All persons are born free and equal in dignity and rights. Everyone, including persons seeking to avoid HIV infection, as well as persons living with HIV/AIDS, is entitled to all the rights and freedoms set forth in the international human rights instruments without discrimination, such as the rights to life, liberty, security of the person, privacy, health, education, work, social security, and to marry and found a family. Yet, violations of human rights in the context of HIV/AIDS are a reality to be found in every corner of the globe. —**Jose Ayala Lasso,** former United Nations high commissioner for human rights, and Peter Piot, executive director of UNAIDS (1997)

Chapter 4

Human Rights and Public Health
in the HIV/AIDS Pandemic

Human rights law is a powerful, but often neglected, tool in advancing the rights, freedoms, health, and well-being of persons living with HIV/AIDS. International law may seem marginal or unimportant in developed countries with democratic and constitutional systems of their own. Yet even democracies often resist legal safeguards of privacy and nondiscrimination, and domestic courts do not always compel changes necessary for the rights and welfare of persons living with HIV/AIDS. Additionally, for countries without democratic and constitutional systems, human rights law may provide the only genuine safeguard against neglect and ill-treatment of persons living with HIV/AIDS.

Human rights law is important in the context of health because of two fundamental ideas unique to global protection of rights and freedoms. First, human rights are the only source of law that legitimize international scrutiny of health policies and practices within a sovereign country. The international system be-

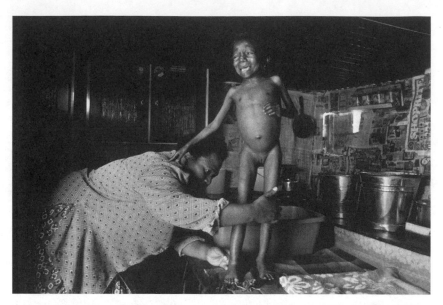

An AIDS patient is washed by a volunteer at a hospice in South Africa in 2001. While pharmaceutical companies fight for patent ownership, developing countries are unable to provide basic health care to people living with HIV/AIDS.

fore World War II focused almost solely on relations between states; human rights violations that occurred within a country's borders were generally deemed an "internal affair." The horrors of that war exposed the vulnerability of the individual in an international system that was based on state sovereignty and demonstrated the gross inadequacy of previous attempts to protect rights and freedoms.[1] One of the first imperatives of the postwar era was to prevent the recurrence of such egregious affronts to peace and human dignity.

The postwar human rights movement permanently altered the scope of international law. It pierced the veil of national sovereignty and elevated human rights as a matter of international import. The idea that individuals possess inherent rights and freedoms was not new. Recognizing these rights under international law was, as was holding states accountable for violations. Human rights, therefore, are not a matter simply between citizens and their government— even if a democratically elected government. Rather, certain basic human rights are a matter of international law enforceable against the state. In theory, although often not in practice, this renders each country's AIDS policies and practices susceptible to international monitoring and control.

The second, related idea is that human rights do not rely on government beneficence. Human rights and freedoms are not granted by governments, nor do governments have the power to deny them. Persons possess rights simply because of their humanity. Thus, persons living with HIV/AIDS, or those groups at special risk, need not prove that they deserve certain rights. Human rights law provides fundamental protections without qualification or exception.[2]

Human rights, then, afford all persons rights and freedoms and place duties on government to respect them. Classic understandings of human rights are limited to government, not personal, obligations to respect rights and freedoms. Human rights law, strictly speaking, does not protect one individual against the harmful actions of another.[3] However, government duties may be conceived quite broadly to include the duty to *protect*, so that states take measures to prevent third parties from interfering with human rights; *respect*, so that states do not interfere directly or indirectly with the enjoyment of human rights; and *fulfill* (facilitate and promote), so that states take positive measures (legislative, budgetary, promotional) to enable and assist individuals and communities to enjoy human rights.[4]

This chapter examines the human rights of persons living with HIV/AIDS. First, it describes three important relationships between health and human rights: the impact of health policies on human rights, the impact of violations of human rights on health, and the inextricable link between health and human rights. This discussion is derived from the classic article of Jonathan M. Mann, Lawrence O. Gostin, Sofia Gruskin, and colleagues in the first issue of the *Journal of Health and Human Rights*.[5]

Second, the chapter considers in closer detail one of the relationships between health and human rights—the effects of public health policies on the rights and dignity of individuals and populations. Here, I propose a "human rights impact assessment" that offers a systematic examination of the effects of public health policies on the dignity and rights of persons living with HIV/AIDS. When public health authorities compel individuals to act, for example, with respect to testing, reporting, partner notification, or isolation, there is often a potential conflict with human rights. This impact assessment helps scholars and practitioners to evaluate the human rights implications.

Third, the chapter reviews the civil and political rights of persons living with HIV/AIDS. There have been many statements of these rights by governments and nongovernmental organizations (NGOs). This section provides an account of the main entitlements and explains their importance.

The final section examines the social, cultural, and economic rights of persons living with HIV/AIDS. Most of the precision and enforceability in human rights have been in the realm of civil and political rights. Human rights scholars and practitioners, until recently, have not thought carefully about how to construct a meaningful set of social and economic rights. This is changing as more scholarship and advocacy are devoted to social and economic rights. The chapter ends with a consideration of the fundamental importance of the right to health in the HIV/AIDS pandemic.

The Fundamental Relationships between Health and Human Rights

All too often, individuals and communities are denied the opportunity to discuss the diffi-cult issues surrounding HIV/AIDS, to organize themselves into self-help groups and to take the necessary measures for protection from HIV infection. In an environment where human rights are not fully respected, the likelihood of vulnerability to infection and further exclu-sion increases dramatically.—Mary Robinson, former United Nations high commissioner for human rights (2001)

Prior to the work of the late Jonathan Mann, founding director of the World Health Organization's (WHO's) Global Programme on AIDS, health and human rights rarely had been linked in an explicit manner. The public health literature seldom mentioned the importance of human rights. Similarly, the human rights literature seldom mentioned health, except perhaps to draw attention to the physical and mental harms of rape or torture. Yet health and human rights are both powerful, modern approaches to defining and advancing human well-being. Mann and his colleagues proposed a three-part framework for consider-ing linkages between health and human rights.

The First Relationship: The Impact of Health Policies on Human Rights

Health policies and practices often have a significant impact on the rights of people and communities. The most obvious illustration is the effect of coer-cive policies: mandatory testing and screening interfere with personal auton-omy, reporting and other forms of surveillance affect privacy, and isolation or quarantine affect liberty. Additionally, selective implementation of AIDS poli-cies can result in discrimination. Consider a policy that criminalizes commer-cial sex workers but not their clients, or a policy that provides treatment for HIV-infected newborns but not their mothers.

Even the simple act of assessment or research can be discriminatory. Think about the early failure of the U.S. government to comprehensively assess the burden of HIV/AIDS on African Americans, Hispanics, and women. Conse-quentially, over half of all new HIV cases in the United States are among African Americans,[6] though African Americans make up only about 13 percent of the total U.S. population.[7]

There are significant human rights implications whenever logistic, financial, or sociocultural barriers impede people's access to health and social services. For example, if women and children living with HIV/AIDS cannot receive adequate care and services due to the unavailability of transportation or child care, or due to language difficulties or limited hours of service, their right to health may be compromised. Human rights violations also occur against those affected but not infected by HIV, such as the millions of children whose parents have died of AIDS.[8] Some governments fail to protect children who are orphaned by AIDS and at higher risk of human rights abuse.[9]

It is essential to recognize that in seeking to fulfill core functions and responsibilities, public health approaches may burden human rights. In the past, when restrictions on human rights were recognized, they were often simply justified as necessary to protect the public's health. Indeed, public health has a long tradition, anchored in the history of infectious disease control, of limiting the "rights of the few" for the "good of the many."

Unfortunately, public health decisions to restrict human rights sometimes have been made in an uncritical, unsystematic, and unscientific manner. There is a prevailing assumption that public health, as articulated through specific policies and programs, is an unalloyed public good that does not require consideration of human rights norms. This characterization must be challenged.

The idea that human rights and public health must inevitably conflict is increasingly tempered with awareness of how each complements the other. It is certainly true that restrictive health policies are sometimes necessary to reduce the burden of HIV/AIDS. More often than not, however, respect for the rights of the individual will actually promote healthy outcomes. If individuals feel secure in their autonomy and dignity, they are more likely to engage in health-promoting activities, cooperate with public health and medical professionals, and disclose their health status to their sex and needle-sharing partners.

The Second Relationship: The Impact of Violations of Human Rights on Health

Severe human rights violations are known to have significant health effects. For example, torture, inhuman and degrading treatment, summary executions, and disappearances affect victims, their families, and the wider community. Torture is often used as a political tool to discourage people from resisting government oppression. Victims of torture explain that their trauma is lifelong and profoundly affects the people who know and love them. Likewise, systematic rape of women is intended to make all women feel vulnerable and powerless; it undermines the stability of the entire community.

For these reasons, health experts concerned about human rights have increasingly made their expertise available to help document such abuses. Examples of this type of public health/human rights collaboration include exhumation of mass graves to examine allegations of executions, examination of torture victims, and entry of health personnel into prisons to assess health status.[10]

Beyond these serious human rights abuses, it is increasingly evident that lesser violations of human rights also adversely affect health. Think about three important human rights infringements and their effects on health: dignity violations, discrimination, and withholding of scientific information.

Violation of the right to individual and collective dignity has a profound effect on health. The Universal Declaration of Human Rights (UDHR) considers dignity, along with other rights, to be inherent, inalienable, and universal. People who are not treated with dignity, such as people at heightened risk for HIV (gay men, injection drug users [IDUS], and sex workers), may have poor health status and difficulty accessing needed services.

People who are subject to discrimination may find it difficult to live safe and healthy lives. Persons living with HIV/AIDS are sometimes denied employment, housing, or insurance because of their HIV status; they may suffer economic hardship, making it difficult to find food, shelter, clothing, and other necessities of life. They may even be denied basic civil privileges such as the right to marry. For instance, the Supreme Court of India suspended the right of HIV-infected persons to marry.[11]

Failure of the government to provide accurate and full scientific information may also affect people's health. Consider a government that withholds valid health information about HIV prevention such as the benefits of using condoms or sterile injection equipment.

Assessment of the health impacts of human rights violations is in its infancy. Progress will require a more sophisticated capacity to document and assess rights violations; the application of medical, social science, and public health methodologies to identify and assess effects on physical, mental, and social well-being; and research to establish valid associations between human rights violations and health impacts.

The Third Relationship: Health and Human Rights—Exploring an Inextricable Linkage

Promoting and protecting human rights is inextricably linked to the challenge of promoting and protecting health. Health advocacy and human rights are complementary approaches to the central problem of defining and advancing human well-being. Modern concepts of health recognize that underlying "conditions" establish the foundation for realizing physical, mental, and social well-being.[12] We now know that adequate levels of income and social status are essential to healthy people and populations;[13] it is also documented that social connections (relationships with family, friends, and community) are important conditions for health.[14] In light of the importance of these conditions, it is remarkable how little priority has been given within health research to their precise identification, modes of action, relative significance, and possible interactions.

The vulnerability of women illustrates the value of using a human rights analysis in public health. Many married, monogamous women in parts of Africa and Asia are infected with HIV.[15] Although these women know about HIV and condoms are accessible in the marketplace, their risk factor is their inability to control their husbands' sexual behavior or to refuse unprotected or unwanted sexual intercourse.[16] Refusal may result in physical harm, or in divorce—the equivalent of social and economic death for the woman. Therefore, women's vulnerability to HIV is now recognized to be integrally connected with discrimination and unequal rights involving property, marriage, divorce, and inheritance.[17] The success of condom promotion for HIV prevention in this population is inherently limited by the absence of legal and societal changes that, by promoting and protecting women's rights, would strengthen their ability to negotiate sexual practice and protect themselves from HIV infection.

More broadly, the evolving HIV/AIDS pandemic has shown a consistent pattern through which discrimination, marginalization, stigmatization, and, more generally, lack of respect for the human rights of individuals and groups heighten the risk of exposure to HIV. In this regard, HIV/AIDS may be illustrative of a more general phenomenon in which individual and population vulnerability to disease, disability, and premature death is linked to the status of respect for human rights and dignity.

The idea that promotion and protection of rights and health are inextricably linked requires creative exploration and rigorous evaluation. At the time of Jonathan Mann's tragic death in 1998, few scholars and advocates were making the connections between health and human rights. That is now changing with important scholarship and advocacy taking place in communities, governments, NGOs, and international agencies.[18]

Human Rights Impact Assessment for Public Health Policies

As we have just seen, there are at least three important relationships between health and human rights. This section focuses on one of these relationships — the effects of public health policies on the rights and dignity of persons living with HIV/AIDS. Public health officials sometimes formulate strategies without carefully considering the goals of the policy, whether the means adopted will achieve the goals, and whether the financial and human rights burdens outweigh the intended benefits. Implementing AIDS policies without seriously considering these dimensions may harm the people affected and the public health strategies themselves.

This section offers a "human rights impact assessment," as developed with Jonathan Mann.[19] Mann and I felt that human rights advocates should have a tool they could use to evaluate the effects of a public health policy on human rights, much as an "environmental impact assessment" evaluates the effects of property development on the environment. Of course, no magic formula exists to understand the effects of public health policies on the human rights of individuals and communities. Still, the basic steps provided here should help decision makers balance competing interests and develop effective public health policies that respect human rights (see Figure 4-1). These steps are intended to complement existing international standards such as the Siracusa Principles.[20]

Step 1: Undertake Fact-finding

The human rights framework dictates that any public health measure be "informed by evidence and openly debated."[21] Scientists understand the importance of carefully gathering and assessing all relevant facts before drawing a conclusion. The unbiased collection of data by the sciences of public health (such as epidemiology, virology, and biostatistics) and health care (such as medicine, nursing, and social services) is a fundamental prerequisite to ethical policy development.

Assessments of the human rights impacts of policy require equally rigorous and impartial fact-finding. Institutions that seek to justify a policy (e.g., Min-

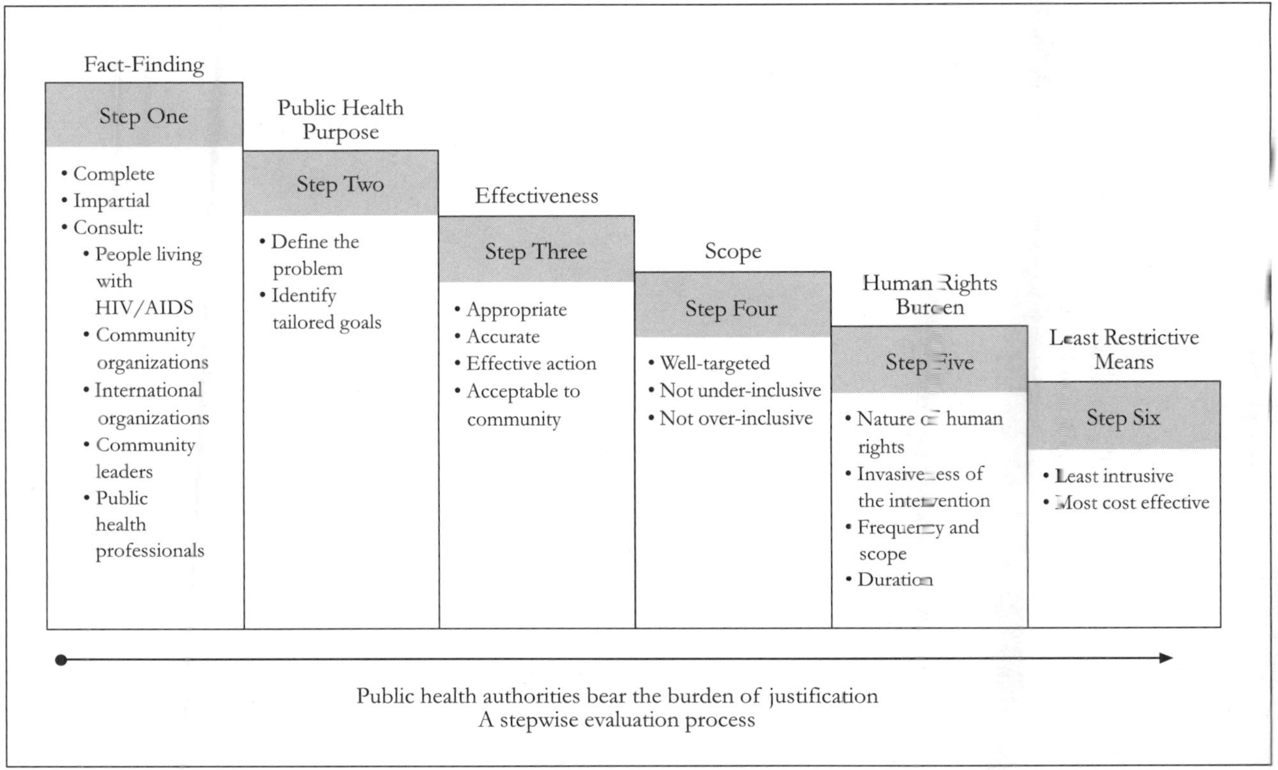

FIGURE 4-1. Steps of a Human Rights Impact Assessment (Lawrence Gostin and Jonathan M. Mann, "Towards the Development of a Human Rights Impact Assessment for the Formulation and Evaluation of Public Health Policies," *Journal of Health and Human Rights* 1 (Fall 1994): 58–81)

istries of Health and Justice) may present seemingly credible arguments supposedly based on evidence. Their "facts," however, may be incomplete or biased. Proper fact-finding entails broad-based consultations with actors outside of the government. International organizations, nonprofit organizations, public health or other professional associations community based or advocacy groups, and community leaders (e.g., elders or tribal leaders) can provide valuable facts and perspectives regarding how health policies affect human rights in their communities. Discussions with individuals living with HIV/AIDS and their advocates are particularly important, since the policies directly and intimately concern them. When consulting these various sources, public health officials should make a special effort to gather material representing all viewpoints to ensure a balanced picture.

Following the fact-finding process, an evaluation of the AIDS policy can begin. The human rights impact assessment involves a step-by-step examination of questions designed to balance the public health benefits of a policy against the human rights burdens.

Step 2: Determine If the Public Health Purpose Is Compelling

An assessment of human rights cannot take place in a vacuum. Policymakers must have a thorough understanding of the public health purposes to be achieved, and these purposes must be substantial. That a government's public health justification is powerful does not warrant disregard of human rights. Most policies, including those with compelling objectives, will affect autonomy, privacy, or equality in some manner. Serious invasions of human rights, such as the right to liberty, weigh heavily in a balance of interests. Any careful assessment of an AIDS policy, then, must begin with the policymakers' objectives.

Public health officials' first step is to define the problem. Defining the objective as combating AIDS is vague and overbroad; a more precise conceptualization at this early stage leads to sound, properly tailored policies. Examples of more narrowly defined public health goals include (1) changing specific behaviors (such as unprotected sex or the sharing of contaminated drug-injection equipment), (2) improving occupational safety (by complying with infection control standards), or (3) safeguarding the blood supply through serological screening.

The objective should be consistent with a country's or a region's priorities. For example, minimizing the occurrence of unprotected sex between men may not be a major public health goal in a developing country where epidemiological evidence shows that HIV is transmitted primarily through heterosexual behavior or needle sharing. Pursuing such a policy might drain scarce resources and restrict the freedoms of men who have sex with men.

Requiring policymakers to define their goals clearly and precisely ensures the presence of a valid public health objective. It also facilitates public debate on the expressed goals. Moreover, this exercise may reveal prejudices, stereotypical attitudes, and irrational fears. This step guards against a policy that, for example, targets sex workers, foreigners, or ethnic minorities. Public health officials should develop their goals critically to avoid basing policy on unsubstantiated fears and discriminatory beliefs.

Step 3: Evaluate How Effectively the Policy Would Achieve the Public Health Purpose

The existence of a valid public health objective does not in itself justify an AIDS policy. Public officials should have the burden of showing that the means used are reasonably likely to achieve the stated purpose. This involves an honest, rigorous scientific investigation into a policy's potential to meet the expressed goals. Developing appropriate questions is one of the most important skills in determining the efficacy of an AIDS policy. Not every policy requires the same questions; however, once public officials formulate a useful set of questions, they will be better positioned to evaluate proposed strategies.[22]

The first question is whether the intervention is appropriate and accurate. If the intervention is unreliable and its effects cannot be measured accurately, it has less utility. For example, HIV screening in a low prevalence population (such as premarital screening) has low predictive value (see Chapter 7). The screening program is likely to lead to false positive and false negative cases, which does not provide a sound basis for an effective policy.[23]

Public health officials also should inquire whether the intervention is likely to lead to effective action. The fact that a government establishes a specific policy such as screening or partner notification does not necessarily mean it is "doing something" about the problem. The real issue is whether the policy leads to effective action. Consider the utility of screening designed to identify and collect "cases" of HIV or AIDS. Policymakers should determine the marginal value of test results. That is, given what is already known about the patient or population, does the test yield new, useful information? More importantly, does the policy respond effectively to that information? One who asks these questions will pursue routine testing only if it leads to preventing transmission of HIV or providing health care that would not otherwise be accessible. Screening or testing, then, emerges as an effective public health policy only if public officials use the information for the benefit of the individual or the community.

Finally, public health officials should determine whether the policy is acceptable to the community and to individuals. Policies are more effective if the community has a say in their development and implementation. If the community is involved from the outset, people are more likely to cooperate with government officials and participate in public health programs.

Individuals, moreover, should have the opportunity to accept or refuse public health interventions—including testing, contact tracing, treatment, and biomedical research. The legal and ethical principle of informed consent requires that individuals be given clear information about the medical and social benefits and risks. They should have the opportunity voluntarily to accept or reject the intervention. Respect for personal autonomy and privacy underlies the doctrine of informed consent. Every competent human being has the right to make decisions regarding her health and well-being and to do so under conditions of privacy and confidentiality.

In sum, policymakers should ask focused questions as they evaluate policy options: Is the form of intervention appropriate and accurate? Is the intervention likely to lead to effective action? Will the policy elicit the cooperation of the people affected? Is informed consent required by individuals? Public health officials who deliberate over these and other issues are most likely to reduce the overall prevalence of HIV infection in their populations while respecting human rights.

Step 4: Determine Whether the Public Health Policy Is Well Targeted

Once public officials determine that a policy would effectively protect the public's health, they should consider how to implement it. Well-conceived policies target the populations in need. Ideally, policymakers will narrowly tailor their approaches to those who will benefit from them, rather than unnecessarily expend resources and interfere with peoples' lives.

Every policy creates a class of people to whom the policy applies and a class to whom it does not. For example, screening policies may target a group such as health care workers (HCWS), patients, marriage applicants, newborns, or foreigners. Similarly, criminal penalties may apply only to IDUS or commercial sex workers but not to others engaging in risk behavior.

Recognizing that all policies create classifications that may discriminate against disfavored people is crucial. This awareness sensitizes policymakers to human rights concerns and helps to ensure that they create only classifications that are related to the public's health. Policies that target individuals because of their race, sex, religion, national origin, sexual orientation, economic status, or homeless status often stem from invidious stereotypes about group members' behavior.

Policymakers should guard against under- and overinclusiveness. A policy is underinclusive when it reaches some, but not all, of the persons it needs to reach. By itself, underinclusiveness is not necessarily a human rights problem. A government may use its limited resources to address part of a public health problem without violating human rights. An example of such a step-by-step approach is a government's provision of special HIV prevention and treatment services to street children, but not to adults. The underinclusiveness of this policy does not necessarily reflect discrimination; it may simply indicate a particular country's public health priorities.

On the other hand, some underinclusive policies may mask discrimination. Providing services to or running clinical trials for men but not women, or for heterosexuals but not homosexuals, may reflect animus rather than legitimate priorities. A government's use of its coercive powers to target politically powerless groups, but not others that engage in similar behavior, may indicate discrimination. Human rights advocates should check for underinclusiveness (either intentional or unintentional) when evaluating public health programs.

Overinclusiveness, or overbreadth, occurs when a policy extends to more people than it must to achieve the objective. Overbreadth with regard to the provision of benefits does not violate human rights, although it may not be cost-effective. For example, counseling or educating persons who are unlikely to engage in high-risk behaviors is consistent with human rights principles. But overinclusiveness with regard to a government's use of power deprives some people of basic rights without proper justification. An example of a misguided, overinclusive policy is one that imposes compulsory screening, isolation, or criminal penalties against groups assumed to be at a high risk of infection. Compulsory measures that apply to all homosexuals, commercial sex workers, IDUs, or foreigners from countries with high rates of HIV infection stem from the erroneous belief that all members of the group engage in unprotected sex or needle sharing. Such policies are overbroad because, although a few individuals may act in a risky manner, most group members act responsibly. To apply compulsory measures to persons who pose little or no risk of HIV transmission is to deprive them of autonomy, privacy, and liberty without justification. From a human rights perspective, violating fundamental rights when the intervention is unnecessary to protect the public's health is inexcusable.

Policies may be both under- and overinclusive. Consider a decision to impose criminal penalties against sex workers but not their male agents (pimps)

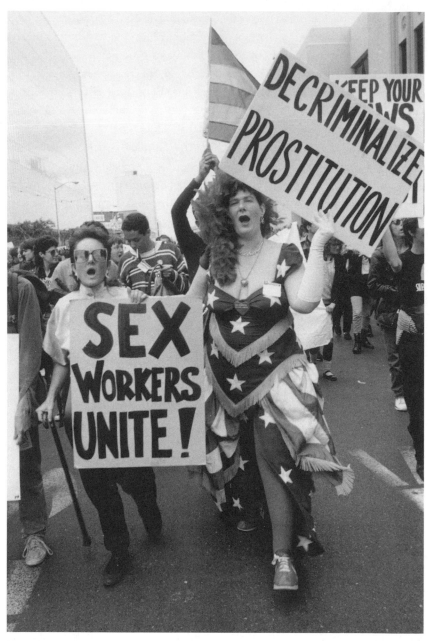

Several organizations, such as the Prostitutes' Education Network, fight for the rights of sex workers at the 1989 World Whores' Summit in San Francisco. Prostitutes are subjected to criminal penalties regardless of safer sexual practices, while underinclusive policies ignore their clients' behaviors regarding safer sex.

or clients (johns). The policy is suspiciously underinclusive because it selectively punishes a vulnerable population and does not punish two other groups that participate in the risky behavior. The policy is also overinclusive because some sex workers inform clients of the potential risks, practice safer sex, and/or are not infected with HIV. The sanctions nevertheless apply to all sex workers (see Figure 4 a).

Well-targeted HIV/AIDS policies are critically important from a human rights perspective. To ensure the protection of human rights, officials should evaluate whether their selected means achieve the public health objective and whether the policy includes appropriate groups in society.

Step 5: Examine Each Policy for Possible Human Rights Burdens

Policymakers should balance the effectiveness of a form of intervention with its impact on human rights. Human rights burdens may outweigh even a well-targeted policy that is likely to achieve its public health goal. Identifying all potential infringements on human rights and evaluating those likely to occur lead to sound government action. Officials should enact policies that protect individuals' rights to self-determination, equal treatment, liberty, privacy, family unity, free expression, free association, and other human rights.

Some policies burden human rights so heavily that their public health benefits do not outweigh such intrusions. That a policy improves public health does not automatically justify the use of any possible means. Indeed, several human rights are considered to be nonderogable, meaning that they can never be infringed, irrespective of the justification. Nonderogable human rights include the prohibition of torture, inhuman or degrading treatment, slavery, and genocide, as well as the freedom to hold opinions including religious beliefs. Minor infringements on privacy or autonomy may be justified where the public health interest is compelling. For example, requiring the immunization of a population by means of a safe and effective AIDS vaccine may undermine the right to self-determination, but the substantial reduction in HIV prevalence may justify it. A blinded (anonymous) survey of HIV prevalence does not seek the individual's consent, but the epidemiological knowledge gained may outweigh the interference.

How does one measure the extent of a human rights burden? I suggest four factors: (1) the nature of the human right, (2) the invasiveness of the intervention, (3) the frequency and scope of the infringement, and (4) its duration.

The "nature" of the human right means that some rights are more important than others. Certain rights are so fundamental that they can never be de-

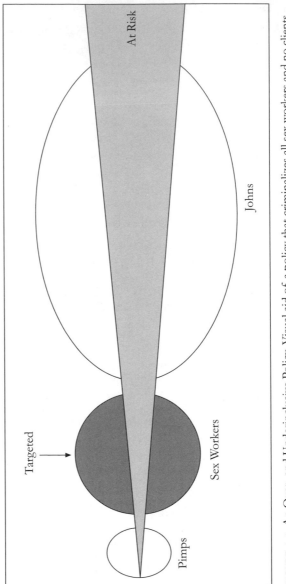

FIGURE 4-2. An Over- and Underinclusive Policy. Visual aid of a policy that criminalizes all sex workers and no clients (johns) or managers (pimps), despite the evidence that a percentage of all three populations practice risky, unsafe behavior while not all sex workers are at risk of HIV infection. Such a policy unduly burdens sex workers who practice safer sex and fails to address the risk behaviors of pimps and johns.

tled—that is, they are nonderogable. Other rights are sufficiently important that any denial is "suspect"—for example, liberty and freedom of movement. Finally, certain rights can be denied if the intrusion is necessary and the effects on the individual are minimal—for example, reasonable privacy invasions that occur in AIDS reporting.

The second factor examines the degree of intrusion on a particular right. Neither liberty nor privacy is an absolute right. All societies tolerate some incursions on these rights, such as the limitations on individual liberty where its exercise would interfere with the fundamental rights of others, or disclosure of private information when protection of it imminently endangers another person. However, the burdens from public health measures that intrude on human rights may well outweigh their potential benefits. A government's decision to grant access to an HIV surveillance registry, for instance, forcefully intrudes on privacy rights of the infected individuals.

A third factor examines whether the deprivation applies to a few people or to an entire population. Restrictions on the liberty of a single individual who intentionally transmits HIV infection (such as by stabbing a person with a contaminated needle) may be justifiable. But restrictions on the liberty of a population (such as a quarantine of persons living with HIV/AIDS) are rarely justified.

Fourth, the duration of a human rights burden is significant. Temporary violations of human rights to achieve a public health objective may be acceptable (such as the exclusion of a child from school until she is vaccinated). However, long-term violations of human rights are unacceptable (such as the permanent exclusion from school of a child living with HIV/AIDS). A child will always remain infected with HIV and the exclusion, therefore, is indefinite.

In sum, evaluating human rights burdens requires assessing all of the potential harms to persons or populations. Human rights advocates should ask (1) What are the core human rights principles involved? (2) How powerfully does a policy invade the rights of a person or population? (3) How many people does the policy affect and how frequently? and (4) What is the duration of the infringement on human rights? A sensitive understanding of what is at stake for the relevant population helps to ensure human rights protections while improving public health.

Step 6: Examine Whether the Policy Is the Least Restrictive, Most Cost-Effective Alternative

The final step in the human rights impact assessment is whether the policy is the least restrictive, most cost-effective option available. This involves comparing a potential policy to other alternatives. Policymakers may find that an initially desirable program, in fact, is less effective, more costly, and/or more invasive than other approaches. The least restrictive alternative does not require public health authorities to adopt policies that are less likely to protect the population's health. Rather, authorities should prefer the least intrusive and least costly policy that achieves their goals as well as, or better than, possible alternatives.

Civil and Political Rights: Principles for Protecting Persons Living with HIV/AIDS

Generally speaking, international treaties protect two broad classes of human rights: civil and political rights on the one hand and economic, social, and cultural rights on the other. These broad, but overlapping, classes of human rights are protected by two binding treaties—the International Covenant on Civil and Political Rights (ICCPR) and the International Covenant on Economic, Social, and Cultural Rights (ICESCR). Both covenants were adopted in 1966 and came into force in 1976. The United States has ratified the ICCPR, but not the ICESCR.[24] The Universal Declaration of Human Rights proclaims the equal significance of these two sets of rights. This section discusses civil and political rights of persons living with HIV/AIDS. The next section considers social, cultural, and economic rights, especially the right to health.[25]

The UDHR, the covenants, and regional human rights accords do not mention AIDS, and international human rights enforcement agencies have rarely dealt with violations of the rights of persons living with HIV/AIDS. However, a wide range of international resolutions and recommendations explicitly address AIDS and human rights. These documents are not legally binding, but they represent a broad international consensus about the rights of persons living with HIV/AIDS.

In May 1987 the United Nations Fortieth World Health Assembly first officially recognized the need for international cooperation in research and education about AIDS.[26] Since then, the World Health Assembly, WHO's Global Programme on AIDS, UNAIDS, and many international public health organizations, human rights groups, and NGOs have passed resolutions concerning the prevention and control of the HIV pandemic. These human rights statements culminated in a major United Nations Declaration of Commitment on HIV/AIDS in June 2001.[27] The declaration, *Global Crisis–Global Action*, called for strong leadership at the national, regional, and global levels; set concrete goals for pre-

vention, care, support, and treatment; and argued for a massive influx of resources. The United Nations General Assembly unanimously endorsed this
declaration, calling upon states, by 2003, to take legal measures to eliminate discrimination and ensure fundamental freedoms.[28] Notably, the United Nations
declared that the realization of human rights and fundamental freedoms for all
is essential to ensure respect for persons living with HIV/AIDS, reduce vulnerability of orphaned children, empower women, and alleviate the social and economic impact of the pandemic.

It is impossible to describe the entire array of AIDS-specific documents that
are relevant to human rights. Perhaps the most important international statement of principles is the Human Rights Guidelines for the Protection of Persons Living with HIV/AIDS (International Guidelines) developed by the United
Nations High Commission for Human Rights and UNAIDS.[29] These guidelines
continue to be amplified as more people speak out about the human rights of
people in the HIV pandemic.[30] In 1999 UNAIDS published a handbook analyzing
each of the International Guidelines on HIV/AIDS and human rights, giving
best practice examples of their implementation.[31]

According to the International Guidelines (par. 10), "HIV/AIDS continues to
spread throughout the world at an alarming rate. Close in the wake of the epidemic is the widespread abuse of human rights and fundamental freedoms associated with HIV/AIDS in all parts of the world." Consequently, protection of
human rights is essential to safeguard human dignity and ensure an effective,
rights-based response to HIV/AIDS. Under the International Guidelines, each
state has an obligation to establish a national framework for undertaking such
a response; ensure that community consultation occurs in all phases of policy
development; reform public health and criminal laws to ensure that they are
grounded in sound public health and do not target vulnerable groups; regulate
HIV-related goods, services, and information to ensure widespread availability, affordability, and quality; provide education and services to promote legal rights;
promote a supportive and enabling environment for women, children, and other
vulnerable groups; educate the public to prevent discrimination and stigmatization; ensure monitoring and enforcement for HIV-related human rights; and
cooperate through national and international organizations to share knowledge and experiences concerning HIV-related human rights.

At the end of 2002, UNAIDS expanded the guidelines to encompass an affirmative right to care and treatment. The world community was bound to regard
health care as a positive human right in light of the fact that antiretroviral treatment was reaching less than 5 percent of persons living with HIV/AIDS.[32] (See
Table 4-1.)

TABLE 4-1. International Guidelines on HIV/AIDS and Human Rights

1   Create an effective national framework.
2   Support community partnerships.
3   Review and reform public health laws consistent with international human rights obligations.
4   Review and reform criminal laws and correctional systems.
5   Enact or strengthen antidiscrimination and other protective laws.
6   Regulate HIV-related goods, services, and information and ensure access to prevention, treatment, care, and support.
7   Implement and assist legal support services.
8   Promote a supportive and enabling environment for women, children, and other vulnerable groups.
9   Change attitudes of discrimination and stigmatization associated with HIV/AIDS to understanding and acceptance through education, training, and the media.
10 Develop public and private sector standards and mechanisms for implementing these standards.
11 Ensure monitoring and enforcement of human rights.
12 Promote international cooperation.

Source: OHCHR and UNAIDS, HIV/AIDS and Human Rights International Guidelines, Third International Consultation on HIV/AIDS and Human Rights, Geneva, July 25–26, 2002, HR/PUB/2002/1 (New York: United Nations, 2002).

The International Guidelines emphasize the civil and political rights to nondiscrimination, equality before the law, privacy, liberty, and freedom of association. Discrimination against groups based on characteristics such as sex, race, economic status, or religion is not only wrong in itself, but also increases the vulnerability of these groups to HIV infection (see Chapter 6). Historical and current discrimination and subordination of women places them at a high risk of infection because they have little control over the factors that cause the spread of HIV.[33] Children are also placed at a high risk of infection when their rights to protection and support are violated by practices such as trafficking, prostitution, or sexual abuse. In Botswana, for example, the HIV incidence among girls aged fifteen to nineteen is 29 percent in some areas, twice that of boys of the same age. The high incidence among girls reflects what is known as "intergenerational sex": older men sleep with girls because they think the girls are less likely to be infected.[34] Policies, laws, and cultural practices should be modified to empower women and to protect children from exploitation that places them at high risk of HIV infection.

Protecting privacy includes respecting the person's right to control how personal information is kept and used by others (see Chapter 5). It also includes the right to engage in intimate behavior without governmental intrusion. For example, people should be free from criminal penalties for private homosexual acts between consenting adults. The protection of privacy advances public health goals by making people feel safe and comfortable using prevention and care services.

The rights to liberty of movement and to seek and enjoy asylum are essential rights that must be protected in the context of HIV/AIDS prevention. There is no public health rationale for restraining a person's liberty to move from one area to another or to seek asylum in another country based on real or suspected HIV status (see Chapter 15). Any law that singles out and restricts the movement of individuals infected with HIV is discriminatory and cannot be justified on public health grounds.

The rights to freedom of assembly and association and to participation in political and cultural life must also be protected in measures designed to prevent or treat HIV/AIDS. First, freedom of assembly is important because it allows the formation of support and self-help groups. Persons living with HIV/AIDS should be protected from exclusion from organizations such as trade unions and collective bargaining groups because such discrimination has no public health justification. Second, political and cultural participation of persons living with HIV/AIDS is important to ensure that policies are effectively tailored to meet their needs.

Adequate protection of civil and political rights is not only an end in itself, but also helps ensure the effectiveness of AIDS prevention and treatment strategies. Civil and political rights, therefore, go hand in hand with social and economic rights, notably the right to health.

The Right to Health in the HIV/AIDS Pandemic

Scholars have developed a sophisticated understanding of civil and political rights but, until recently, have failed to examine systematically the meaning and enforcement of social and economic rights.[35] Perhaps the most important social and economic entitlement is the right to health. The right to health is derived from multiple sources including the UDHR, the ICESCR, regional treaties, and national constitutions.[36]

Article 25 of the Universal Declaration of Human Rights expressly recognizes a right to health: "Everyone has the right to a standard of living adequate for the health and well-being of himself and his family, including food, clothing, housing and medical care and necessary social services, and the right to security in the event of unemployment, sickness, disability, widowhood, old age or other lack of livelihood in circumstances beyond his control."[37] Article 12 of the ICESCR imposes a binding obligation on governments to secure "the right of everyone to the highest attainable standard of physical and mental health." Regional systems for the protection of human rights exist in several areas of the world, including the Americas, Europe, and Africa. The American Convention on Human Rights includes the Pact of San Jose (1969)[38] and the later Protocol of San Salvador (1988), both of which contain provisions guaranteeing the right to health. The Protocol of San Salvador defines health as the "enjoyment of the highest level of physical, mental and social well-being."[39]

The right to health is also recognized in national constitutions in many countries. (Figure 4-3 shows the number of nations using different legal methods to recognize a right to health).[40] For example, the Constitutional Court of South Africa ruled that the government has a constitutional obligation to provide antiretroviral medication to HIV-infected pregnant women at all public hospitals to ensure the health of the women and their babies (see Chapter 16).[41] Chief Justice Chaskalson announced that the government's drug allocation policy was unreasonable and infringed on the rights of all those who would otherwise have access to this particular form of healthcare. "The drug is available to the government at no charge and its administration is simple, efficacious and potentially lifesaving."[42] The court made clear that its principal concerns were for indigent women who could not afford treatment and newborns who were entitled to special protection: "Protecting the child against the transmission of HIV is . . . essential. Their needs are 'most urgent' and their inability to have access to nevirapine profoundly affects their ability to enjoy all the rights to which they are entitled. Their rights are 'most in peril' as a result of the policy that . . . excludes them from having access to nevirapine."[43]

Although the right to health may be enshrined in global or regional treaties and in national constitutions, it is still vital to understand the meaning and parameters of the entitlement. Considerable disagreement exists as to whether "health" is an identifiable, operational, and enforceable right, or whether it is merely aspirational or rhetorical. A right to health that is too broadly defined lacks clear content and is less likely to have a meaningful effect. For instance, if health is, as suggested by WHO, "a state of complete physical, mental and social well-being and not merely the absence of disease or infirmity," then it can never be achieved.[44] Even if this definition were construed as a reasonable—as opposed to an absolute—standard, it remains difficult to implement and is unlikely to be justiciable.

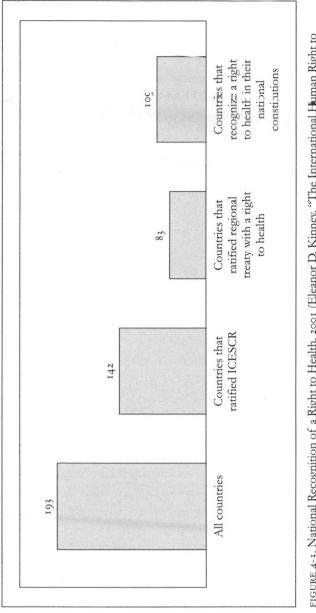

FIGURE 4-3. National Recognition of a Right to Health, 2001 (Eleanor D. Kinney, "The International Human Right to Health: What Does This Mean for Our Nation and World?," *Indiana Law Review* 34 [2001]: 1457, 1465.)

It is important to develop a clear definition of the human right to health that helps clarify state obligations, identify violations, and establish criteria and procedures for enforcement. To achieve this goal, the United Nations Committee on Economic, Social, and Cultural Rights (CESCR), which monitors the implementation of the ICESCR, issued *General Comment No. 14: The Right to the Highest Attainable Standard of Health.*[45] The *General Comment* represents the most authoritative statement on the meaning of the right to health.

General Comment No. 14 proclaims that "health is a fundamental human right indispensable for the exercise of other human rights. Every human being is entitled to the enjoyment of the highest attainable standard of health conducive to living a life in dignity." The right to health is not confined to health care but embraces a wide range of socioeconomic conditions necessary for people to lead healthy lives, including the underlying determinants of health (such as nutrition, housing, uncontaminated drinking water, sanitation, safe workplaces, and a healthy environment). The CESCR categorizes the right to health in terms of norms, obligations, violations, and implementation.

Normative Content

The normative content of the right to health is expressed in terms of "availability, accessibility, acceptability, and quality" of public health and health care facilities, goods, and services. "Availability" requires healthy conditions (such as safe drinking water and sanitation) and functioning health services (such as hospitals, clinics, trained HCWs, and essential drugs). "Accessibility" requires health services to be accessible to the entire population, without discrimination or physical, geographic, or economic barriers. "Acceptability" requires adherence to medical ethics and culturally appropriate health services. "Quality" requires health services to be scientifically and medically appropriate and of good quality.

An inherent tension exists between health and human rights.[46] In fact, Article 4 of the ICESCR permits the limitation of individual rights on the grounds of public health. The CESCR, however, stresses that states have the burden of justifying each element of Article 4: powers must be in accordance with the law, including international human rights; in the interest of legitimate aims; and strictly necessary for the general welfare in a democratic society. Public health powers also must be the least restrictive necessary, of limited duration, and subject to review.

Core Obligations

General Comment No. 14 imposes "core obligations" to ensure minimum services, including (1) access to health services on a nondiscriminatory basis, especially for vulnerable or marginalized groups; (2) essential food that is nutritionally adequate and safe; (3) basic shelter, sanitation, and safe and potable water; and (4) essential drugs. To fully realize the right to health, states must adopt and implement a national public health strategy and plan of action, on the basis of epidemiological evidence, addressing the health concerns of the whole population. The CESCR also gives priority to reproductive and maternal, immunization, infectious disease control, and health information services.

Violations

In determining which actions or omissions violate the right to health, it is important to distinguish the inability to comply (due to lack of resources) from the unwillingness to comply. Violations through *acts of omission* include the failure to take appropriate steps to realize everyone's right to the enjoyment of the highest attainable standard of physical and mental health. Violations through *actions* include state policies that contravene the standards set in the *General Comment* and are likely to result in injury, disease, or premature mortality (such as denial of access to health services or deliberate withholding of information vital to health).

Implementation

The *General Comment* contains detailed standards for implementing the right to health, including the duty to (1) adopt framework legislation (such as a national strategy and plan of action, with sufficient resources), (2) identify appropriate right-to-health indicators and benchmarks (such as to monitor improvements in community health), and (3) establish adequate remedies and accountability (such as access to courts, ombudsmen, or human rights commissions).

The *General Comment* mandates that states adopt legislation to ensure that everyone has access to appropriate medical care. The framework should take into account the nation's available resources and the most effective way of using those resources. Effective community action is essential to accomplishing this goal. The community must be allowed to set priorities, make decisions, plan, implement, and evaluate health-promoting strategies. The people's participation is essential for the state to provide effective health services.

Next, the *Comment* requires that states identify right-to-health indicators and benchmarks. The indicators should be designed to monitor the nation's progress in achieving compliance with its obligations under Article 12. Further, the state should set national benchmarks with respect to each of these indicators. This system will assist the state in monitoring its implementation of Article 12 and identifying the reasons for the difficulties that it may have encountered.

Further, the state is obliged to provide appropriate and adequate remedies for any violation of the right to health. Individuals must have access to appropriate remedies at both the national and international levels. The victims of violations should be entitled to reparation, which may be in the form of restitution, compensation, satisfaction, or guarantees of nonrepetition. States should encourage judges and legal professionals to pay greater attention to violations of the right to health in the exercise of their duties. Finally, states should encourage the work of human rights advocates assisting vulnerable or marginalized groups in the realization of their right to health.

The United Nations Commission on Human Rights appointed a Special Rapporteur in 2002 with a mandate to focus on "the right of everyone to the enjoyment of the highest attainable standard of physical and mental health."[47] In his preliminary report in 2003, the Special Rapporteur identified three primary objectives: to promote, and encourage others to promote, the right to health as a fundamental human right; to clarify the contours and content of the right to health; and to identify good practices for operationalization of the right to health at the community, national, and international levels. The Rapporteur will explore these objectives in two interrelated themes: the right to health and poverty and the right to health, discrimination, and stigma.[48]

Conclusion

Human rights and public health are complementary strategies for achieving the well-being of people and populations. People who are denied their rights and dignity are unlikely to lead lives of contentment, and people who do not have their health are unlikely to be able to assert their basic rights. Complex interactions exist between health and human rights including the influence of public health policies on rights, the influence of human rights violations on people's health, and the synergistic relationship between health and rights.

This chapter has sought to provide basic tools for human rights advocates. In particular, it should enable advocates to carefully evaluate the human rights impacts of public health policies, identify the primary violations of human rights experienced by persons living with HIV/AIDS, and begin an exploration of the right to health in the context of the AIDS pandemic. Human rights have become a powerful method of discourse and analysis in public health. This new way of thinking about public health policies has considerable potential in safeguarding individual dignity and securing the common good. The next two chapters consider two fundamental aspects of human freedom and dignity: privacy and fair treatment.

The right to privacy is a right that is mediated by class. The poor do not have the right to privacy. When everyone is required, as a matter of routine, to go through tests, and when health delivery systems of the State are required to conduct them and maintain detailed and accurate records of these tests, the issue of privacy becomes redundant.
—**Kalpana Kannabiran,** professor of law, NALSAR University, India (2001)

Chapter 5

Health Informational Privacy
in the HIV/AIDS Epidemic

The collection, storage, and disclosure of HIV/AIDS data are pervasive throughout the health care and public health systems. In the health care system, HIV/AIDS data serve numerous purposes such as clinical care, quality assurance, utilization review, and reimbursement. In the public health system, data are used for surveillance, outbreak investigations, program evaluations, and prevention and control of injuries and diseases in the population. The government draws on HIV/AIDS data to meet a variety of nonhealth-related objectives in such areas as immigration, law enforcement, litigation, and commercial marketing.

Although the collection and sharing of data are necessary to achieve important public purposes, the vast acquisition, storage, and disclosure of HIV/AIDS data raise significant privacy concerns. HIV/AIDS data are highly intimate. They not only reveal a person's health status but also may associate the person with stigmatized groups such as gay men and injection drug users. Wrongful disclo-

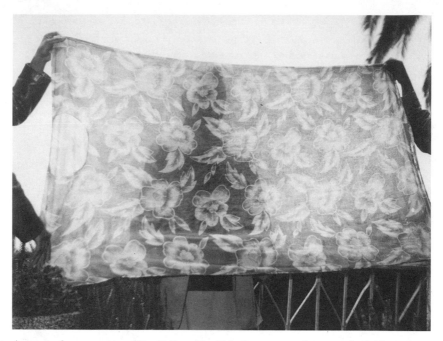

As part of a 1999–2000 Hart Fellowship, Eric Gottesman photographed this twenty-year-old Ethiopian woman who was diagnosed with HIV when she was thirteen. She said, "I'm not married. I had a boyfriend but he tested negative. I don't know how I got it. I don't want to talk to my friends. I fear being rejected. When I was in the hospital, the doctor asked me, 'Who should I tell?' I said he might tell my mother. She teaches the other children about HIV indirectly but they don't understand my situation. They ask me, 'Where are you going?' when I go to counseling. I say I'm going to the hospital where they teach us about AIDS, but my brothers and sisters don't understand. It is my mother who doesn't want to tell. I don't know why. Only my mother knows about it. She did not respond negatively when I told her. She accepted it as a simple fact. I was afraid but she was good to me. She comforts me and tells me not to worry. She said it is in God's hands."

sure of HIV/AIDS information can also result in discrimination in health insurance, employment, and housing (see Chapters 3 and 6).

The collection and use of HIV-related information involves two important goals. On the one hand, it is essential to gather and disseminate accurate and timely information to track the epidemic, prevent new infections, and treat persons living with HIV/AIDS. On the other hand, it is important to protect health information from uses or disclosures that cause embarrassment or harm to individuals to whom the information pertains. A tension exists in the use of HIV/AIDS data between common goods (health and safety) and individual interests (privacy and nondiscrimination). This chapter examines this tension in the context of the health care and public health systems. Since the flow of information, risks to privacy, and legal safeguards vary depending on whether data are collected for health care or public health purposes, each are examined separately.

Privacy in the Health Care System

Health information privacy has fundamental importance in American society. Yet public opinion surveys suggest that people feel a loss of privacy, with over 80 percent of consumers saying that they had "lost all control over their personal information.[1] Public concern about erosion of privacy reflects marked changes in the health care system. First, there has been a transition from written to electronic records for many medical and financial transactions.[2] Computerization makes it efficient to acquire, manipulate, and disseminate vast amounts of information. Second, systematic flows of highly sensitive data are evident in the daily operation of employer-sponsored health plans, managed care organizations, hospitals, pharmacies, and laboratories (see Figure 5-1 under "Proposals for Law Reform on Public Health Information Privacy" below).

The legal system has been ill-prepared for these changes in the health care system. The Privacy Act of 1974 protects only "systems of federal records," such as Medicare and Veterans Administration data; it does not apply to the private sector.[3] Special protections are applicable to certain alcohol and drug treatment records,[4] research that qualifies for a certificate of confidentiality,[5] or research funded by the Agency for Health Care Research and Quality.[6]

Many state and local medical privacy laws exist, but the U.S. Department of Health and Human Services (HHS)[7] and independent scholars characterize those safeguards as inadequate and highly variable. Often these laws apply specifically to state government records, but not to privately held records.[8]

Federal Health Informational Privacy Regulations

Congress recognized the need for national health information privacy standards when it enacted the Health Insurance Portability and Accountability Act of 1996 (HIPAA).[9] Under section 264 of HIPAA, Congress created a self-imposed deadline of August 21, 1999, to adopt comprehensive health information privacy legislation. HIPAA required the secretary of HHS to promulgate privacy regulations if Congress failed to act by the deadline. Secretary Donna Shalala issued a proposed rule in November 1999[10] and a final rule late in President Clinton's term of office.[11] Tommy Thompson, secretary of HHS under President George W. Bush, issued proposed modifications to the Privacy Rule on March 21, 2002,[12] and issued the final rule on August 14, 2002.[13] The compliance date for the new rule for most entities was April 14, 2003. Certain small health plans have until April 14, 2004, to comply. The final rule covers personally identifiable health information including HIV/AIDS data.

Scope of the National Privacy Rule

The national Privacy Rule provides the first systematic nationwide privacy protection for personally identifiable health information (unidentifiable data are not protected). The rule reaches virtually all those who use medical and financial information in the health care system. "Covered entities" include (1) health plans that provide or pay for the cost of medical care in the private sector (e.g., health insurers or managed care organizations) or public sector (e.g., Medicaid, Medicare, or Veterans Administration), (2) health care clearinghouses that process health information (e.g., billing services), and (3) health care providers who conduct certain financial and administrative transactions electronically (e.g., billing and fund transfers). The standards for covered entities apply whether its patients are privately insured, uninsured, or covered under public programs such as Medicare or Medicaid. HIV/AIDS data pervade the record systems of covered entities, including health insurers, hospitals, and managed care organizations.

Notice of Privacy Practices and Consumer Access to Records

The rule affords consumers the right to adequate notice of privacy and information practices. Providers and health plans must give patients a clear written explanation of allowable uses and disclosures of protected health information and patients' rights. Covered entities must also disclose personal information to the individual when requested. Individuals have a right to inspect their records and may request amendments.

These provisions implement "fair information practices" that give patients the right to be notified of data uses, request confidential communications, gain access to personal data, request corrections of inaccurate or incomplete data, and understand to whom their data has been disclosed. Fair information practices are particularly important for persons living with HIV/AIDS because they build trust. If persons at risk of HIV trust a health care provider's privacy practices, they are more likely to seek testing, counseling, and treatment. Therefore, privacy policies benefit individuals, who are more likely to receive AIDS treatments, as well as society at large, which is better protected from the spread of HIV infection.[14]

Acknowledgment of Privacy Notice: Disclosure for Treatment, Payment, or Health Care Operations

When the privacy regulations were originally published, they required health care providers to obtain the individual's written consent prior to disclosure of health information for the "routine" uses of treatment, payment, or health care operations (e.g., quality assurance or utilization review). Although privacy advocates strongly supported this provision, providers argued that the consent requirements would interfere with pharmacists filling prescriptions, referrals to specialists and hospitals, provision of treatment over the telephone, and emergency medical care. Additionally, "informed consent" was not truly voluntary because the rule specifically permitted the provider to condition treatment, and the health plan to condition enrollment, on the signing of the consent.

The Bush administration's modifications to the rule abolished the consent requirement. Instead, direct treatment providers must make a good-faith effort to obtain a patient's written acknowledgment that the patient received the covered entity's notice of privacy rights and practices. This change gives patients the opportunity to consider a provider's privacy policies before making health care decisions, but it does not allow them to consent (or withhold consent) to the uses of their personal data for treatment, payment, or health care operations.

Most persons living with HIV/AIDS understand the importance of disclosing medical records to health care workers (HCWs) to ensure high quality care. However, they might be less satisfied with losing control over disclosure of identifiable data for nontreatment purposes such as reimbursement of health care costs or review of hospital operations. Sharing of information for reimbursement requires disclosure of sensitive information to third-party payers, leaving persons living with HIV/AIDS vulnerable to discrimination. There are many recorded instances where health insurance coverage for HIV/AIDS was discontinued or reduced by self-insured employers or third-party insurers.[15] Similarly, the sharing of information for quality assurance or other hospital operations requires disclosure to lawyers, risk managers, and others within the institution, as well as disclosure to government regulators. Thus, individuals within and outside the health care institution would gain access to sensitive named HIV data.

Authorization: Disclosure for Purposes Not Related to Health Care

Covered entities may not use health information for purposes unrelated to health care (e.g., employment or mortgage eligibility) without explicit patient authorization. The rule has detailed standards for authorization for nonroutine uses: the authorization must contain a "specific and meaningful" description of the information and the name of the person or class of persons authorized to make the use.

The authorization model for nonroutine uses of health information offers a valuable safeguard. It is informed because the covered entity must apprise the patient of the specific use to be made of the data. It is also voluntary because covered entities generally cannot condition treatment, payment, enrollment, or eligibility on a patient's agreement to disclose health information for nonroutine purposes.

The right to authorize disclosures provides strong protections for persons living with HIV/AIDS because it gives them control over information that could be used to embarrass or victimize them. Disclosure of HIV information to employers, mortgage brokers, family, and friends may be stigmatizing and harmful.[16] The rule safeguards against such uses of data by empowering individuals to refuse to permit disclosure of data for nonroutine uses of health information.

The Minimum Disclosure Standard

Covered entities and their business associates must not use or disclose protected health information beyond what is reasonably necessary for the purposes of the use or disclosure. This standard does not apply to the disclosure of medical records for treatment purposes because health care professionals need access to the full record to provide quality care. The final rule also exempts from the minimum necessary standard any use or disclosure for which the covered entity has received an authorization or that is required by law.

The minimum disclosure standard is important to prevent unnecessary disclosure of HIV/AIDS data. For example, if a physician was seeking reimbursement for an office visit, he or she would not have to give the insurer the entire medical record, but only the precise information needed to process the claim. This means that physicians often may not have to disclose to the insurance company that the patient is infected with HIV.

Incidental Disclosures

The final rule exempts incidental disclosures of health information from being in violation of the Privacy Rule, provided that the covered entity has met reasonable safeguards and minimum requirements. Thus, health care professionals may continue to use waiting room sign-in sheets, hospitals may keep charts at the bedside, and physicians may talk to patients in semiprivate rooms and may confer at nurses' stations. The rule was modified to encourage communications about patient treatment and reduce fear of liability.

Privacy and Security Policies

Covered entities have detailed responsibilities for privacy and security. They must (1) designate a privacy official responsible for policies and procedures, (2) train members of the workforce, (3) adopt written procedures describing who has access to information and the circumstances in which information will be disclosed, and (4) accept inquires and complaints from consumers. The rule gives the health care industry flexibility in devising policies and procedures but ensures that covered entities have adequate measures in place to safeguard privacy and security.

Privacy, of course, is not the only important value in health policy. Health information can be used to accomplish many public goods. Consequently, the rule permits disclosures of health information without individual consent or authorization under specified guidelines for a variety of public purposes.[17] Many of these exceptions to the rule of consent or authorization are not specifically relevant to HIV/AIDS, such as national security, child abuse, and fraud prevention. However, many other exceptions directly impact persons living with HIV/AIDS, such as uses and disclosures for research, law enforcement, commercial marketing, and public health. The provisions for parents' access to children's records may also affect persons living with HIV/AIDS.

Research

The rule closes gaps in privacy protection for records-based research. A covered entity must obtain a waiver from an Institutional Review Board (IRB) or privacy board before using or disclosing information. The waiver criteria include findings that there are only minimal risks that are outweighed by the anticipated benefits. Personally identifiable HIV/AIDS data are often used for records-based research. This poses a concern for human subjects because personal data may be shared with researchers without their knowledge or consent. The new rule ensures that an independent body reviews whether the privacy risks are reasonable. But the rule does not ensure that persons living with HIV/AIDS will always be given the opportunity to consent to records-based research. The final rule does require researchers to enter into a data use agreement in which the recipient would agree to limit the use of the data to the purpose for which it is given.

Law Enforcement

A covered entity may disclose protected health information to a law enforcement official without the person's permission pursuant to a court order or subpoena. This disclosure of sensitive HIV data weakens public trust in the health care system. The police may seek HIV records to investigate a crime, even in the absence of probable cause. Since many states make it an offense for persons living with HIV/AIDS to not inform their sex partners (see Chapter 10), this sharing of data between HCWS and the police is deeply worrisome to civil libertarians.

Commercial Marketing

Under the original Privacy Rule, a covered entity could use or disclose protected health information without the person's permission for marketing communications in many specified circumstances. Based on consumer concerns that the marketing provisions were ineffective to protect privacy, the final rule explicitly requires pharmacies, health plans, and other covered entities to first obtain the individual's specific authorization before sending him or her marketing materials. A covered entity is prohibited from selling lists of patients to third parties or from disclosing protected health information to third parties who intend to use the information for marketing purposes without the patient's permission.[18] Marketing does not include communicating with patients about treatment options or the covered entity's own health-related products and services.

Privacy protection is essential, as most people would not want to be targeted for marketing based on their HIV status. The idea that a health care provider could sell lists of names of patients living with HIV/AIDS to businesses presents a gross invasion of personal privacy.

Parents' Access to Minors' Records

Under the original rule, parents could not routinely obtain access to the health records of their children. The Bush administration changed this, so that state law now governs parental access to their children's medical records. Generally, the final rule provides parents with new rights to control the use and disclosure of health information about their minor children, with limited exceptions that are based on state or other applicable law and professional practice. In states that have specific laws on parental access to a child's medical record, that state law prevails. But in states where there is no clear requirement about the ability of a parent to access the child's health information, the health care provider can exercise discretion to grant or deny access.

AIDS advocates express concern about these new provisions because mature minors may want to keep their health status confidential. Not all parents are supportive and may react negatively to news that their child is HIV-infected.

The parent, for example, may not be aware of the child's sexual orientation. The new rule violates the principle of confidentiality between a physician and a minor patient. It may also have detrimental effects on the public's health as minors may be discouraged from seeking testing, counseling, and treatment for their HIV infection.

Public Health

A covered entity may disclose protected health information for most public health purposes without the person's authorization or consent. Public health authorities often have a strong desire for HIV/AIDS information, but many individuals do not wish to see their data released to government agencies (see Chapter 8). For instance, public health agencies may seek identifiable HIV/AIDS data from health care providers for monitoring, interventions, postmarketing surveillance of medications, and occupational health and safety. The HIPAA rule gives health care providers considerable discretion to release named HIV information to public health agencies.

Government collection of sensitive health information (e.g., named HIV reporting) raises serious privacy concerns. Yet the rule leaves public health information virtually unprotected at the federal level. The rule assumes that the states will protect public health informational privacy. This assumption, as discussed below, is not well founded.

Privacy Safeguards in the States: HIV/AIDS Specific Statutes

The federal privacy regulations preempt, or supercede, all state health care privacy laws if those laws provide less protection than the national standard.[19] This means that state laws that offer stronger privacy protection usually are not preempted. Virtually every state has enacted HIV-specific privacy laws. In many cases, these laws are sufficiently strong and, therefore, are not preempted.

State HIV privacy laws are so extensive and variable that they defy orderly categorization. These laws may apply to all HIV information irrespective of how it was acquired, to HIV test results only, or to HIV information collected for certain purposes such as reporting, partner notification, or epidemiological investigations.

The scope of these state laws also varies widely. Some states have near blanket prohibitions on unauthorized disclosure of HIV data. However, most states authorize disclosure for specified circumstances. Depending on the state, common permissible disclosures are to HCWs involved in the patient's care; parties with a subpoena or court order; blood banks or organ donors; researchers; correctional facilities; school officials; HMOs, health care institutions, or mental health facilities; and insurance companies.

Some disclosures are permitted only in the event of a potential exposure to blood or other bodily fluids. For example, many states allow, or require, disclosure to sex or needle-sharing partners; victims of sexual assaults; and emergency workers such as police, firefighters, or emergency management personnel.

Some disclosure provisions require that patient-identifying information be removed, but most allow personally identifiable data. Persons holding the data usually have discretion whether to make the permitted disclosure, but in some statutes the disclosure is mandatory. In states that allow multiple disclosures, privacy is not well protected and persons living with HIV/AIDS may have to rely on federal protections.

Privacy protection in the health care system relies on a patchwork of laws and regulations at the national, state, and local levels. The federal privacy rules provide more uniform protection then ever before. They contain critical safeguards against disclosure to those outside the health care system such as employers, landlords, and, to a lesser extent, commercial marketers. However, the federal rules leave gaping holes in privacy protection for many uses of health information including law enforcement and, as the following discussion demonstrates, public health.

Privacy in the Public Health System

One of the core functions of the public health system is the collection, storage, and use of information about the population's health.[20] Public health agencies have sophisticated surveillance systems to identify and track HIV infection and AIDS in populations across the United States. The benefits of HIV/AIDS surveillance to the population, such as better targeting of resources for prevention, care, and treatment are undeniable (see Chapter 8).

Despite the advantages of effective HIV/AIDS surveillance, citizens (often with support from the medical profession) may object on privacy grounds to governmental acquisition of the HIV status of individuals.[21] Many forms of HIV/AIDS surveillance, notably reporting, require physicians, allied HCWs, and laboratories to disclose patient information to health departments. This raises several concerns. First, persons living with HIV/AIDS divulge intimate details of their lives to their physician; medicine's paternalistic traditions have long recognized that the patients' weakened position compels assurances of strict confidentiality even in the face of governmental demands. Second, both law and ethics in the late twentieth century emphasized autonomy as a theoretical justification for privacy; individual autonomy encompasses the right to control the dissemination of personal health information.[22] Third, respecting confidences promotes candor about health and disease risks; failure to respect informational privacy could lead to decreased disclosures, less frank revelations, or, worse, reluctance to seek care.[23]

For their part, health departments have a strong history of maintaining the confidentiality of personal information, particularly information relating to HIV/AIDS. Disclosure to health departments (as opposed to family, friends, employers, or insurers) seldom produces tangible harm such as stigmatization, embarrassment, loss of employment, or denial of insurance. Yet patients may feel wronged simply because the government—without their permission—maintains databases containing intimate and identifiable health information. Patients may worry that no matter how strong the public health commitment to maintaining privacy is, a change in the political climate could result in laws that compel public health officials to disclose such information for nonessential uses. For example, in 2003 the South Dakota legislature passed a statute authorizing public health officials to disclose a person's medical records to law enforcement officials if the Department of Health suspects that the person intentionally exposed another to HIV.[24]

Justifications for privacy are based primarily on respect for the individual. In contrast, justifications for collecting and using HIV/AIDS data are based mainly on attaining societal or collective goods. The law tries to mediate between these individual and collective interests. Virtually all states have laws designed specifically to safeguard the privacy of data held by governmental public health agencies. Most of these states have statutes that protect public health data generally or communicable or sexually transmitted disease (STD) information particularly, including HIV/AIDS.[25]

In many states, health data collection is done through special registries and databases. Registries often include HIV/AIDS information, which may receive special protection by law. Although most states guarantee access to public records, the majority explicitly exempt medical records from public inspection.[26]

Virtually all state public health privacy laws permit disclosure of public health information under specified circumstances. Just as in the case with health care privacy, common justifications for disclosure include statistical purposes, contact tracing of persons exposed to an infectious disease, spousal or partner notification of an STD, epidemiologic investigations, and subpoena or court order. In South Dakota, public health officials may disclose a person's medical records to law enforcement officials if the Department of Health suspects that the person intentionally exposed another to HIV.[27] These permitted disclosures significantly undermine privacy because they enable many individuals and organizations to gain access to sensitive HIV/AIDS data.

States vary greatly in the degree of disclosure authorized. A few states have crafted strict criteria for permissible disclosure, such as requiring written consent, requiring a showing that data are needed to enforce public health laws, or requiring that data are released only in aggregate form.

Most states have numerous exceptions to privacy protections. They do so either by relying on broad general disclosure provisions or by extensively listing permissible disclosures. For example, many states grant the health officer broad discretion to release information if he or she believes that an individual poses a public health risk. States that permit specified disclosures often include release of HIV/AIDS information to emergency workers, funeral home directors, HCWs, and others.

Existing state privacy law neither facilitates effective public health information systems nor adequately protects privacy. Although most states have nominal safeguards of public health privacy, they are often incomplete or inadequate. Statutes may be silent about the degree of privacy protection afforded, confer weak privacy protection, or grant health officials broad and unreviewable discretion to disseminate personal information. Notably, statutes seldom both specify a narrow group of individuals who are entitled to access and explain why the group has a need for the information. Rather, the statutes may provide wide definitions of who may have access. Alternatively, legislation may authorize access to so many groups that it undermines the right to privacy.

In contrast to weak or erratic protections, some states restrict information access so much as to thwart public health responses. Some states do not expressly permit disclosure to other state and local health departments for the control of communicable diseases. Certain state legislation can even be construed to restrict the intrastate transfer of communicable disease data to public health officials and HCWs. Consequently, persons with HIV, STDs, or tuberculosis (TB) may be lost to follow-up services when they move from state to state, or to different programs within the same state, due to the difficulty in releasing patient identifying information.

Proposals for Reform of Public Health Information Privacy Law

Although there has been fundamental reform of privacy law in the health care system, no national reform has taken place in the public health system. The

HIPAA rule does not preempt state public health privacy law and continues to look to the states for adequate protection. This results in two related problems. First, state legislation is so erratic that it does not adequately safeguard health informational privacy. Second, HIPAA regulations do not clarify the obligations of hospitals, managed care organizations, and pharmacies to share information with public health officials. This sharing of data is especially important outside of the HIV/AIDS context, such as in the early identification of bioterrorism.

To ensure a rational privacy policy for public health data, Georgetown University Law Center convened a multidisciplinary team of privacy, public health, and legislative experts to propose a model public health information privacy statute.[28] The Model State Public Health Privacy Act (Model Act) would provide, for the first time, strong and consistent privacy safeguards for public health data, while still preserving the ability of state and local health departments to act for the common good. The Centers for Disease Control and Prevention (CDC) has recommended that states consider adopting the model legislation to "strengthen the current level of protection of public health data."[29]

The Model Act's approach is to maximize privacy safeguards where they matter most to individuals and facilitate data uses where they are necessary to promote the public's health. Consider the sequence of events when government collects public health data through, for example, reporting or other forms of surveillance. First, the agency *acquires* the data, typically after the patient has disclosed information to a HCW (e.g., a positive HIV test). Providing there is a strong public health interest, most people believe that patients should accept this privacy invasion for the collective good. Next, the agency *uses* the data strictly within the confines of the public health department. Again, providing the agency has a strong public health interest and the data are shared only with agency officials who have a need to know, data uses should prevail over privacy. When public health authorities acquire and use data strictly within the agency, public health benefits are at their highest and privacy risks are at their lowest. The agency needs the freedom to use the data to monitor and to prevent health risks. If public health authorities do not disclose the identifiable data outside the agency, patients face few social risks.

Finally, the agency may be asked to or, under unusual circumstances, may seek to disclose personally identifiable information to persons outside the agency—for example, to employers, insurers, commercial marketers, family, or friends. These kinds of disclosures are not important for the public's health, but they do place patients at considerable risk of embarrassment, stigma, and discrimination. For these reasons, the law ought to provide maximum privacy protection from outside disclosures. The Model Act, therefore, would give government flexibility to acquire and use data strictly within the mission of the public health agency, providing it could demonstrate an important public health purpose. However, it would afford public health authorities little discretion to release personally identifiable data outside the agency and imposes serious penalties for disclosure without the patient's informed consent. For this reason, the proposed act has been supported by a broad coalition ranging from public health and health care organizations to AIDS and civil liberties organizations.

The Model Act is structured to protect privacy and security interests without thwarting public health goals underlying the acquisition, use, disclosure, and storage of identifiable health data at the state and local levels. Figure 5-1 provides a flow chart image of the act, the design of which is based on several core assumptions.

Public Health and Privacy Are Synergistic

The debate surrounding public uses of identifiable data and individual privacy assumes that these interests are mutually exclusive. Yet this is not invariably the case. Public health agencies have significant interests in protecting the privacy of health-related information. Protecting their privacy encourages individuals to voluntarily participate in public health and individual health care programs and freely divulge personal information, thus improving the reliability and quality of data. Persons living with HIV/AIDS benefit from a well-functioning, efficient public health system that works to improve population health outcomes. In these ways, public health and privacy are synergistic, suggesting that the Model Act, if passed, would improve public health outcomes, not thwart them.

All Identifiable Health Information Deserves Legal Protection

The Model Act applies to all "protected health information" held by public health agencies. This includes any public health information—whether oral, written, electronic, or visual—that relates to past, present, or future physical or mental health status, including an individual's condition, treatment, service, products purchased, or provision of care. This broad definition of protected health information recognizes that any identifiable data (e.g., HIV, STD, or immunization status) can be sensitive.

Nonidentifiable Health Information Requires No Protection

The definition of "protected health information" specifically incorporates another core assumption: nonidentifiable health data do not merit privacy protection. When health data do not reveal a person's identify, individual privacy

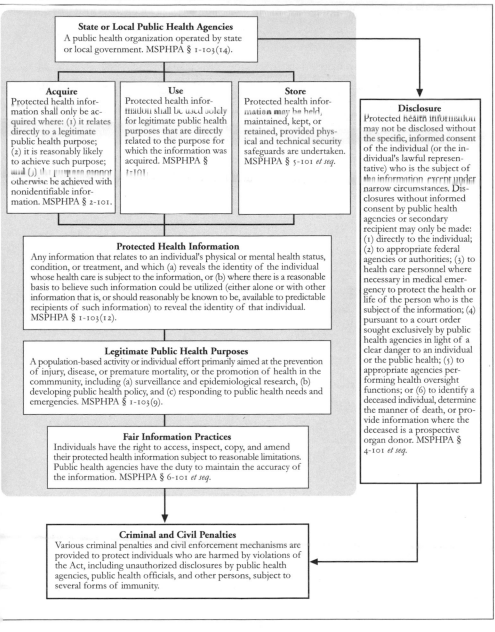

State or Local Public Health Agencies
A public health organization operated by state or local government. MSPHPA § 1-103(14).

Acquire
Protected health information shall only be acquired where: (1) it relates directly to a legitimate public health purpose; (2) it is reasonably likely to achieve such purpose; and (3) the purpose cannot otherwise be achieved with nonidentifiable information. MSPHPA § 2-101.

Use
Protected health information shall be used solely for legitimate public health purposes that are directly related to the purpose for which the information was acquired. MSPHPA § 3-101.

Store
Protected health information may be held, maintained, kept, or retained, provided physical and technical security safeguards are undertaken. MSPHPA § 5-101 et seq.

Disclosure
Protected health information may not be disclosed without the specific, informed consent of the individual (or the individual's lawful representative) who is the subject of the information, except under narrow circumstances. Disclosures without informed consent by public health agencies or secondary recipient may only be made: (1) directly to the individual; (2) to appropriate federal agencies or authorities; (3) to health care personnel where necessary in medical emergency to protect the health or life of the person who is the subject of the information; (4) pursuant to a court order sought exclusively by public health agencies in light of a clear danger to an individual or the public health; (5) to appropriate agencies performing health oversight functions; or (6) to identify a deceased individual, determine the manner of death, or provide information where the deceased is a prospective organ donor. MSPHPA § 4-101 et seq.

Protected Health Information
Any information that relates to an individual's physical or mental health status, condition, or treatment, and which (a) reveals the identity of the individual whose health care is subject to the information, or (b) where there is a reasonable basis to believe such information could be utilized (either alone or with other information that is, or should reasonably be known to be, available to predictable recipients of such information) to reveal the identity of that individual. MSPHPA § 1-103(12).

Legitimate Public Health Purposes
A population-based activity or individual effort primarily aimed at the prevention of injury, disease, or premature mortality, or the promotion of health in the community, including (a) surveillance and epidemiological research, (b) developing public health policy, and (c) responding to public health needs and emergencies. MSPHPA § 1-103(9).

Fair Information Practices
Individuals have the right to access, inspect, copy, and amend their protected health information subject to reasonable limitations. Public health agencies have the duty to maintain the accuracy of the information. MSPHPA § 6-101 et seq.

Criminal and Civil Penalties
Various criminal penalties and civil enforcement mechanisms are provided to protect individuals who are harmed by violations of the Act, including unauthorized disclosures by public health agencies, public health officials, and other persons, subject to several forms of immunity.

FIGURE 5-1. The Model State Public Health Privacy Act

interests are not threatened. Notwithstanding the interests of societal groups (e.g., ethnic, racial, or religious minorities) in the protection of some non-identifiable information, the act only regulates in favor of individual privacy.

Protected health information includes only health information (1) that reveals the identity of the individual whose health care is the subject of the information (e.g., the name, Social Security number, or any other information about the person who is the subject of the data), or (2) where there is reason to believe such information could be utilized (either alone or with other information that is known to be available to predictable recipients of such data) to reveal the identity of that individual. Under the latter category of protected health information, even aggregate statistical data may be identifiable. Consider, for example, statistical data that reveal that a Native American female in a small county has HIV. If this information may be used to identify this individual because the ethnic group membership is sufficiently small in the county, the data are individually identifiable under the Model Act. Since nonidentifiable information cannot infringe individual privacy, the act requires public health agencies, whenever possible, to use data stripped of personal identifiers.

*Acquisition and Use Are Contingent upon
Legitimate Public Health Purposes*

The Model Act regulates the ways in which public health agencies acquire, use, disclose, and store protected health information. It safeguards privacy, in part, by requiring public health authorities to demonstrate a legitimate public health purpose for the acquisition and use of data. The act defines "legitimate public health purpose" to mean a population-based activity or individual effort primarily aimed at the prevention of injury, disease, or premature mortality, or the promotion of health in the community (see Figure 5-1 above). This includes conducting public health surveillance, doing epidemiological research, developing public health policy, and responding to public health needs and emergencies.

Although interpretation of a "legitimate public health purpose" may admittedly narrow or broaden the scope of the act, it allows flexibility in prioritizing various state public health activities across jurisdictions. Public health authorities use information for many purposes, and it is necessary to clearly delineate which purposes are lawful and appropriate. To accomplish this task, the CDC has established a consultation process to specify which data uses conform with a legitimate public health objective. This process will lead to the publication of recommendations in the *Morbidity and Mortality Weekly Report* by 2004.

Disclosures Must Be Strictly Limited

Although the act affords public health agencies the power to acquire and use health data for important public health purposes, it grants little authority to disclose identifiable data outside the public health system. The act clarifies that protected health information is not subject to public review (e.g., inspection, dissemination, or investigation by members of the public) and may not be disclosed without the informed consent of the individual who is the subject of the information (or the individual's lawful representative) except under narrow circumstances.

Disclosures without informed consent may only be made

1. Directly to the individual. For example, a public health agency may contact an individual about identifiable health information it has about that individual.
2. To appropriate federal agencies or authorities. As a model state law, the act cannot restrict federal demands for identifiable information under constitutional principles.
3. To health care personnel in a medical emergency to protect the health or life of the person who is the subject of the information from serious, imminent harm. This exception is exceedingly narrow. It would not allow, for example, a disclosure to protect the health of a person who is not the subject of the information, such as a HCW who may have suffered a needlestick injury from an individual infected with HIV.
4. Pursuant to a court order sought exclusively by public health agencies in light of a clear danger to an individual or the public health that can be averted or mitigated only through a disclosure by the agency. This is the only exception for the disclosure of protected health information pursuant to a court order.
5. To appropriate public or private agencies performing health oversight functions relating to the public health agency as authorized by law.
6. To identify a deceased individual, determine the manner of death, or provide information where the deceased is a prospective organ donor.

Secondary disclosures by recipients of protected health information from public health agencies are specifically prohibited absent individual informed consent or authorization. Naturally, this prohibition does not apply to (1) the individual subject of the information, (2) persons authorized to make health care decisions for the individual, or (3) any person who is specifically required by federal or other state law to disclose the information.

Finally, the Model Act permits the exchange of data among public health agencies within and outside the state. These information exchanges are viewed as data acquisitions or uses, not disclosures. As such, public health agencies may exchange identifiable health data with other state or local agencies provided the exchanges are necessary for the public's health. For example, comparing HIV and TB registries among state and local health agencies is an important public health function given the strong relationship between these two diseases.

Safeguarding privacy requires data holders to engage in a range of fair information practices. These practices ensure strong security and privacy of public health information but do not unreasonably burden public health authorities. The act incorporates the following fair information practices.

Justifying the Need for Data Collection

Acquiring identifiable data is not an inherent good. Rather, public health authorities must substantiate the need for identifiable data. The Model Act affirms that public health agencies shall only acquire identifiable health information that (1) relates directly to a legitimate public health purpose and (2) is reasonably likely to achieve such a purpose. When information is no longer needed to fulfill the purpose for which it is acquired, it must be expunged or made nonidentifiable.

Informing Data Subjects

The act acknowledges that individuals are entitled to know how information about them is being used. Public health agencies may not acquire identifiable data without public knowledge. Prior to acquiring such data, public health agencies must provide public notice (through written information distributed in such a way as to reasonably inform the public) concerning their intentions to acquire the data and the purposes for which the data will be used. Individuals are entitled to view records of disclosures of their protected health information that public health agencies are required to maintain.

Access to One's Own Data

Subject to reasonable limitations, individuals are entitled to access, inspect, and copy their health data. Public health agencies are required to explain to individuals any code, abbreviation, notation, or other marks appearing in the information, as well as to ensure the accuracy of such data and to amend any errors.

Public health agencies have a duty to adhere to privacy and security safeguards. Specific protections are administered by a designated health information officer appointed by each public health agency and enforced through significant administrative, criminal, and civil penalties. These protections apply to identifiable health data, regardless of their holder, through various provisions of the act that (1) require an affirmative statement of privacy protections to accompany the disclosure of protected health information and (2) apply similar criminal and civil sanctions for unlawful disclosures to public health officials as well as secondary recipients.

Conclusion

The Model State Public Health Privacy Act is a product of consensus building among nationally prominent experts in privacy and public health. The act provides a balance between the social good of data collection (recognizing its substantial value to community health) and the individual good of privacy (recognizing the normative value of respect for persons). It authorizes public health agencies to acquire, use, and store identifiable health data for public health purposes while simultaneously requiring them to respect individual privacy and to impose stiff penalties for failure to comply with the act. Individuals are afforded various privacy rights and remedies for breaches of these duties. The community generally is sympathetic to data collection for public health purposes but seeks strong legal protection against potentially harmful uses of personal information. States that adopt the act, or laws consistent with its structure, can stabilize and modernize public health information practices. If the act serves as a model across multiple jurisdictions, it will reduce variability of existing protections among states, allow for the responsible exchange of health data within a national public health information infrastructure, and ultimately improve public health outcomes.

We cannot deal with AIDS by making moral judgments or refusing to face unpleasant facts—and still less by stigmatizing those who are infected and making out that it is all their fault. In the ruthless world of AIDS, there is no them and there is no us.—**Kofi Annan,** secretary general, United Nations (2001)

Chapter 6

Stigma, Social Risk, and Discrimination

Early in the HIV/AIDS epidemic, a consensus emerged among U.S. public health practitioners and community-based organizations that effective legislation prohibiting discrimination on the basis of HIV/AIDS was crucial to the nation's fight against the disease. Government,[1] medical,[2] public health,[3] legal,[4] and civil liberties[5] organizations all condemned discrimination.[6] Recommendations for antidiscrimination legislation relied on four justifications: justice, economic and social harms, public health, and the normative and educative functions of civil rights law.

First, discrimination against persons with HIV violates basic tenets of individual justice. The Supreme Court has long recognized that discrimination on the basis of an infectious condition is just as inequitable as discrimination based on race, gender, or disability. In *School Board of Nassau County v. Arline* (1987), Justice William Brennan wrote: "Society's accumulated myths and fears about disability and disease are just as handicapping as are the physical limitations

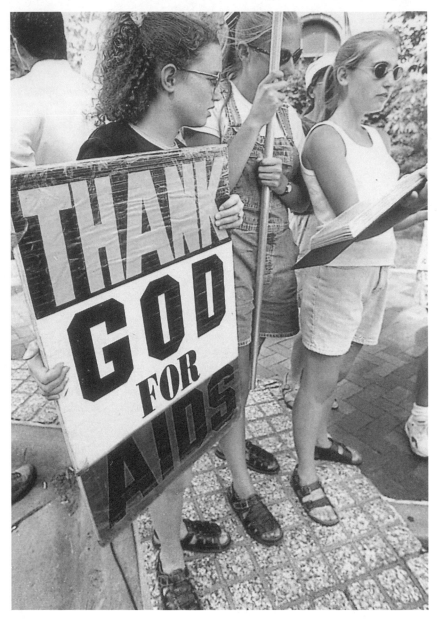

Three young followers of the Reverend Fred Phelps, ages 12, 15, and 17, protest against a gay former city official in Duluth, Minnesota, on July 24, 1998. Members of Phelps's Westboro Baptist Church in Topeka, Kansas, travel the country to voice their views in stark, often explicit, language. Homophobia and ignorance dominated the first phase of the AIDS epidemic in the United States. (Reprinted with the permission of the *Duluth News Tribune*)

that flow from actual impairment. Few aspects of handicap give rise to the same level of public fear and misapprehension as contagiousness."[7] On a daily basis, persons living with HIV/AIDS face the myths and stereotypes that concerned Brennan. Not only must HIV-infected persons endure unfounded fears that they present a health threat, but also the public's association of HIV/AIDS with traditionally disfavored groups—like gay men, injection drug users, and commercial sex workers—stigmatizes and isolates people and communities.

Second, discrimination against persons living with HIV/AIDS has serious economic and social consequences for the nation. It renders talented individuals unemployable or uninsurable and impairs their ability to secure housing or receive health care or other services. In the 1980s the ACLU documented 13,000 instances of HIV-related bias.[8] The sheer number of lawsuits brought in the 1990s by individuals who had been dismissed from their jobs, denied health care and insurance, or excluded from housing because of their HIV status indicates that discrimination against persons with HIV continues to be prevalent. (For more on the types of discrimination lawsuits brought by persons living with HIV/AIDS, see Chapter 3.)

Third, discrimination undermines public health efforts to identify persons infected with HIV, prevent transmission, and provide care and treatment.[9] The public health strategy is to encourage persons at risk to be tested, to educate the population to avoid risk behaviors such as unprotected sex and the sharing of drug-injection equipment, and to provide opportunities for humane care and effective treatment for all persons living with HIV/AIDS. From the beginning, it has been clear that if individuals fear the personal, social, and economic consequences of being diagnosed with HIV/AIDS, they may forego testing, fail to discuss their health and risk behaviors with counselors or health care professionals, and refrain from entering the health care system for treatment.

Finally, civil rights legislation has important normative and educative functions. Antidiscrimination laws mark society's disapproval of unfair treatment of persons living with HIV/AIDS. By enacting these laws, government signals its expectation of decent and civilized behavior. For example, the civil rights movement, aided by antidiscrimination laws, had the effect of humanizing gay men and lesbians in the eyes of the American public during the 1990s.[10] Civil rights legislation also has an educative function. The law forces employers, landlords, and others to learn the facts about HIV transmission because only by doing so can they comply with the law's mandate. As people in society learn more about the disease and its methods of transmission, they will adjust their behavior and policies to ensure respect and dignity for persons living with HIV/AIDS.

The need for law reform to protect vulnerable people against discrimination emerged as one of the most important public health strategies in the early years of the epidemic. The Presidential Commission on the Human Immuno-deficiency Virus Epidemic, in 1988, was particularly insistent about the tran-scending importance of federal legislation to safeguard against invidious dis-crimination: "As long as discrimination occurs, and no strong national policy with rapid and effective remedies against discrimination is established, individ-uals who are infected with HIV will be reluctant to come forward for testing, counseling, and care. This fear of potential discrimination . . . will undermine our efforts to contain the HIV epidemic and will leave HIV-infected individuals isolated and alone."[11]

The social, economic, and public health effects of the HIV/AIDS epidemic in the 1980s[12] set in motion a series of events that would lead to the enactment of the most significant civil rights legislation since the Civil Rights Act of 1964. A coalition of organizations and people committed to the rights of persons with disabilities and persons with HIV/AIDS formed to lobby for federal legislation to proscribe discrimination.[13]

The result of these efforts was the Americans with Disabilities Act of 1990 (ADA). The National Commission on the Acquired Immune Deficiency Syn-drome, in 1991, applauded this legislation: "The landmark Americans with Dis-abilities Act . . . is a significant step toward protecting the rights of all disabled Americans, including people with HIV disease. The passage of the ADA with the inclusion of protections for people with HIV disease is a victory worth celebrating."[14]

That celebration was not long-lived. Over the years the courts have substan-tially eroded the protection afforded by the ADA by narrowing the definition of disability, limiting the scope of protection, and removing the right to sue states for disability discrimination. This chapter offers an overview of disability dis-crimination law—its history, principal provisions, and application to the field of public health generally and to HIV/AIDS specifically; explains how the courts have diminished ADA protection; and analyzes HIV-specific antidiscrimination legislation at the state and local levels.

Disability Discrimination Law: An Overview

In 1973, in the process of amending the federal Rehabilitation Act, Congress added a brief sentence stating: "No otherwise qualified handicapped individ-ual in the United States . . . shall solely by reason of his handicap, be excluded from the participation in, be denied the benefits of, or be subjected to discrimination under any program or activity receiving Federal financial assistance."[15] For almost twenty years, until the passage of the ADA, this sentence (section 504 of the Rehabilitation Act) was the most important source of civil rights protection for persons with disabilities. Professor Chai Feldblum, director of the Georgetown Law Center's Federal Legislation Clinic and a pioneer in disability law, explained the significance of the Rehabilitation Act:

> In one respect, the statement of non-discrimination in section 504 is clear and simple: no otherwise qualified individual with a disability may be subjected to discrimination solely on the basis of his or her disability. But, in many respects, this simple sentence leaves many questions unanswered. What does "discrimination" on the basis of disability actually mean? Does it mean *ignoring* the fact that a person has a disability? That approach to anti-discrimination [would] be insufficient to ensure true, equal opportunity for people with disabilities. Is it not possible that a non-discrimination mandate on the basis of disability might actually require some *affirmative* efforts . . . to create a system that would offer *real*, equal opportunity for people with disabilities?[16]

In the 1980s persons with disabilities successfully used section 504 to challenge discrimination by various recipients of federal funding—among them, educational systems, public welfare departments, and state zoning agencies.[17] There began a movement that cut across groups of persons with disabilities and united them in fighting for causes such as fair opportunities for persons with disabilities to buy or rent housing and increased access to public transportation. In 1988 the Fair Housing Act was expanded to prohibit discrimination on the basis of disability in housing. Still, advocates and persons with disabilities saw gaps in antidiscrimination law. Most strikingly, while section 504 of the Rehabilitation Act protected individuals with disabilities against discrimination by federal fund recipients, it provided no protection against discrimination by private employers and businesses.

The ADA was enacted in 1990 to provide a "clear and comprehensive national mandate for the elimination of discrimination against individuals with disabilities."[18] It does not replace the body of federal disability law that predated it, including the Rehabilitation Act, Fair Housing amendments, and Individual with Disabilities Education Act, or state disability statutes. Additionally, many states and localities have laws proscribing discrimination against persons with particular health statuses such as HIV/AIDS or genetic diseases.

The jurisprudence on the ADA is vast and complex, well beyond the scope of a text on HIV/AIDS. Nevertheless, it is important to understand the act's basic provisions. The ADA proscribes discrimination against persons with disabilities in employment (Title I),[19] public services (Title II),[20] public accommodations (Title III),[21] and telecommunications (Title IV).[22] Although the specific requirements under the ADA vary, a finding of discrimination generally requires adverse treatment of a person with a "disability" who is "qualified" (or "eligible"), or who would be qualified if "reasonable accommodations" (or "modifications") were made.[23] In most circumstances, reasonable accommodations are not required if they would impose an "undue hardship."[24]

Person with a Disability

A "person with a disability" is defined as someone who (1) has a physical or mental impairment that substantially limits that person in one or more major life activities, or (2) has a record of such a physical or mental impairment, or (3) is regarded as having such a physical or mental impairment.[25] Under the first prong of the definition, the person must have a physical or mental impairment that "substantially limits" her in a "major life activity" (e.g., caring for herself, performing manual tasks, walking, seeing, hearing, speaking, breathing, learning, reproducing, or working).[26] The definition of disability covers most serious medical conditions ranging from communicable diseases (like TB, hepatitis, or syphilis) to chronic illnesses (like cerebral palsy, diabetes, or schizophrenia).[27]

The second prong of the definition of disability covers a person with a "record" of an impairment, extending protection to persons who once had a physical or mental impairment but have since recovered (e.g., a cancer survivor).[28] The third prong covers people who are "regarded as" having an impairment. These are individuals who have minor impairments or no disability at all, but who are regarded by others as having a physical or mental disability that substantially limits a major life activity.[29] For example, if a gay man is perceived to be HIV-infected and is adversely treated for that reason, he should be protected under the ADA even if he is perfectly healthy.

"Qualification" Standards: "Direct Threat" or Significant Risk

Persons with disabilities are protected under the ADA only if they are "qualified" or "eligible." A person is qualified or eligible if he or she is capable of meeting the essential performance or eligibility criteria for the position, service, or benefit.[30] "Essential functions" are those necessary to perform the major tasks of employment, not marginal tasks.[31]

Qualification standards can include a requirement that the person with a disability does "not pose a direct threat to the health or safety of others." The "direct threat" standard means that people can be excluded from jobs, public accommodations, or public services if necessary to prevent a "significant risk" to
others.[32] The Supreme Court in *School Board of Nassau County v. Arline* (1987) held
that a person suffering from the contagious disease of tuberculosis can be disabled within the meaning of section 504 of the Rehabilitation Act of 1973.[33]
The Court enumerated the basic factors to be considered in determining whether
a person with an infectious disease poses a significant risk: (1) the nature of the
risk (how the disease is transmitted), (2) the duration of the risk (how long the
carrier is infectious), (3) the severity of the risk (what the potential harm is to
third parties), and (4) the probability that the disease will be transmitted and
will cause varying degrees of harm. In making these findings, courts should
defer to the reasonable medical judgments of public health officials.

Applying the factors stated in *Arline*, courts have reached varying conclusions regarding whether persons living with HIV/AIDS pose a significant risk to
others. In *Doe v. County of Centre* (2001), a county youth services agency prohibited foster parents from taking in an additional foster child because one of the
children currently living with them was infected with HIV. The Third Circuit
Court of Appeals found that the county wrongly discriminated against the foster parents in denying their request for another child because there was little
risk of HIV transmission from one young child to another.[34] This is an appropriate way to construe the "significant risk" doctrine because the probability of
transmission is negligible.

In contrast, the Sixth Circuit found in *EEOC v. Prevo's Family Market* (1998)
that a grocery store did not discriminate when it dismissed an employee who
claimed to be HIV positive but refused to submit to a medical examination as
a condition of continued employment. The employee, who worked in the produce department, testified that he and other produce workers often got cuts
at work. The court found that although there was only a small risk of infection,
the worker posed a direct threat to the health and safety of others because "we
are dealing with a profession and environment where there is continuous
blood exposure. It is undisputed that [the plaintiff's] condition presents potential transmission opportunities."[35] The same court ruled that an HIV-infected
surgical technician posed a direct threat to patients' safety even though the
technician rarely touched their wounds or body cavities during surgery and the
risk of HIV transmission was quite small.[36] The court stated, "The uncontra-
dicted fact that a wound causing an HIV-infected surgical technician to bleed
into the body cavity could have catastrophic results and near certainty of death,

indicates that [the technician] was a direct threat."[37] This kind of ruling perverts the ADA because it tolerates discrimination where the risk is remote and speculative.

The Supreme Court has constricted ADA qualification standards to deny individuals protection if their work poses a risk to their *own* health. In *Chevron U.S.A. Inc. v. Echazabal* (2002), the Court affirmed Equal Employment Opportunity Commission (EEOC) guidelines finding that employers may lawfully fire an individual whose work poses a direct threat to his or her own health.[38] The Court's decision is legally questionable because it seems, on its face, contrary to the language of the ADA itself, which explicitly refers to a "direct threat to the health or safety of *other individuals* in the workplace."[39]

From an ethical perspective, the "threat-to-self defense" may be justified in contexts where the work environment poses a high level of risk to employees. But in the context of HIV/AIDS, it opens the door to unfair treatment. Since persons living with HIV/AIDS have compromised immune systems, employers simply may claim that they are more vulnerable to infections. For example, hospitals may discriminate against HIV-infected health care workers (HCWS) even if they are not engaged in invasive procedures. This paternalistic reasoning could threaten the employment security of persons living with HIV/AIDS in a wide range of jobs.[40]

Reasonable Accommodations or Modifications

The ADA requires employers or operators of public accommodations to provide reasonable accommodations or modifications to enable persons with disabilities to perform the job or participate in the activity.[41] Reasonable accommodations or modifications are designed to address the unique needs of a person with a disability.[42] The objective is to identify aspects of the disability that make it difficult or impossible for the person to perform the job or engage in the activity and then to provide the appropriate adjustments in environment, schedule, or equipment. For instance, persons living with HIV/AIDS may require flexible working hours to enable them to receive treatment. Reasonable accommodations or modifications must also be provided if they would reduce a significant health threat. For example, employers might have to provide training and equipment to HCWS to reduce the probability of blood-borne transmission of infection.

Fundamental Alterations and Undue Hardships

The ADA requires the provision of reasonable accommodations or modifications unless the changes would "fundamentally alter" the nature of the job or activity. For example, the Supreme Court held that allowing Casey Martin, a golfer with a disability, to ride a golf cart during tournament play would not fundamentally alter the nature of professional golf.[43] Additionally, employers are not required to provide reasonable accommodations if doing so would impose an "undue hardship." The term "undue hardship" means an action requiring significant difficulty or expense which considered in light of such factors as the nature of the job and the employer's overall financial resources.[44]

HIV/AIDS as a Disability under the ADA: Bragdon v. Abbott

In the first AIDS case considered by the Supreme Court, the Court held that Sidney Abbott, a woman with asymptomatic HIV infection, was protected against discrimination by the ADA; the Court indicated that all people with HIV infection may be protected.[45] In 1994 Sidney Abbott disclosed her HIV infection to her dentist, Dr. Randon Bragdon, at his private office in Bangor, Maine. Bragdon performed an examination and determined that Abbott had a dental cavity. Although it was Bragdon's customary practice to fill cavities in his office, he informed Abbott that he would only fill her cavity in a hospital setting. Any additional costs beyond his standard fees would have been Abbott's responsibility.

In *Bragdon v. Abbott*, the Supreme Court inquired whether Abbott's asymptomatic HIV infection constituted a (1) "physical impairment" that (2) "substantially limits" one or more of the (3) "major life activities." The scientific evidence was sufficient to satisfy the Court that asymptomatic HIV infection is a physical impairment with immediate, constant, and detrimental physical effects.[46]

A more troubling issue for lower courts had been how to characterize the "major life activities" that are affected by asymptomatic HIV infection. The Supreme Court found that the life activity on which Sidney Abbott relied—her ability to reproduce and to bear children—constitutes a major life activity: "Reproduction and the sexual dynamics surrounding it are central to the life process itself." The Court rejected the idea that Congress intended the ADA to cover only those aspects of a person's life that have a public, economic, or daily character. Reproduction and sexual intimacy cannot be regarded as any less important than working and learning. One troubling implication of this reasoning is that reproduction may not be an issue for many persons such as older women and gay men. This could leave the door open for future courts to exclude certain people living with HIV/AIDS from the protection of the ADA. For example, the Fifth Circuit Court of Appeals held that a person living with HIV/AIDS was not impaired in the major life activity of reproduction because he and his wife had decided not to have more children before the alleged discrimination took place.[47]

Finally, the Court found that HIV infection "substantially limits" the major life activity of reproduction. First, the risk of sexual transmission of HIV impedes reproductive choices. The Court cited studies showing that 20 percent, or more, of long-term male partners of infected women contracted HIV.[48] Second, the risk of perinatal transmission limits reproduction. Certainly, antiretroviral treatment of the mother and infant significantly reduces this risk,[49] but the Court found that, even with mitigating treatment, the risk is sufficiently substantial to limit reproduction.[50]

The Court confined its inquiry to the major life activity raised by the parties —reproduction—but strongly signaled that its decision should not be read to focus narrowly on reproduction. Instead, Justice Anthony Kennedy emphasized that asymptomatic HIV infection imposes substantial limitations on many major life activities: "Given the pervasive, and invariably fatal, course of the disease, its effect on major life activities of many sorts might have been relevant to our inquiry . . . [HIV infection has a] profound impact on almost every phase of the infected person's life."[51] HIV infection, indeed, has a transcendent effect on a person's life: the disease and the medical regimen can have debilitating physiological and psychological effects; the social stigma transforms the way a person is seen in the family, at work, and in the community; and the person's health and life span potentially are severely impacted. As Justice Ruth Bader Ginsburg said in her concurring opinion: HIV infection "inevitably pervades life's choices: education, employment, family and financial undertakings, . . . and the ability to obtain health care."[52]

The *Bragdon* decision makes it more likely that, in the future, the courts will find persons with asymptomatic HIV infection protected under the ADA. Nevertheless, there are disturbing signs that the judiciary may limit the scope of *Bragdon*. New data demonstrating dramatic reductions in perinatal transmission could undercut the Court's reasoning that HIV infection substantially limits reproduction. Additionally, since treatment can significantly improve functioning, the courts could find that persons living with HIV/AIDS can engage in most, if not all, major life activities.

The Judicial Dismantling of the Americans with Disabilities Act

The Rehnquist Court has dismantled the ADA by narrowing the definition of disability and removing the right to sue states for discrimination. Emblematic of the Court's judicial philosophy, Justice Sandra Day O'Connor, in a speech at Georgetown University Law Center in Spring 2002, criticized the ADA as "ambiguous and poorly drafted." She said that the Supreme Court's 2001–02 term might be remembered as "the Disabilities Act term." For persons with disabilities and civil rights advocates, the term will remain a painful memory—a time when the Supreme Court was unfaithful to Congress' broad aspirations for the rights of persons with disabilities.

Narrowing the Definition of Disability

Courts deciding cases under the Rehabilitation Act (the ADA's predecessor) did not view the definition of disability as a strict obstacle for plaintiffs. The issues did not turn on whether an individual had a disability, but rather on whether the disability was the cause of the adverse action, or on whether the action was justified because a person's disability rendered her unqualified for a job or ineligible for a service. The judicial approach in disability cases was similar to the approach in discrimination claims based on race or gender. When making decisions regarding race or gender discrimination, courts do not engage in searching inquiries into whether the individual is "really a woman" or "really an African American." Rather, these cases are often lost because individuals are unable to prove that they have been discriminated against because of their race or gender.

Nothing during the passage of the ADA suggested that courts would adopt a narrow definition of disability. In fact, the ADA's definition of disability is derived from the Rehabilitation Act, which courts interpreted broadly. Congress explicitly said that the ADA should not "be construed to apply a lesser standard than [applied under the Rehabilitation Act]."[53] However, the legal landscape has changed dramatically. For example, in approximately 87 percent of ADA cases from 1992 to 2000, federal appellate courts favored employers, usually on grounds that individuals failed to meet the statutory definition of disability.[54] The definitional barriers to access to the courts meant "what was once touted as 'the most comprehensive civil rights legislation . . . since the 1964 Civil Rights Act' has become increasingly narrowed to the point where it is in danger of becoming ineffective."[55] By 2002 Justice O'Connor, writing for a unanimous Court, declared that the ADA must "be interpreted strictly to create a demanding standard for qualifying as disabled."[56] The Court strictly construed several concepts in the ADA to significantly narrow the definition of disability.

Major life activity. The Court narrowly construed the definition of "major life activity" in *Toyota Motor Mfg. Ky Inc. v. Williams* (2002).[57] The Court focused on the major activity of performing manual tasks. A woman with carpal tunnel syndrome was fired because she could not perform the manual tasks associated with her car assembly-line job; she claimed that, with reasonable accommodations, she was able to work. The Court found that a medical diagnosis of carpal tunnel syndrome was insufficient to qualify as disabled, as was evidence that the person cannot perform "isolated, unimportant, or particularly difficult manual tasks."

The finding that a major life activity must be centrally important to daily life (not to work-related tasks) may seem reasonable, but it flies in the face of congressional aspirations. Suppose a person is fired because she cannot perform the functions of her job *because* of a disability. Her claim is that, with reasonable accommodations, she would be able to remain at her employment. This is precisely the kind of discrimination that Congress set out to address because it would afford opportunities for persons with disabilities to work. However, according to the Court, if tasks centrally important to a person's job are not also important to daily life, she is excluded from any protection under the ADA.

This problem might be remedied if the Court were prepared to conceive of "working" as a major life activity as discussed in the congressional history of the ADA and in its implementing regulations. Yet, in *Williams*, the Court explicitly declined to examine the major activity of working, which is critical in employment discrimination cases. Justice O'Connor said that there are "conceptual difficulties" inherent in the argument that working could be a major life activity. Earlier, the Court noted that even assuming that working is a major life activity, a claimant would be required to show an inability to work in a "broad range of jobs," rather than in a specific job.[58]

Once the argument is framed in this way, courts often conclude that the impairment is not sufficiently limiting because there is a range of jobs that the individual can still perform. The idea that an individual must be unable to work in a range of jobs to meet the ADA's definition of disability inappropriately suggests that persons with disabilities are unable to function and work. This image of disability may make sense in certain limited circumstances — for example, when determining if an individual should receive cash payments under a disability benefit plan. But the ADA was designed to prohibit discrimination against people with disabilities who *can* work. For these individuals, a different concept of disability is desirable — one that recognizes that there is a spectrum of physical and mental impairments among all members of society, with many impairments not actually limiting the individual's ability to work effectively but for the fears and biases held by others.[59]

Substantial limitation. Courts have restricted coverage under the ADA by a second method. Courts scrutinize whether the individual's impairment of a major life activity is sufficiently "substantial." The Supreme Court requires that the impairment be "considerable." In *Albertsons, Inc. v. Kirkingburg* (1999), the Court held that a person with monocular vision is not disabled because the condition is not serious enough to substantially restrict his life activities.[60] The Court explained that it is not sufficient to find a "significant difference" between the manner in which the plaintiff sees and the manner in which most people see. The person must have a substantial impairment in a major life activity to gain the protection of the ADA.

Mitigating measures. The Supreme Court not only requires a substantial limitation in a major life activity, but it also requires that corrective and mitigating measures be considered in determining whether an individual is disabled. In *Sutton v. United Air Lines, Inc.* (1999), the Court held that severely myopic job applicants for airline pilot positions are not disabled because eyeglasses or contact lenses mitigate their impairment.[61] Similarly, in the companion case of *Murphy v. United Parcel Service, Inc.* (1999), the Court held that a driver with high blood pressure is not disabled because his condition could be mitigated with medication.[62] The Court did not claim that individuals with myopia or high blood pressure are not qualified to be pilots or drivers. Rather, it held that since the plaintiffs were not disabled, their qualifications for the job were not even relevant considerations under the ADA. Thus, in an ironic twist, although the ADA's goal is to provide antidiscrimination protection to individuals who (perhaps because they are taking medication) are qualified for jobs and eligible for services, such individuals are denied protection precisely because their medical conditions are under control. These rulings are particularly troubling to persons with disabilities who can control their symptoms with medication, such as persons living with HIV/AIDS. Under the Court's theory, an employer might lawfully fire an employee taking antiretroviral medication based on unreasonable fears or biases, claiming that the employee was not truly disabled.

"Regarded as" disabled. The definition of disability includes individuals who are "regarded as" having a substantially limiting impairment. The "regarded as" provision was thought to be important because it protects those who are perceived as disabled and subjected to discrimination, even though they are not, in fact, substantially impaired. Under the "regarded as" criterion, the simple act of terminating a person's employment, or denying medical care, be-

cause of a disability should result in a finding that the person was perceived as having a disability.

The courts, however, rarely find that a person who is not, in fact, disabled is protected under the third prong of the definition. Indeed, the Supreme Court in *Sutton* suggested that the employer or service provider must actually believe that the person is substantially limited in a major life activity before she receives protection against discrimination. Thus, a person fired due to bigotry and animus may not receive protection under the ADA provided the employer does not think the individual has a substantial physical or mental limitation. This is a perverse interpretation of civil rights legislation, which is designed to combat irrational fears and hatred.

In sum, the judiciary is whittling away the ADA's protection by narrowing the definition of "disability."[63] The courts' principal methods are to insist that the major life activity must be centrally important to daily life, not just a work-related activity; that the impairment substantially limits the activity; and that the disability is not mitigated by medical treatment. At the same time, the courts have significantly narrowed the meaning of being "regarded as" disabled by requiring evidence that the defendant actually believes that the individual has a substantial impairment in a major life activity. Even if the courts find that the person is disabled, she can be adversely treated under the paternalistic guise that she poses a risk to her own health or safety. The new conservative mood in the courts does not bode well for protecting persons living with HIV/AIDS and other disabilities from discrimination. The ADA, it appears, is reserved for the "truly disabled." As a result of these judicial decisions, we are in a sense being thrown back to a time when there was no uniform federal standard, with disabled persons dependent on the vagaries of state and local law. This was precisely the problem that the ADA was supposed to address.

Disability Discrimination by States:
The Ugly Specter of Sovereign Immunity

Congress made the ADA enforceable through private causes of action. This is an important provision because it gives individuals access to the courts to vindicate their rights. The Supreme Court has already held that municipalities are not liable to private plaintiffs for punitive damages in actions arising under the ADA. In *Barnes v. Gorman* (2002), the Court overturned a jury award of punitive damages after a paraplegic suffered serious injuries when, after arrest, he was transported to a police station in a van that was not equipped to accommodate the disabled.[64] The Supreme Court, more importantly, is severely limiting congressional power to authorize individuals to sue the states for violating their rights under antidiscrimination legislation.[65] In *Board of Trustees of University of Alabama v. Garrett* (2001), the Court held that suits in federal court by state employees to recover money damages because of the state's failure to comply with Title I of the ADA (employment) are barred by the Eleventh Amendment.[66] That case is troubling because it means that qualified individuals cannot sue states that fire them from employment because of their disability.

In its 2003 term, the Court was scheduled to hear an even more important case. In *Medical Board of California v. Hason*,[67] the Court was set to decide whether states are immune from suit under Title II of the ADA (public service) for refusing to give a mentally ill physician a license to practice medicine. Title II is particularly important to persons with disabilities because it binds the government itself to the principles of fair treatment. The number of activities covered by Title II is vast, including voting, education, public transportation, and conditions of confinement in public institutions for people with mental or physical disabilities. In a highly unusual decision, the Supreme Court dismissed the case and canceled the oral argument for March 25, 2003. California's governor asked the state medical board to withdraw the appeal, calling the ADA "a cornerstone of our nation's civil rights protections." The disability community rightly believed that the Supreme Court was poised to yet again undermine the ADA.

Garrett and a future Title II case could deal a potentially severe blow to the ability of persons with disabilities to vindicate their rights. That is the opposite of the result Congress intended and potentially represents an enormous loss for the public interest. It means, moreover, that Congress will often be unable to enforce civil rights legislation of all kinds by authorizing private suits against the states.

The judicial dismantling of federal protection makes it imperative that the states enact adequate antidiscrimination laws. Many states have done so, as the next section indicates.

A Fifty-State Survey of Disability Discrimination Law

The ADA envisages that states and localities have, and will, provide antidiscrimination protection to persons with disabilities. Congress expressed its will not to interfere with these state statutes and local ordinances, provided they afford as much, or greater, protection against discrimination.[68] This survey examines antidiscrimination protection under state and local laws, and how *Bragdon* affects the interpretation of these laws. The survey was originally conducted through library and electronic searches of disability statutes in the fifty states in 1999 and has been updated through July 2002 (see Table 6-1).

Although federal antidiscrimination laws are comprehensive, state and local laws frequently provide significant additional protection against discrimination. These laws, for example, often apply to employers of fewer than fifteen persons[69] (the minimum necessary to be covered by the ADA).[70]

All states have statutes that prohibit discrimination on the basis of disability, and some also have HIV-specific statutes. Disability discrimination laws protective of individuals with HIV are also found at the local level, often in communities with large populations of persons living with HIV/AIDS (e.g., New York City,[71] Los Angeles,[72] and San Francisco[73]). Jurisdictions can be characterized by their antidiscrimination statutes as (1) states that incorporate the federal statutory definition of disability, (2) states that use definitions of disability other than the federal definition, often in broader, more protective ways than the federal law, (3) states that have HIV-specific statutes, explicitly listing HIV or related conditions as a protected class, and (4) states that prohibit discrimination based on HIV test results (see Table 6-1).

State Laws Incorporating Federal Disability Standards

Forty states have at least one statute that incorporates the federal definition of disability in some form. Additionally, among the twenty-two states with partial protection based on HIV-specific statutes or statutes that prohibit discriminatory use of HIV testing, seventeen states also use the federal standard to define "disability" for at least some purpose.[74] As a result, the federal disability standard significantly affects the rights of individuals with HIV in at least thirty-three states. Although state courts have sole discretion to interpret state law, they will likely conform to the reasoning in *Bragdon*, given the similarity of statutory language and purpose. In some states, in fact, reliance on *Bragdon* and other definitive interpretations of federal law is statutorily mandated. California, for example, requires that state law must provide as much or more protection than the ADA.[75]

State Statutory Definitions of Disability
Not Adopting the Federal Standard

Fourteen states and Puerto Rico employ a definition of disability in at least one nondiscrimination statute that either departs significantly from the federal

TABLE 6-1. HIV Infection as Protected by State Statute in the United States
(including Guam, Puerto Rico, and the U.S. Virgin Islands)

STATE	A	B	C	D	E	F	COMMENTS
Alabama			x	x		→	No disability protection in private employment
Alaska			x				
Arizona			x				
Arkansas		→	x	x			Prohibits health care provider discrimination based on HIV test result
California		→	x				Prohibits employment discrimination based on HIV test result
Colorado			→				Legislature has declared policy of HIV nondiscrimination
Connecticut				→			State definition of disability broader than federal
Delaware			x	→			State definition of disability broader than federal for employment
District of Columbia			x				
Florida	→	x	x				HIV explicitly incorporated in handicap definition
Georgia			x			→	No coverage of public accommodations, housing, other areas
Guam			x				
Hawaii	→	x	x				HIV protected in housing discrimination statute
Idaho			x				
Illinois				x	→		Ill. Court of Appeals ruled that HIV is a disability
Indiana				x	→		State definition of disability broader than federal for housing
Iowa	→						HIV explicitly incorporated in handicap definition
Kansas		→	x				HIV case reporting data may not be used to discriminate
Kentucky	→	x	x				Prohibits employment discrimination based on HIV status
Louisiana			x				
Maine		x	x			→	1st Cir. Ct. of Appeals ruled HIV is disability under state law and ADA
Maryland	→	x		x			HIV discrimination by public safety personnel prohibited
Massachusetts			x				
Michigan				x	→		Federal district court ruled that HIV is protected under state law

Table 6-1. (continued)

STATE	A	B	C	D	E	F	COMMENTS
Minnesota		x			→		Court of Appeals ruled HIV a disability
Mississippi			x			→	No coverage of private employment and other areas
Missouri	→		x				No coverage for "regarded as" HIV-infected
Montana	→		x				Health care facilities may not refuse to admit persons with HIV
Nebraska	→		x				Broad protection from discrimination based on HIV
Nevada			x				
New Hampshire			x				
New Jersey	x			→			Superior Ct. ruled persons viewed at risk to develop AIDS covered
New Mexico		→	x				HIV test results may not be used to discriminate in employment
New York				→	x		State definition of disability broader than federal
North Carolina	→					x	Statute offers significantly less protection than federal law
North Dakota			x				
Ohio		→	x				No HIV discrimination in government services and government-funded services
Oklahoma			x				
Oregon				→			State definition of disability broader than federal
Pennsylvania			x				
Puerto Rico				→			Only condition of "motor or mental nature" covered
Rhode Island		→	x				Discrimination based on "positive AIDS test" prohibited
South Carolina			x				
South Dakota			x				
Tennessee			x				
Texas		→	x	x			HIV testing for employment purposes prohibited
Utah			x				
Vermont	→		x				HIV discrimination in public and private employment prohibited
Virgin Islands, US						→	No prohibition against HIV discrimination

Table 6-1. (continued)

STATE	A	B	C	D	E	F	COMMENTS
Virginia	→		x				HIV discrimination by public safety personnel prohibited
Washington	→			x			HIV discrimination in public and private employment prohibited
West Virginia			x		→		W. Va. Supreme Ct. has ruled HIV a disability
Wisconsin	→		x				HIV discrimination by public safety personnel prohibited
Wyoming				→			"Federal disability" definition adopted by state agency

Key:

A = Statute explicitly includes protection for HIV
B = Statute bars discriminatory use of HIV testing or test information
C = Statute uses "federal disability" standard
D = Statute uses disability definition other than federal standard (or does not define term)
E = Judicial precedent interprets statute as covering HIV infection
F = No disability nondiscrimination law in at least one significant category
Arrow symbol (→) indicates column referred to in comment

standard or does not set forth any definition. Although these statutes are open to varying interpretations, eight of these states appear to define "disability" more broadly than does federal law,[76] while one state—Texas—and Puerto Rico appear to define it more narrowly. The remaining four states do not include any comprehensive statutory definition.[77]

HIV-Specific State Statutes

The issue of whether asymptomatic HIV infection is protected for the purposes of antidiscrimination law may be answered by inclusion of that term in the statute itself. Fourteen states have antidiscrimination statutes that include the term "HIV infection" or equivalent terminology denoting that symptomatic illness is not required.[78] Of these fourteen states, five include HIV as a disability with protection equivalent to that of other disabilities.[79] The other nine states offer more limited protection than accorded other disabilities.[80] The five states in which HIV is defined as equivalent to other disabilities do so by simply incorporating HIV in the definition of "disability."

North Carolina's HIV-specific statute purports to grant protection from discrimination, yet it authorizes many forms of discrimination. The law prohibits discrimination in *continued* employment, housing, public services, public accommodations, and public transportation.[81] Yet the statute permits HIV testing of job applicants, denial of employment to HIV-infected applicants, and HIV testing as part of employment-related annual medical examinations. Health care providers are also allowed to refuse treatment if they fear the risk of exposure.[82]

In sum, of the fourteen states with HIV-specific statutes, only five provide across-the-board protection;[83] eight offer coverage equivalent to other disabilities but limit that coverage to certain contexts or settings,[84] and one state allows significant discrimination against persons living with HIV/AIDS.[85] Finally, some HIV-specific state statutes cover HIV-infected individuals, but not those perceived to be infected.[86] If read literally, this could exclude from protection individuals who are discriminated against as a result of the erroneous belief that they are infected.

State Law Limitations on the Use of HIV Testing or Test Results

After a reliable test for HIV antibodies became widely available in 1985 and the evils resulting from the misuse of that test became known, some states adopted statutes that prohibit the use of HIV test results for discriminatory purposes, or prohibit HIV testing for purposes such as employment, where testing is not fully voluntary.[87] As a result, these "information restrictive" statutes prohibit discrimination based on knowledge of test results but may not prohibit discrimination based on actual HIV status or perceived status. For example, if an employer discriminates on the basis of a person's HIV status, the employer may not have violated state law if there is no knowledge of an HIV test result.

Twelve states have statutes that limit the use of HIV testing or HIV test results for discriminatory purposes.[88] Of the twelve states in this category, only Hawaii, Kansas, and Rhode Island impose broad restrictions on the use of such information in employment, public accommodations, housing, and other areas. Six states impose restrictions only in the employment context.[89] Two states impose limits on HIV testing and the use of results in health care settings.[90] One state prohibits discrimination by health care providers and in public (or publicly funded) services.[91]

Although these testing and confidentiality statutes may offer protection in many instances, if read literally they provide significantly weaker protection than nondiscrimination enactments that define discriminatory conduct more broadly. For example, statutes that restrict the use of HIV test results in employment may be interpreted by the courts to deny protection to a job applicant who is discriminated against because the potential employer, who is unaware of a specific test result, is aware only of rumors that the applicant is HIV-infected.

Judicial Interpretations of State Nondiscrimination Law

The highest courts of appeal in only three states have addressed the issue of asymptomatic HIV infection.[92] Two of those rulings involved state laws that were changed by subsequent legislation, so they are of limited precedential value.[93] But in a third ruling, *Raintree Health Care Center v. Illinois Human Rights Comm'n* (1996), the Illinois Supreme Court held that HIV infection is a disability under the Illinois Human Rights Act, given that statute's definition of disability as "a determinable physical characteristic resulting from a disease."[94]

Several state intermediate appellate and federal courts, applying state law, have addressed the issue of HIV infection as a disability.[95] In the most prominent ruling, *Beaulieu v. Clausen* (1992), the Minnesota Court of Appeals interpreted the state Human Rights Act to cover asymptomatic HIV infection in a case of dental care discrimination.[96] The court concluded that individuals infected with HIV are materially limited in several major life activities, including social participation (because of emotional or psychological problems such as depression, as well as ostracism by others), sexual and reproductive activities, and employment.[97]

The Demographics of State HIV Nondiscrimination Standards

Given this interpretation of relevant statutes, states can be placed into three categories: first, those with clearly established protection for HIV infection (either from HIV-specific laws, judicial precedent, or a combination of both); second, those in which coverage of HIV as a disability can be reasonably inferred, given state reliance on the federal definition of disability and the Supreme Court's ruling in *Bragdon*; and third, those that provide little or no protection for HIV infection.

Due to widespread reliance on the federal definition of disability, roughly half (47 percent) of the persons with AIDS in the United States and its territories live in jurisdictions where there is now a reasonable basis to infer that asymptomatic HIV infection is a disability, given the Supreme Court's ruling in *Bragdon*.[98] Additionally, the states in which protection for individuals with asymptomatic HIV infection can be said to be clearly established as a result of explicit statutory language or state court precedent include an additional one-third (29 percent) of the reported AIDS cases. Jurisdictions that significantly limit or have no protections from HIV-related discrimination include only about 1.5 percent of the reported AIDS cases.[99] Thus, there is a clear national trend to protect individuals with asymptomatic HIV infection from discrimination under federal law, as now interpreted by the Supreme Court, and under state and local laws.

The Future of Disability Discrimination Law in America

With the exception of the *Bragdon* case, the judiciary has whittled away federal protection afforded to persons with a broad range of injury and disease by constricting the definition of disability under the ADA and limiting the right to sue. State and local laws often fill some, but certainly not all, of the gaps in antidiscrimination protection.

The AIDS epidemic has often caused conflict and dissent. However, the one area that almost all responsible people agree on is the evil of discrimination. Discrimination is unfair, socially and economically damaging, and detrimental to the public's health. Rather than eroding the safeguards afforded by disability discrimination law, this nation should renew its commitment to combat the stigma, social isolation, and adverse treatment of persons living with HIV/AIDS and other disabilities.

Having considered important entitlements to privacy and fair treatment, this book now examines specific government policies relating to the HIV/AIDS epidemic. Those in public health, AIDS advocacy, and politics have bitterly contested AIDS policies throughout the last two decades, including screening, reporting, partner notification, and criminal penalties. These policies reflect on the humanity and decency of society and are crucial to persons living with HIV/AIDS. It is important to understand the history, science, and politics of these disputes. Above all, it is essential to develop neutral principles for formulating public health policies and evaluating their fairness and effectiveness. That is the task to which we turn in Part III of this book.

Part 3 Policy, Politics, and Ethics

Prevention is the most effective tool in our arsenal. No matter the cultural or religious factors to overcome, families must talk about the facts of life before too many more learn about the facts of death. —**William Jefferson Clinton,** former president of the United States (2000)

Chapter 7

Testing and Screening in the HIV/AIDS Epidemic

A Public Health and Human Rights Approach

Testing and screening have become major public health policy tools in the HIV/AIDS epidemic. The Centers for Disease Control and Prevention (CDC) advise that individuals at risk for HIV should have access to anonymous as well as confidential HIV testing and counseling, that testing should be informed and voluntary, and that individuals should be notified of test results.[1] Early knowledge of HIV infection is now recognized as a critical component in HIV prevention and treatment.[2]

Client-centered counseling, as an adjunct to testing, seeks to prevent the spread of HIV. Armed with knowledge, individuals can take precautions to avoid acquisition and transmission of infection. Individuals also can receive help in identifying the specific behaviors that put them at risk and commit to reducing their risk. Researchers have demonstrated the efficacy of HIV prevention counseling models aimed at behavioral risk reduction.[3]

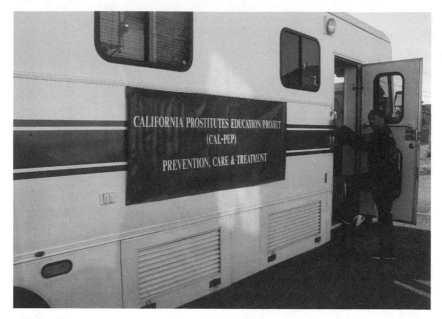

Mobile clinics, such as this one belonging to the nonprofit California Prostitutes Education Project (CAL-PEP), allow service providers to bring HIV testing and counseling into communities and expand access to HIV prevention and care. CAL-PEP was chartered in 1984 in San Francisco to provide health education and HIV/STD testing services to commercial sex workers. Since then, CAL-PEP has expanded its services and its client population.

HIV counseling and testing can also serve as a pathway to treatment. Medical treatment that lowers HIV viral load is useful in prevention because it may reduce a person's infectiousness.[4] More importantly, treatment for HIV disease has been demonstrated to reduce illness and premature death.[5] Consequently, screening has the potential to benefit individuals clinically and improve the public's health. It is not surprising that screening for HIV is uniformly supported by public health policymakers and AIDS advocates.[6]

Programs to encourage testing are particularly important because of the lack of awareness among persons at risk for HIV. An estimated 25 percent of persons living with HIV do not know they are infected.[7] Indeed, most young gay men infected with HIV are unaware of their serological status. They fail to be tested because they misunderstand the risk factors, fear a positive test result, worry about breaches of privacy and discrimination, and lack an expectation of benefit.[8] These barriers can be overcome by raising awareness of the benefits of treatment, offering testing as part of standard care, and providing a cheap and convenient test.[9]

In April 2003 CDC announced a new initiative on testing, "Advancing HIV Prevention: New Strategies for a Changing Epidemic."[10] The new initiative is aimed at reducing barriers to early diagnosis of HIV infection, making testing part of routine medical care (e.g., de-emphasizing pretest counseling), implementing new models for HIV diagnosis outside medical settings (e.g., in correctional populations), preventing new infections among persons with HIV/AIDS and their partners (e.g., prevention and treatment services), and further reductions in perinatal transmission (see Chapter 13).[11]

Although testing is very important, it is not an unmitigated good. Identification of a person's HIV status poses health and social risks, including invasion of privacy and discrimination. HIV testing information is acquired and shared throughout the health care, public health, and health insurance systems. If information is disclosed to family, friends, or employers, it could result in stigma and discrimination (see Chapters 5 and 6). Although the CDC recommends fully informed and voluntary testing, some laws and policies have coercive elements. Involuntary testing is problematic because it interferes with the autonomy and dignity of the individual. Further, if individuals fear coercion, they are less likely to seek diagnosis and treatment.

This chapter offers a systematic evaluation of testing and screening in the HIV epidemic. It thus considers the technical aspects of HIV screening—the principal methods of testing and their predictive value; the various forms of screening, ranging from fully voluntary to compulsory; and compulsory screening from a legal perspective—the constitutional right to avoid unreasonable searches and seizures, and the statutory right to be free from discrimination. In conclusion, the chapter proposes a series of criteria for evaluating screening policies from a public health and human rights perspective.

Although the words are often used interchangeably, a distinction exists between "testing" and "screening." Testing refers to a medical procedure that determines the presence or absence of disease, or its precursor, in an individual patient.[12] Individuals are often selected for testing because of a history of risk behavior (e.g., multiple sex or needle-sharing partners) or clinical symptoms (e.g., opportunistic infections). In contrast, screening is the systematic application of a medical test to a defined population (e.g., pregnant women, infants, immigrants, or prisoners).[13] Typically, medical testing is administered for diagnostic or clinical purposes (e.g., to determine if a person is infected with HIV and to provide early treatment), whereas screening is undertaken for broader public health purposes (e.g., identifying previously unknown or unrecognized cases of HIV infection in apparently healthy or asymptomatic persons).[14] This chapter primarily discusses screening because populations are deliberately chosen as a matter of public policy, thus raising interesting issues of potential co-ercion, injustice, and ineffectiveness. Personal testing, on the other hand, is usually voluntary and a critical part of diagnosing and treating persons infected with HIV.

Scientific Aspects of HIV Testing: Test Technologies and Predictive Value

Several HIV test technologies have been approved by the U.S. Food and Drug Administration (FDA) for diagnostic use in the United States and are used inter-nationally.[15] These tests enable evaluation of different fluids (e.g., whole blood, serum, plasma, oral fluid, and urine) with varying degrees of accuracy.[16] Stan-dard HIV testing (enzyme immuno-assay [EIA] confirmed with the Western blot or immuno-fluorescence assay [IFA]) is highly accurate and produces few false positives (affirmative results for persons not actually HIV-infected). However, it requires a phlebotomy (extraction of blood), and individuals must return for a second visit to obtain test results. Rapid tests (rapid EIA) hold promise for im-proving testing and increasing early detection.[17] At the end of 2002, the FDA authorized the use of the OraQuick rapid diagnostic test kit. OraQuick returns HIV test results in twenty minutes, can be stored at room temperature, requires no special equipment, and can be used outside clinical settings. OraQuick has an accuracy rate of 99.6 percent but requires a confirmatory test.[18] Finally, home sample collection tests allow convenient and anonymous testing, but individ-uals cannot receive face-to-face counseling.[19] Although the FDA has approved home collection kits, it has not approved home-use HIV test kits, which allow consumers to interpret their own test results. The Federal Trade Commission has warned that some home-use HIV test kits supply inaccurate results and do not ensure effective counseling.[20]

Standard HIV tests are highly accurate, but a test's accuracy is not a sufficient reason for engaging in screening. Ideally, HIV screening should identify a signifi-cant amount of previously unrecognized disease in the population at a reason-able cost. Screening in a low-prevalence population identifies very few cases at high cost. It identifies few cases of infection because relatively few cases actu-ally exist, and it is resource-intensive because the entire population must be screened irrespective of their individual risk. The screening program, more-over, will produce some false positive cases, which can have profound psycho-logical consequences.[21]

The state of Illinois powerfully illustrated the problems with screening in a low-prevalence population by mandating premarital HIV screening in the late 1980s. The legislature assumed that HIV could be prevented by screening marriage applicants who would then be counseled on the risks of unprotected sex. However, during the first six months of the program, screening identified only eight HIV positive persons at a cost of $2.5 million ($312,000 per infected individual). The annual cost was nearly 1.5 times the state appropriation for all other AIDS surveillance and prevention programs combined. At the same time, the marriage rate dropped in Illinois and rose in adjacent states.[22] This suggests that policymakers need to think carefully about the likely costs and benefits of screening in low-prevalence populations.

The Problem of Compulsion and Consent: A Taxonomy of Screening

AIDS historians have developed the idea of a "voluntaristic consensus" in the HIV epidemic, meaning that public health authorities and community groups both favor cooperation rather than compulsion.[23] It was not always this way, and, though voluntarism in public health may be currently fashionable, pressures for increased restrictions of the person are likely to reemerge. The politics of HIV screening are volatile since policymakers are often attracted to the notion that identifying persons living with HIV/AIDS promotes the public's well-being. At the same time, groups that bear the burden of compulsion vigorously insist on maintaining their personal autonomy—a claim that civil liberties organizations strongly support.

The terms "voluntary" and "compulsory" appear simple enough: the former connotes unfettered freedom to choose and the latter the absence of freedom. Between these two extremes, however, is a gradation of different kinds of screening that warrant explanation. It is possible to identify at least five forms of screening: compulsory, conditional, routine with advance notification (opt-in), routine without advance notification (opt-out), and voluntary.[24]

Compulsory Screening

Pursuant to their police powers, states may compel citizens to submit to HIV screening without informed consent. Compulsory HIV screening requires legislative authority, and many statutes provide that authority. Statutes often define a class of persons to which the compulsory power applies, such as sex workers,[25] newborns,[26] sex offenders,[27] or inmates.[28] Alternatively, statutes define a set of circumstances that triggers a screening requirement, such as when a person is "exposed" to HIV.[29]

Conditional Screening

The government can make access to certain privileges or services contingent upon undergoing medical screening. For example, the law mandates HIV screening to immigrate to the United States (see Chapter 15). Additionally, persons living with HIV/AIDS may not donate blood or other tissue for use in humans. Conditional screening is not mandatory in the strict sense of the term, because persons can avoid the test by foregoing the privilege or service sought. But if the privilege or service is important to the individual, the screening requirement may be perceived as highly coercive.

Routine Screening with Advance Notification ("Opt-In")

There are few concepts used with less care and precision than "routine" screening. Sometimes routine screening simply refers to population screening whereby each member of a defined population is routinely tested. However, this definition fails to explain the essential characteristics of the screening—whether persons are informed that they are being tested, how they are informed (e.g., individually or by public notice), when they are informed (before testing or after the fact), and whether they can withhold consent.

There are at least two forms of routine screening: with advance notification ("opt-in") and without advance notification ("opt-out"). In opt-in screening, all individuals in the defined population are routinely "offered" testing (e.g., they are notified that a certain test is a standard part of the treatment they are about to receive). As part of the informational process, individuals are told that they have the right to give, or to withhold, consent; they are not actually tested until they have consented. A clearer term for this kind of program would be "routine offering" with informed consent.

Routine Screening without Advance Notification ("Opt-Out")

In opt-out screening, all individuals in the defined population are routinely and automatically screened unless they expressly ask that the test not be performed. This meaning of routine screening is a hybrid between mandatory and voluntary. It verges on compulsory because individuals may not be aware that they are being screened, and, even if they are aware, they may not fully understand the purposes of the test or their right to withhold consent. Yet opt-out screening does not expressly coerce because it theoretically respects a person's expressed desire not to be tested.

There are important policy implications in choosing between these two forms of routine screening. Opt-in screening is far more respectful of individual autonomy and the importance of informed consent. Opt-out screening, however, reaches a larger population and is less expensive.[30] In opt-out screening, health care workers (HCWs) do not have to provide pretest counseling, thereby rendering the program less time-consuming and costly.

The differences between opt-in and opt-out screening are powerfully illustrated in policies relating to the screening of pregnant women. The Institute of Medicine (IOM)[31] and the CDC[32] recommendations on HIV screening of pregnant women represent a complicated hybrid between opt-in and opt-out screening. Both sets of guidelines recommend HIV testing as a routine part of medical care, and both emphasize the importance of informed consent. However, the IOM and CDC want to dismantle barriers to widespread screening and, therefore, do not recommend pretest counseling or other complex information requirements. This may mean that some patients are tested without a complete understanding of the benefits and risks.

Voluntary Screening

Voluntary screening is the norm in medicine and public health, and any deviation from the norm requires careful justification. Information about the nature of the test must be provided in advance and be fully understood by a competent person, who has the freedom to choose to be tested or to decline. Nondirective counseling is thought to be the "best-practice," whereby individuals are informed of the options and the choice is left to them.

Even in the absence of legislation explicitly safeguarding voluntariness, the common law affords individuals a right to consent.[33] Since testing involves physical contact with the patient, physicians technically commit an intentional tort if they perform a test without consent or another legally sufficient justification; physicians are also negligent if they fail to provide adequate information so that the patient can make an informed decision.[34] Physicians sometimes bristle at such a stark legal requirement, arguing that hospitals routinely perform serological screening without asking each patient for permission.[35] Physicians insist, by analogy, that it should not be necessary to seek the patient's consent before screening for HIV. For example, health care workers frequently argue that they should be permitted to test patients if a HCW has sustained a needle-stick injury. The analogy does not hold because it assumes that the physician does not need consent for routine serologic screening. In law, she does need consent, but, because screening is sufficiently routine and expected, consent is implied. HIV screening, however, is far from routine or inconsequential; screening is essential to the diagnosis of a serious chronic disease, so the patient would wish to be informed. A better analogy is to compare HIV screening with diagnostic tests for cancer or Huntington's chorea, where physicians usually respect patients' choices.

Compulsory Screening from a Constitutional Perspective: Unreasonable Search and Seizure

Since the guarantees of the U.S. Constitution constrain actions by the state, the legal battleground over screening has centered on government agencies as well as private entities acting on federal or state rules that require or authorize testing. The primary constitutional impediment to testing is the Fourth Amendment's right of people to be "secure in their persons" and not be subjected to "unreasonable searches and seizures."[36] Although the Fourth Amendment is popularly perceived as applying solely to personal or residential searches, the Supreme Court has long recognized that the collection and subsequent analysis of biological samples are "searches."[37] The invasion of bodily integrity involved in the collection of the sample and the ensuing chemical analysis that extracts personal information threatens privacy and security. The constitutional issue is whether the analysis of blood, urine, or other tissue is "unreasonable." In most criminal cases, a search is unreasonable unless it is conducted pursuant to a judicial warrant issued upon probable cause. If the warrant requirement is impracticable, the courts require, minimally, "reasonable suspicion" based on an individualized assessment.

In drug screening cases, the Supreme Court has held that when the state has "special needs beyond the normal need for law enforcement," the warrant and probable or reasonable cause requirements may not apply.[38] The courts have often found that screening falls within the "special needs" exception, unless the screening program is devised in close cooperation with police (such as when a hospital hands over drug testing results to law enforcement).[39] For example, in 2002 the Supreme Court held that public schools could require drug testing of all students who participate in competitive extracurricular activities. The Court saw the intrusion to be minimal and found that students have diminished expectations of privacy.[40] Some courts have even held that mandated

HIV screening for persons accused or convicted of sexual assault fits within the special needs exception because the results are not used as evidence in a criminal trial (see Chapter 11).

If screening is for public health rather than criminal justice purposes, the courts balance the governmental and privacy interests to determine the reasonableness of the search. On one side of the balance is the government's interest in public health, and on the other is the individual's expectation of privacy. The courts weigh the state's interests in public health and safety quite heavily but perceive individual interests as nominal: "Society's judgement [is] that blood tests do not constitute an unduly extensive imposition on an individual's privacy and bodily integrity."[41] As a result, most courts have assumed a permissive posture when reviewing government screening programs.[42] Even for highly stigmatized diseases such as HIV, the courts have upheld screening of firefighters and paramedics,[43] military personnel,[44] overseas employees in the State Department,[45] immigrants,[46] sex offenders,[47] and prisoners.[48] In most of these cases, the public health justification is illusory and the screening program imposes burdens on those affected.

The Supreme Court's Fourth Amendment jurisprudence does not fairly balance the benefits and burdens of screening. The judiciary tends to accept government assertions of a strong public health interest without a searching inquiry as to whether the screening will, in fact, achieve those objectives. Public health guidelines have not supported any of the mandatory HIV screening programs upheld by the courts.[49] Compulsory screening, rather than furthering the government's interests, may dissuade individuals at risk from accessing the health care system. At the same time, by focusing on the physical intrusion of the blood test, the courts do not sufficiently weigh the informational privacy interests and social risks entailed in compelled disclosure of sensitive HIV information.[50]

Compulsory Screening from a Disability Discrimination Perspective

Society's accumulated myths and fears about disability and disease are as handicapping as are the physical limitations that flow from . . . impairment. Few aspects of . . . a handicap give rise to the same level of public fear and misapprehension as contagiousness.
—William J. Brennan, former justice of the U.S. Supreme Court (1987)

The Americans with Disabilities Act of 1990 (ADA) and the corpus of antidiscrimination legislation appear to be unlikely sources of law to fill the doctrinal void left by deferential constitutional standards.[51] Disability law, however, is highly relevant to screening, because the information acquired can be used to discriminate based on health status. Although the specific titles to the ADA have different provisions, a finding of discrimination requires adverse treatment of a person with a "disability" who is "qualified" or would be qualified if reasonable "accommodations" or "modifications" were made. For more on the ADA, including recent Supreme Court opinions that narrow the ADA's scope, see Chapter 6.

Employment Screening

The ADA's prohibition against discrimination in employment (Title I) specifically includes medical screening, physical examinations, and inquiries:[52] an employer is not permitted to screen applicants for HIV before offering a job (*pre-offer*); an employer is permitted to screen for HIV after a job offer is made, provided that all entering employees are screened and the medical information is kept confidential (*post-offer*); and an employer may screen current employees only if screening is job related and consistent with business necessity (*current employees*). It is difficult to conceive of any context where HIV screening would be job related and consistent with business necessity, although the courts have upheld testing of HCWs suspected of being HIV-infected (see Chapter 12). Even where employers are permitted to screen, they may not withdraw a job offer or adversely treat a current employee if the person is qualified.

Government-Conducted or -Authorized Screening

The ADA's prohibition against discrimination applies to all government-conducted or -authorized screening. For example, health department screening of its own employees (Title I), patients in HIV, STD, or TB clinics (Title III), or populations pursuant to public health powers (Title II) are all covered by the ADA.[53]

Health Care Screening

The ADA's prohibition on discrimination includes screening in public accommodations, including hospitals, managed care organizations, and physicians' offices (Title III).[54] For example, hospital decisions to compulsorily test patients for HIV would be viewed through the lens of disability discrimination. Indeed, the Supreme Court has invalidated HIV screening of dental patients on grounds that the patient poses no direct threat to the dentist.[55]

In summary, the courts review compulsory HIV screening programs under

TABLE 7-1. Criteria for Assessing Population Screening

High reservoir of infection

Compelling public health objective
- Prevent transmission
- Clinical benefits
- Monitor the epidemic

Effective use of test results ("means-ends" inquiry)

Human rights burdens
- Autonomy
- Privacy
- Discrimination
- Liberty

Justice

No less restrictive or intrusive means

---

the Fourth Amendment (if it is a government program) and/or the Americans with Disabilities Act (if it fits within one of the titles to the ADA). The courts have been highly deferential to public health agencies under the Fourth Amendment, rarely finding that screening is unconstitutional.[56] The courts have been less consistent when reviewing screening under the ADA. Here, the Supreme Court has found that HIV infection is a covered disability, but the courts have been progressively narrowing the scope and applicability of the ADA (see Chapter 6). In particular, the courts have been largely unwilling to invalidate HIV testing of HCWs, believing (wrongly) that they pose a significant risk to patients (see Table 7-1 and Chapter 12).

Criteria for Screening: A Public Health and Human Rights Approach

Policymakers sometimes assume that any acquisition of knowledge about a population's HIV status must promote the public's health. For instance, legislators proposed screening as an immediate response to publicized cases of HIV transmission from HCWs to patients, mothers to infants, and rapists to victims. These legislative initiatives, on their face, may appear to be appropriate responses to an epidemic, but screening should not be regarded as an inherent good. Policymakers should have an important public health purpose and demonstrate that the screening program actually will achieve the stated purpose. What is the marginal usefulness of the test? Given what is known about the population, will the test yield new information and are effective responses available based on that information? Is the screening program acceptable to the population and will it deter individuals from seeking testing, counseling, and treatment?

This chapter has already emphasized the importance of technical standards in evaluating screening: Is the test instrument valid, and does it have positive predictive value in the population? According to these technical standards, screening is usually most cost-effective when targeted to high-prevalence populations. In this section, I propose additional criteria for evaluating screening programs from a public health and human rights perspective: (1) a substantial public health objective, (2) the means-ends inquiry (the degree to which screening is likely to achieve the public good), (3) the human rights burdens, (4) justice and fairness, and (5) public acceptability.

A Substantial Public Health Objective

Since screening invades personal privacy and can lead to discrimination, it can be justified only by a substantial interest. The primary health objectives of HIV screening are to prevent a significant risk of transmission, to serve as a pathway to needed treatment, and to help monitor the epidemic.

Screening theoretically could be justified if it focused on particular populations or settings where transmission of infection is likely to occur—perhaps bathhouses or shooting galleries where clients engage in unprotected sex or needle sharing. Public health authorities recommend screening of pregnant women because there is a significant risk of perinatal transmission in the absence of treatment (see Chapter 13). But screening in low-risk settings, such as schools or nursing homes, rarely would be justified. Public health authorities do not recommend universal screening in the health care system (e.g., for all physicians and patients) or among marriage applicants because the prevalence of HIV among these groups is quite low.

Screening could also be warranted if it serves as a pathway to treatment. Screening that results in clinical benefits for patients is usually justified. Thus, it is important to examine whether the policy simply screens or whether it provides assurances of treatment backed by sufficient resources. Too often, policymakers imply that clinical benefits justify screening but do not assure that those who test positive will have full access to treatment.

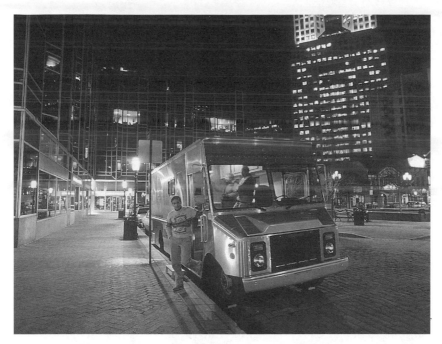

Many hospitals reach out to communities by offering mobile health care services at night and on weekends. Operation Safety Net is run in collaboration with Pittsburgh Mercy Hospital and provides HIV testing and counseling to people who are homeless. Individuals who test positive are linked to a case manager and HIV care and treatment services. (Reprinted courtesy of Operation Safety Net and Pittsburgh Mercy Hospital System)

Finally, screening could be justified by the need for sound epidemiologic data. For example, for many years the CDC conducted a blinded newborn screening program. This provided much needed epidemiologic data while not interfering with the rights of mothers and their infants. Congress discontinued the program due to concerns that the mothers of newborns who tested positive would not be informed of the results. Nevertheless, anonymous screening (i.e., without a patient identifier) can help monitor the epidemic and thereby provide a strong justification for the screening policy. On the other hand, named testing, with or without consent, is seldom justified from an epidemiological perspective. If individuals do not go to testing sites, or simply refuse testing, the sample is skewed. Accordingly, public health authorities seldom rely on named HIV screening of targeted populations as a reliable method of obtaining epidemiologic data.

Effective Use of Test Results: The "Means-Ends" Inquiry

Policymakers often assume that information collection is an inherent good. Why wouldn't public health authorities want to know who in the population is living with HIV/AIDS? This information is thought to be necessary to effectively monitor and intervene in the epidemic. The public may even claim that failure to screen for HIV, especially among groups at higher risk, is an unacceptable form of "AIDS exceptionalism."[57]

Despite these claims, collection of HIV data for their own sake may not produce any tangible benefits. If all persons within a selected population are to be screened, the resulting information must be used effectively to achieve a public good, such as a significant reduction in the burden of HIV disease. If the actions that could be taken based on the data are ineffective, there is no purpose to the screening. Further, if the proposed action *should* be taken whether or not the population is screened, the screening is unnecessary. Consider a policy of screening all HCWs to exclude those who test positive from continuing to practice invasive procedures. The proposed action (excluding HCWs) will not achieve any important public purpose because the risk of transmission to patients is already minuscule (see Chapter 12). At the same time, there are actions that hospitals should take irrespective of the screening program—for example, adoption of universal infection control procedures to prevent transmission of blood-borne infections such as HIV, hepatitis B, and hepatitis C.

The need to ensure the effective use of test results represents a "means-ends" inquiry. Even if policymakers have a compelling public health objective, they still need to demonstrate that screening is reasonably likely to achieve the objective. That is, what is the marginal usefulness of obtaining the information to be collected given what is already known about the population? If the data provide little added value to what is already known, or what could be accomplished without those data, screening is not justified.

Human Rights Burdens

Screening, as emphasized throughout this chapter, imposes social risks on vulnerable populations. It is essential to think carefully about those risks. Where the risks outweigh the benefits, screening should not be undertaken. The major human rights implications of screening include autonomy, privacy, discrimination, and liberty.

Screening can undermine autonomy unless it is completely voluntary with full disclosure to patients in advance of the testing. Persons should provide uncoerced, fully informed consent appropriate to their culture and educational level. Given the multiple forms of screening (ranging from voluntary and routine to compulsory), the more coercive the program, the greater the public benefit needed to justify screening.

Screening inherently undermines privacy because it involves collection, use, and disclosure of sensitive data. When a person is tested for HIV, the results will almost always be shared with persons in the health care and health insurance systems and will be mandatorily reported to the state public health agency. There is also the potential for disclosure to persons outside the health system, including family, friends, employers, and mortgage companies. Thus, there are significant privacy concerns. Moreover, to the extent that information is widely disseminated, there are risks of discrimination. Persons living with HIV/AIDS face discrimination in many aspects of their lives, and most discrimination begins with unauthorized disclosure of test information.

Screening programs can be designed to reduce risks of privacy invasion and discrimination. Policymakers can create legal and operational safeguards by limiting allowable disclosures. They can also require security measures (e.g., sign-on codes, audit trails, and encryption) to prevent tampering with data systems. The greater the privacy and security safeguards, the fewer the burdens on human rights.

Screening often is structured (directly or indirectly) so that there are critical consequences for persons who test positive. Those consequences might be exclusion from a livelihood (e.g., HCWs), loss of privileges (e.g., segregation of prisoners), or loss of liberty (e.g., persons who face criminal penalties for knowingly risking transmission of HIV). Some screening is undertaken in conjunction with other public health programs such as partner notification. In these cases, the consequences might even include physical or emotional abuse by a partner (see Chapter 9). The "critical consequences" must be factored into any screening policy.

Justice

Public health policymakers should carefully consider whether screening of a specific population is just. A fair program distributes benefits and burdens equitably. The question needs to be asked—are the individuals to be screened receiving sufficient advantages to outweigh the burdens? Further, are there sufficiently sound reasons for screening this particular population compared with other populations that could be screened? Sometimes, it makes more sense from a scientific perspective to target high-risk populations because screening is likely to be more cost-effective. Yet screening a vulnerable, high-risk population may be unfair and send the wrong message.

Consider policies for screening pregnant women to prevent perinatal HIV transmission (see Chapter 13). Health care providers could either screen pregnant women in high-prevalence geographic areas or they could screen all pregnant women. The screening of high-risk women would be more cost-effective, but targeting high-risk populations would be considered unfair. These populations often contain higher proportions of African Americans, Latinas, and women of lower socioeconomic status. Targeting them for screening would be stigmatizing and associate everyone in the community with HIV risk behaviors. As a result, the CDC and the IOM recommended HIV screening of all pregnant women.[58] This was regarded as a policy that was less cost-effective but fairer to all concerned. It sent the right message—that everyone is at risk for HIV, regardless of race or socioeconomic status. The IOM explained why justice is an important factor in deciding whether to screen:

> In practice when screening is conducted in contexts of gender inequality, racial discrimination, sexual taboos, and poverty, these conditions shape the attitudes and beliefs of health system and public health decision-makers as well as patients, including those who have lost confidence that the health care system will treat them fairly. Thus, if screening programs are poorly conceived, organized, or implemented, they may lead to interventions of questionable merit and enhance the vulnerability of groups and individuals.[59]

No Less Restrictive or Intrusive Alternative

Policymakers should protect the health of the community with a minimum of restrictions on the rights of individuals. This criterion is important because individuals should be allowed as much freedom as possible without imposing significant risks to the public's health. The principle of the least restrictive alternative can also promote public health interests. A major strategy in combating the spread of HIV is to foster voluntary cooperation, such as through notification of contacts and reduction of risk behavior. The use of involuntary, highly restrictive measures may deter people from attending public health programs, such as clinics for the treatment of sexually transmitted diseases or drug dependency.

HCWs may have difficulty with the principle of the least restrictive alternative because public health measures traditionally have been predicated on the notion that it is best to err on the side of caution. Under this philosophy, public health takes precedence over individual rights, and if a control measure *might* promote the public's health, it should be implemented. But the principle of the least restrictive alternative is not necessarily inconsistent with this view. It does not require a less effective measure merely because it is less intrusive. It requires a less intrusive measure only if it is equally, or more, efficacious.

Public Acceptability

One of the most important measures of a successful screening program is whether it is acceptable to the population.[60] AIDS advocates have resisted HIV screening, particularly if it is involuntarily imposed. Public acceptance is important because individuals are unlikely to cooperate unless they understand the purpose and benefits of screening. Also, democratic support is crucial to the legitimacy of public health activities. Public acceptance, of course, is far from simple—in urgent situations the general public may clamor for strong measures, while persons at risk resist compulsion. Wherever possible, screening works best if it is accepted within the community that will be subject to testing. As a result, public health programs should be planned and implemented in close consultation with representatives of the community.

The Paradigm for Testing and Screening: Counseling, Confidentiality, and Consent

The paradigm for HIV testing has been set from early in the epidemic. Any person who has engaged in risk behavior (e.g., sex with multiple partners or sharing drug-injection equipment) should be tested. Testing should be confidential and with fully informed consent. For individuals who choose not to have their identity disclosed, states should make available "alternative" sites for anonymous testing. Individuals should be offered client-centered counseling and, where appropriate, partner notification and treatment referrals. And they should always receive their test results in a timely manner.

This paradigm for voluntary testing has worked well, but there are still social and political pressures to implement "tougher" screening programs. Some screening is explicitly involuntary, such as for the military and prisoners. Other screening may be conditional, such as testing HCWs to see if they can continue to practice (Chapter 12). In still other cases, individuals may not receive pretest counseling, such as pregnant women who undergo routine screening (Chapter 13). Finally, some states have steadfastly refused to offer anonymous test sites (Chapter 8).[61]

This chapter has offered criteria for population screening: technically superior tests in a high-prevalence population, a substantial public health interest, effective use of test results, minimal burdens on human rights, justice, the least restrictive alternative, and public acceptability. These criteria should help guide screening policy so that it is scientifically effective, beneficial, nonburdensome, fair, and welcomed in the community.

Once individuals test positive for HIV infection, their records may be sent to the state health department. This "reporting" of HIV data to the government has been deeply controversial, as the next chapter explains.

Using names discourages testing only for those who don't understand the system. . . . What they see as a risk is greatly exaggerated. —**David Satcher,** U.S. surgeon general (1998)

Chapter 8

National HIV/AIDS Reporting

Reporting patients with AIDS by name (AIDS surveillance) has formed the cornerstone of the nation's efforts to monitor and characterize the HIV epidemic. AIDS surveillance tracked the growth of the disease from a small number of cases in a few large cities on the East and West Coasts to a national epidemic with over 340,000 individuals living with AIDS.[1] Public health officials and legislators have used AIDS surveillance data to measure the size and character of the epidemic through ongoing collection, analysis, and evaluation of population-based information, which is then used to determine where to best spend the limited resources available.[2] AIDS surveillance data, however, have proved increasingly ineffective for these purposes. The surveillance focuses on the most advanced stage of HIV disease, which—in the absence of effective treatment—develops on average ten years after initial infection. Consequently, the AIDS reporting system provides a snapshot of a distant epidemic. The widespread use of antiretroviral therapy, which further delays the progression of HIV, has

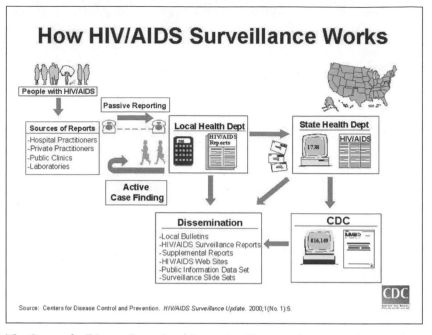

How HIV/AIDS Surveillance Works

People with HIV/AIDS

Passive Reporting

Sources of Reports
-Hospital Practitioners
-Private Practitioners
-Public Clinics
-Laboratories

Active Case Finding

Local Health Dept
HIV/AIDS Reports

State Health Dept
HIV/AIDS
1738

CDC
816,149
MMWR

Dissemination
-Local Bulletins
-HIV/AIDS Surveillance Reports
-Supplemental Reports
-HIV/AIDS Web Sites
-Public Information Data Set
-Surveillance Slide Sets

Source: Centers for Disease Control and Prevention. *HIV/AIDS Surveillance Update.* 2000;1(No. 1):5.

The Centers for Disease Control and Prevention illustrates the process for named HIV/AIDS reporting in the United States. Health care professionals, clinics, and laboratories report the names of persons with HIV infection and/or AIDS (depending on the state) to the state health department. That department then notifies the CDC, which maintains the data in coded form. This system is intended to promote understanding of the scope of the epidemic, while protecting individual privacy.

significantly diminished the ability of AIDS surveillance to show trends in HIV infection or the impact of the epidemic on the nation's health care system.[3] The compelling need for accurate monitoring of HIV infection led the Centers for Disease Control and Prevention (CDC), in December 1999, to recommend that all states develop systems for named reporting of HIV.[4]

A History of AIDS Surveillance and HIV Reporting

AIDS reporting can be understood only by examining its unique history.[5] In 1981, shortly after case clusters were reported of unusual pneumonia and rare cancer among gay men, the CDC determined that the syndrome's likely cause was a transmissible agent spread via the same routes as hepatitis B.[6] Even before the virus was discovered and an antibody test was approved, however, states instituted reporting of AIDS cases with names, a measure that generated little public or political controversy. Not until late 1983 did researchers identify the causative agent for AIDS, then called the Human T-Cell Lymphotropic virus–Type III (HTLV-III) in the United States and Lymphadenopathy-associated virus (LAV) in France.[7] The U.S. Food and Drug Administration did not license an antibody test until two years later, in 1985, and then only to screen the nation's blood supply.[8] Thus AIDS surveillance can be explained historically: it was predicated on epidemiologic investigations of an end-stage syndrome and implemented before antibody testing for the causative agent was available.

AIDS surveillance was, and still is, broadly accepted among the community of persons living with HIV/AIDS. The relatively short period of patient survival once diagnosed with AIDS and the need for health and human services were thought to offset the social risks of surveillance. In contrast, the reporting of HIV cases where those infected can often live long and healthy lives has generated bitter political controversy and impassioned community resistance. The first HIV reporting requirement in Colorado and the early public health proposals for HIV surveillance in the mid-1980s ignited a firestorm of community protest.[9] Civil libertarians and gay organizations opposed HIV case reporting due to distrust of the government to maintain the privacy of information contained in sensitive HIV registries and due to fears of political retribution, potential invasions of personal privacy, and discrimination in employment, housing, and insurance.

In the late 1990s the United States entered an era of ever more sophisticated advances in the knowledge and treatment of HIV disease. Instead of being a latent infection as previously believed, HIV pathogenesis is now known to produce high rates of viral replication and CD4+ cell death soon after transmission.[10] A treatment regime of HIV reverse transcriptase inhibitors and protease inhibitors reduces mortality and delays disease progression.[11] Persons on highly active antiretroviral therapy (HAART) have demonstrated lower levels of circulating virus, suggesting that treatment not only benefits the individual, but also may reduce the risk of transmission.[12] Antiretroviral therapy has been shown to markedly decrease perinatal transmission of HIV (see Chapter 13).[13] Although the long-term benefits are unknown and much research remains to determine the role of HAART in reducing infectiousness, delaying or preventing clinical manifestations of disease, and developing resistant strains of HIV, innovative therapies are already dramatically affecting AIDS surveillance trends.

Population-based data indicate that new therapies significantly impede the progression of HIV disease. The number of AIDS deaths in the United States fell dramatically from 1995 through 2001, from 50,877 in 1995 to 15,603 in 2001. During the same period, the number of persons living with AIDS increased steadily from 216,010 to 362,827 (the annual number of incident AIDS cases and deaths, however, have remained stable in recent years).[14] Finally, data show that new AIDS cases are increasingly diagnosed among persons not previously tested for HIV. These figures suggest that persons who test for HIV before they develop AIDS symptoms are receiving life-prolonging treatment.[15]

Reported AIDS cases no longer reflect trends in HIV infection because many people infected with HIV now receive life-prolonging therapy.[16] Although the number of new AIDS cases in the United States has declined dramatically, the CDC estimates that there are still over 40,000 new HIV infections in the nation each year.[17] The disparity between HIV infection rates and numbers of AIDS cases is even greater in subpopulations where the incidence of HIV is increasing most rapidly. For example, a CDC study in twenty-five states that use named HIV reporting found that between January 1994 and June 1997, 14 percent of new HIV cases were diagnosed in persons aged thirteen to twenty-four. In the same states, only 3 percent of reported AIDS cases occurred among persons thirteen to twenty-four years old. Similarly, 57 percent of new HIV infections were diagnosed in African Americans as compared with only 45 percent of AIDS cases. In states that do not report HIV, decreasing AIDS trends may be mistakenly viewed as reflecting a similar decline in HIV infection. The inability of AIDS surveillance data to accurately show the progression of the epidemic among subpopulations such as young adults, communities of color, and women makes the implementation of a national HIV reporting system all the more important.

We are at a defining moment in the HIV/AIDS epidemic. With therapy that delays the progression to AIDS-related illnesses and death, HIV/AIDS is now a complex chronic disease that does not lend itself to monitoring based only on end-stage illness. Unless all states adopt reliable HIV reporting systems, health authorities will not possess reliable information about the prevalence, incidence, and future directions of HIV infection, the contemporary risk behaviors for HIV transmission, and the heightened impact on specific subpopulations such as communities of color and women.

HIV/AIDS Surveillance: The Current Status

During most of the HIV/AIDS epidemic, national, state, and local monitoring of the scope and impact of the epidemic was based on AIDS surveillance. Every state has a statute or regulation requiring laboratories and physicians to report to health departments the names of persons newly diagnosed with CDC-defined

AIDS.[18] Unfortunately, recent research has shown that physicians report less than 60 percent of new HIV and AIDS cases, in violation of the legal mandate.[19] For those who do notify health departments, case reports follow uniform standards to provide complete, timely, and accurate data. Personal information includes demographics, diagnostic facility, patient risk history, laboratory analysis, clinical status, and treatment/service referrals. State health departments, in turn, forward cases to the CDC using a soundex code, wherein patient and provider identifiers are deleted and the data are encrypted for aggregation at the national level. From 1981 through December 2001, state and local health departments reported to the CDC a cumulative total of 816,149 AIDS cases.[20]

HIV surveillance reports are recorded locally and forwarded to the CDC using the same system as for AIDS cases.[21] Forty-eight states require confidential HIV case surveillance for those who test positive for HIV infection (see Map 8-1). California, Illinois, Kentucky, Maryland, Massachusetts, New Hampshire, Rhode Island, Vermont, and Puerto Rico report HIV infections using unique identifier codes. In Maine, Montana, Oregon, and Washington, HIV cases are initially reported by name, but names are later removed and replaced with codes.[22] California and Pennsylvania, two of the states that did not report HIV through 2001, accounted for approximately 18 percent of AIDS cases. In July 2002, after great debate, the California legislature approved the use of numerical codes, rather than names, to report new cases of HIV. Still, though HIV surveillance is increasingly common, gaps remain in the nation's understanding of the disease's current impact.

Justifications for National HIV Case Reporting in the United States

Multiple methods of HIV/AIDS surveillance covering the full spectrum of the disease would promote the public's health. These methods include reporting, in-depth interviews, medical record reviews, unlinked seroprevalence surveys, and sampling of representative populations.[23] A national system of confidential HIV case reporting would (1) improve monitoring of the epidemic, (2) enhance the ability to target prevention and other public health services, (3) link HIV-infected persons with treatment opportunities and educational services, including partner notification support services, and (4) lead to more equitable resource allocations for AIDS programs. HIV reporting is not unequivocally beneficial; nor is it a panacea for the multidimensional problems arising from the HIV/AIDS epidemic. Yet HIV reporting is likely to help public health agencies

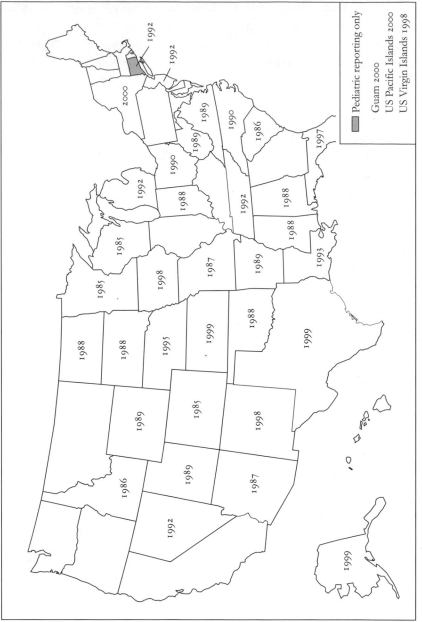

MAP 8-1. Year of Initiation of Confidential HIV Case Surveillance as of April 2002

track the epidemic more accurately and intervene in a more specific and effective manner.

Monitor the Epidemic

A national HIV surveillance system would improve epidemiological assessments of the epidemic and help answer vital public health questions such as how many people in America are infected with HIV? How many of these infections are newly acquired and diagnosed? How were these newly diagnosed infections contracted? Are persons living with HIV receiving appropriate medical and social services? How effective is treatment? What strains of HIV are becoming resistant to treatment? Which communities have the highest rate of new infections?

A national HIV surveillance system, as recommended by the CDC, would fulfill the need for accurate data on various aspects of the epidemic. First, the system would monitor the methods by which HIV infection is acquired and transmitted by measuring the precursors to infection such as risk behaviors and modes of transmission (sexual, perinatal, multiperson use of drug-injection equipment, accidental needle sticks, etc.). Second, data collection on recent HIV infections would offer a window into the emerging trends of the epidemic. Third, monitoring HIV-related deaths would improve understanding of the number of persons living with HIV infection and the characteristics of those for whom treatment fails. Finally, a national HIV surveillance system would collect laboratory markers of disease severity (HIV RNA, CD4+ values) and monitor preventable opportunistic illnesses, thus enabling health authorities to characterize the natural history of HIV disease and to evaluate the access to, and efficacy of, medical treatment.

Target and Evaluate Effective Public Health Services

An improved monitoring system would help target and evaluate effective prevention services, including population-based testing, counseling, and education. By directing scarce resources to geographic areas and subpopulations with the greatest needs, health authorities could most efficiently reduce HIV transmission. Research suggests that targeted HIV prevention services are effective in both averting infections in high-risk populations and reducing costs.[24] A study among patients at STD clinics in five cities with high rates of HIV showed that after receiving interactive client-centered HIV/STD counseling approximately 30 percent fewer study participants were infected with an STD within six months, and 20 percent fewer were infected within one year.[25] Enhanced surveillance assists in community planning for HIV prevention, implementing public health strategies, and evaluating their efficacy. For example, a CDC analysis found that states conducting HIV surveillance were able to identify 49 percent of children born to infected mothers, compared with 5 percent in states that reported AIDS alone.[26] These types of data could enable states to develop more effective strategies (including testing, counseling, and treatment) to reduce perinatal transmission and provide services for HIV-infected mothers and children. A recent CDC study confirmed the need for HIV outreach and testing among young men who have sex with men (MSM) in the United States. Of young black MSM who tested positive, 93 percent were unaware of their positive status and, therefore, had not sought treatment and care.[27] Targeted testing and counseling services can increase awareness among high-risk populations and prevent the further spread of HIV.

Link to Health Education, Treatment, and Partner Notification

HIV surveillance benefits people with HIV infection or AIDS by connecting them to health education, treatment, and support services. Where HIV infection is reportable, public health authorities have greater ability to ensure timely referrals for health and social services including counseling, education, treatment, and voluntary partner notification. Studies suggest that client-centered counseling and health education reduce risks for HIV transmission.[28] Persons with HIV/AIDS who receive early treatment have an increased likelihood of living longer and higher-quality lives.[29] Moreover, as the CDC reports, "ensuring timely access to HIV-care services for HIV-infected persons remains important because in many persons HIV infection is not diagnosed until AIDS is diagnosed."[30] Furthermore, HIV case reporting facilitates notification of and treatment referral for the sex and needle-sharing partners of HIV-infected persons.[31]

Improved surveillance, of course, will not ensure that persons with HIV infection receive services. Many barriers to health and social services exist, notably those related to cost, geographic accessibility, and culture. Still, HIV reporting can facilitate access to services. Public health authorities have long provided government-funded counseling, treatment, and partner notification services for persons with sexually transmitted diseases. HIV surveillance would receive more enthusiastic community support if it too were explicitly linked to reliable health and human services.

Just Resource Allocation

Historically, resource allocation for HIV/AIDS prevention programs has been based on AIDS surveillance data. This is particularly true for programs under the purview of the Ryan White CARE Act and other federally authorized expenditures. In 2000 Congress appropriated over $1.8 billion for HIV/AIDS prevention and treatment under the Ryan White CARE Act.[32] Much of this money was distributed to metropolitan areas based on how many AIDS cases those areas reported.[33] AIDS data have been used to decide the federal appropriations because they are universally available and provide a standardized, representative accounting of the number of persons with severe HIV disease.

Health care planning based on HIV rather than AIDS trends, however, would provide a more accurate assessment of the distribution of the infected population and the number of people needing access to treatment. Accurate estimates of the current status and future directions of HIV infection could mobilize political opinion in favor of more adequate and enduring funding for surveillance, prevention, research, and treatment. Political efforts to protect the health of women, children, and communities of color would be best served by surveillance that reveals the nature and extent of HIV infection in those groups.

The Behavioral and Social Impact of Named HIV Reporting

Most objections to HIV surveillance are behavioral and social, and relate to voluntary testing, privacy, and discrimination.[34] Public health authorities and community representatives share one core concern about HIV case reporting: that it might deter at-risk individuals from seeking testing and care.[35] Persons at risk for HIV are advised to undergo testing to receive needed counseling and treatment.[36] If persons at risk for HIV infection are required by law to report their names to health officials, will they decline to be tested or delay seeing a physician?

The Risk of Deterrence

Although the data are mixed, there are good reasons to believe that HIV case reporting does not provide a distinct disincentive to testing. Studies suggest that most persons at risk for HIV do not know their state's case reporting requirements.[37] If individuals are unaware of the law, it is unlikely to affect their behavior.

In states with named reporting, few individuals who delayed or avoided testing reported that fear of named reporting was their primary reason for not getting tested. More people delay or avoid testing because they are afraid of finding out that they are HIV positive.[38] Additionally, a review of health department data from six states showed that in the six months after the states implemented named reporting, the number of HIV tests per month increased in four states. Testing rates declined in two states, but these declines were not statistically significant. Critics contend that because these studies were conducted in states with a low HIV prevalence, they cannot accurately predict the deterrent effect of named reporting of HIV in areas where HIV is more prevalent.

A survey conducted in San Francisco among men who have sex with men found that 47.7 percent of participants said that they would not test if named reporting were required; 42.3 percent stated that they would still test; and 10 percent did not know. Of those who would test even if named reporting were required, 42 percent stated that they would not give their real name.[39]

The available data thus appear to be mixed. Most studies suggest that persons at risk will not delay or avoid seeking an HIV test if their state requires named reporting; in fact, the great majority of respondents were unaware of their state's reporting laws. However, in large cities like San Francisco, individuals indicated that the potential invasion of privacy could keep them from testing (for more on privacy and the risk of discrimination, see Chapters 5 and 6).

Anonymous Testing

"Alternative" test sites are locations where individuals can be tested without having to provide a name or other personal identifier. Empirical studies demonstrate that alternative test sites encourage voluntary testing.[40] In these studies, respondents reported an increased likelihood of seeking HIV testing if anonymous testing were available.[41]

Good public health policy demands that states provide opportunities for anonymous testing to individuals concerned about the confidentiality of reported test results. Substantial evidence indicates that anonymous testing is widely used, especially by members of the at-risk populations that have most vocally opposed named reporting. After South Carolina eliminated anonymous testing in the late 1980s, 51 percent fewer MSM sought HIV testing in the state.[42] In contrast, demand for HIV testing in Oregon increased 125 percent when that state began offering anonymous testing. More recently, data from the Multistate Evaluation of Surveillance of HIV showed that 25 percent of persons who tested positive for HIV chose to test anonymously; compared with persons who received confidential tests, the time between diagnosis of HIV and diagnosis of AIDS was generally a year and a half longer for persons who had tested anonymously.[43] This was a result of earlier diagnosis and treatment of HIV. Finally, a 1997 study of testing patterns at publicly funded testing sites concluded that more than half of MSM chose to test anonymously.[44]

Recognizing the importance of anonymous testing, the CDC requires states to provide such testing as a condition of receiving HIV prevention funding unless prohibited by state law. Eleven states, however, do not provide anonymous testing.[45] The potential health consequences of failing to offer anonymous HIV testing include delays in testing and care, increased blood donations by individuals at risk for HIV who seek anonymous testing, and reduced quality of HIV surveillance because of false identifying information given at confidential testing sites.[46]

Even in states where anonymous testing is not offered, individuals may purchase home collection test kits over the counter at major drug stores to be tested anonymously (see Chapter 7).[47] Individuals who buy home collection kits possess the means to be tested anonymously, but those who are indigent may not be able to afford them. Considerations of equity, as well as public health, militate in favor of public access to anonymous HIV testing in all jurisdictions.

Privacy and Security of HIV Registries

Strict privacy and security of HIV data are necessary to ensure the success of a national HIV case reporting system (see Chapter 5). Persons living with HIV/AIDS have potent reasons for desiring privacy. Not only is HIV infection a serious and costly disease, but its disclosure may also expose intimate information about an individual's sexual or drug-using behavior. In addition, both physicians and patients may perceive the reporting of test results, demographics, and risk behaviors to a government agency as a breach of trust.[48] Unauthorized disclosures, moreover, may embarrass the patient and result in discrimination in housing, employment, and health care.

Public health departments have a strong history of maintaining the confidentiality of reported information, but community anxieties have been heightened by well-publicized invasions of privacy. For example, thieves stole a computer containing the names of sixty persons with AIDS in Sacramento, California,[49] and a log of hundreds of people tested for HIV "vanished" from a public health clinic in New York.[50] In Florida, a health official publicly revealed names from an HIV registry without authorization.[51] Courts have occasionally ordered HIV data to be disclosed for the purposes of litigation.[52] A few state legislatures have abused HIV surveillance for political purposes. Illinois enacted, but never implemented, legislation requiring the state health department to identify HIV-positive HCWs by cross-matching the state AIDS registry against health care licensure records.[53]

Although worrisome, these examples are the exception rather than the norm. The Supreme Court requires that states provide reasonable levels of privacy and security for reported health data.[54] Virtually all states statutorily protect the privacy of government-held data.[55] In addition, most states have enacted HIV-specific privacy legislation that imposes stricter standards for HIV information (see Chapter 5). Finally, the federal government offers a confidentiality assurance for HIV/AIDS surveillance, prohibiting the use of personally identifiable information for any purpose other than that for which it was provided (unless the supplier of the information has consented to an alternate use).[56] Failure to maintain the confidentiality of individuals in reporting registries in violation of these legal protections may subject responsible persons to criminal and civil sanctions.

The CDC requires states to comply with its security standards as a precondition for receiving federal funds for HIV surveillance (see Chapter 5). Privacy problems with HIV data already exist, suggesting that issues relating to HIV reporting are hardly unique. The names of persons with HIV infection are entered into multiple databases, such as those of Medicaid, drug-assistance registries, and public health registries for other reportable conditions. Sensitive HIV data are also collected, stored, and widely used by insurers, managed care organizations, and researchers.

An Alternative to Named HIV Surveillance: Unique Identifiers

Most public health authorities and civil liberties groups agree that HIV reporting is important for the public's health.[57] At the heart of the debate is the means through which HIV reporting is accomplished—whether by name or unique identifier (UI). Named reporting relies on the disclosure of an individual's name and other identifying characteristics. Reporting by UI strips identifying information from a reporting record. Instead, it relies on a numeric code (intended to be unique for each person) to report cases of HIV infection.

Public health authorities (with some exceptions) advocate the use of named HIV reporting for several reasons. First, named reporting has successfully been used for other STDs, as well as AIDS reporting. Second, authorities argue that privacy protections for reported data are sufficient. Third, reporting by name is more efficient, more reliable, and less costly than by UI.

Many civil liberties organizations reject the use of named reporting in favor of reporting by UI.[58] Named reporting, they contend, is "bad policy" because it discourages individuals from being tested for HIV. They support UI reporting because it better protects the privacy of HIV-infected persons, virtually eliminating the need for other privacy protections of government-held HIV data.

Advocates of UI reporting argue that HIV surveillance that could be conducted as, or more, effectively without revealing an individual's identity is preferred to named reporting. The problem is that UI systems have not been shown to work as well or provide the same level of privacy protection for the same cost as named reporting systems in the United States.[59]

In the mid-1990s two states, Maryland and Texas, began conducting HIV surveillance for all populations using non-named UIs. These identifiers consisted of four distinct components: (1) the last four digits of the Social Security number, (2) the numerical birth date (MM/DD/YY), and (3, 4) numerical indications of a person's gender and race based on coding schemes used by the CDC. Results from both states demonstrated that these systems are more costly to implement than named reporting and that their data contain a significant number of duplicate and difficult-to-match records.

UI systems are not as simple to operate as named reporting systems. The lack of simplicity was exacerbated by the poor acceptance of the reporting methods among medical providers and testing laboratories. Medical providers experienced difficulty in correctly completing the UI form and in obtaining sufficient information from individuals to complete it. In 34 percent of cases reported in Texas and 22 percent of cases in Maryland, health care workers failed to provide a key element of the UI—the four-digit component of the individual's Social Security number.[60]

Failures in supplying the Social Security component do not necessarily prevent medical workers from providing other UI components that are easier to determine.[61] Over a two-and-a-half-year period, only 71 percent of the UI reports in Maryland and 61 percent of the reports in Texas were fully completed.[62] Based on these results, Texas decided to discontinue its UI system in favor of named HIV reporting,[63] and the CDC decided to recommend named reporting rather than the UI method.

Advocates nevertheless contend that the reporting information obtained from UI systems is accurate enough. They argue that named reporting results in duplication as well, and the purpose of HIV reporting is not to count every last person, but to compute reliable prevalence and incidence rates in communities; UIs accomplish this end. Maryland officials point out that the state's UI system has improved substantially.[64] Moreover, in the last few years, several more states and Puerto Rico have adopted UI systems, suggesting that some jurisdictions find these systems both palatable to the community and sufficiently accurate to meet their surveillance needs.[65]

Although these arguments have considerable merit, there are strong reasons to believe that UI systems cannot at present provide adequate surveillance data. UI surveillance complicates the ability of public health authorities to obtain complex data about risk behavior and natural history—the type of information that is available from physician and patient interviews and medical record review and currently accessed through the patient's name.

UI systems, moreover, may actually create increased privacy risks. Because they rely on physicians and laboratories to keep individual logs of reported cases to cross-check for duplicates, private information about persons living with HIV must be centrally kept in many thousands of private health care provider offices. Each of these locations must separately maintain adequate security to prevent breaches. Security violations, even on a limited basis, can result in the dissemination of intensely private information within local communities where affected individuals may reside.

Four states, Maine, Montana, Oregon, and Washington, have attempted to resolve the conflict between community support for non-named reporting and the privacy and security advantages of named-reporting by implementing hybrid surveillance systems.[66] In those states, persons living with HIV are first reported to the health department by name, but the health department then replaces the name with a code. By eliminating the need for health care providers to report by code, these states hope to achieve the same level of accuracy in surveillance as named reporting states and eliminate the need for multiple lists of persons with HIV.[67] At the same time, by destroying records naming individuals with HIV, they hope to address community privacy concerns. These programs are relatively new and there has been no evaluation of their success. For these reasons, maintaining reportable health information at local and state health departments through named reporting should still be considered the most accurate and secure surveillance method.

The Future of HIV Surveillance

Reporting requirements pose an enduring conflict of values between individual rights to privacy and the collective good of society. Perhaps the initial resistance to HIV case reporting was warranted by the sensitivity to a new and frightening disease that posed a disproportionate hardship on stigmatized populations. Battling science for years, the disease left persons living with HIV and their partners without the benefit of effective treatment. Given the need for privacy and the near absence of viable interventions, individual rights were thought to outweigh the societal benefits of HIV surveillance.

With advances in science, medicine, epidemiology, and law, however, we are now at a very different point in the history of the epidemic. Collective justifications for a national system of HIV case reporting are compelling. HIV reporting would improve epidemiological understanding of the epidemic; prevent infections by targeting scarce resources for testing, counseling, education, and partner notification; benefit persons with HIV/AIDS and their partners by providing a link to medical treatment and other human services; and promote more equitable allocation of government funding.

One of the purposes of HIV testing and reporting is to inform the individual of his or her serologic status and provide an opportunity to notify sex or needle-sharing partners. But notification of partners can be socially and politically controversial. The next chapter describes the various forms of partner notification, offers an ethical analysis, and reviews the empirical evidence of their effectiveness.

In no other respect is the [medical] practice in this country more reprehensible than in the failure of physicians, and even of public health clinics, to make diligent inquiry as to sources of infection and to use all available methods to bring these persons under treatment.
—**Thomas Parran,** U.S. surgeon general, 1936–48

Chapter 9

Piercing the Veil of Secrecy

Partner Notification, the Right to
Know, and the Duty to Warn

At least since their appearance in Western Europe in the late fifteenth century,[1] sexually transmitted diseases (STDs), or "venereal diseases" as they were once called,[2] have been characterized by a remarkable paradox. Despite their endemic nature in Europe and North America, STDs were, and still are, a "secret malady."[3] Persons have endeavored to keep their sexually transmitted infections hidden from the social world—from their sex partners, families, and communities. At the same time, prevailing social mores have kept STDs from the public consciousness and consequently from public action and effective intervention.

Secrecy nurtures disease because it provides a social environment conducive to the spread of infection. If the social construction of sexuality and disease condones secrecy, sex partners will be unaware of the risks and public health

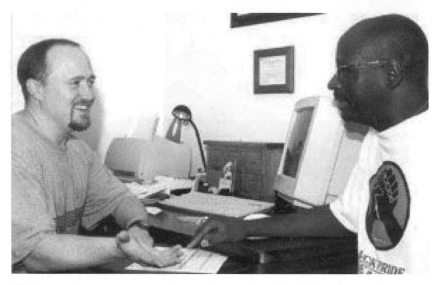

This image shows an HIV counseling session at the California Prostitutes Education Project (CAL-PEP) in Oakland, California. CAL-PEP began HIV counseling services in 1984. California encourages newly diagnosed individuals to take advantage of the anonymous partner notification service to prevent the further transmission of HIV.

authorities will be unable to effectively monitor the epidemic. Not surprisingly, one of the earliest recorded public health strategies for STD prevention was to pierce the veil of secrecy surrounding these hidden diseases by notifying sex partners ("contacts") of infected patients. The rationale behind "contact tracing" was that sex partners could take precautions and seek medical treatment if the risks of infection were disclosed.[4] Once the risks of infection were identified, the incidence of STD infection would decline as infected persons received treatment or reduced behaviors that placed them at risk for contracting or further spreading disease.[5]

Sexual contact tracing was probably practiced years before it became a formal means of STD control.[6] Originating from the reglementation[7] of prostitutes in sixteenth-century Europe, the earliest reference to contact tracing in contagious disease law dates to the mid-nineteenth century in Europe[8] and to the 1930s in the United States.[9] Buttressed by federal financial support and a decade of state STD laws, "contact epidemiology" became a central public health strategy in America to combat the syphilis epidemic.[10]

Since its widespread use during the 1930s, the notification of sex partners with the assistance of public health authorities remained an accepted part of the law and practice of STD control throughout the twentieth century. This concept of tracking sexual contacts would later be equated with the term "partner notification." Partner notification has recently expanded to include a range of services, including substantial counseling and medical treatment in addition to notification.

The social construction of STDs, however, changed during the HIV/AIDS epidemic.[11] Infected persons and public health authorities questioned the theory of disclosure that justified partner notification. During the AIDS epidemic, secrecy and individual privacy reemerged as the prevailing social construct of public health, much as it was in the early days of the syphilis epidemic. As Susan Sontag writes, "More than cancer, but rather like syphilis, AIDS seems to foster ominous fantasies about a disease that is a marker of both individual and social vulnerabilities."[12] Within this context, there was a question whether partner notification is an acceptable public health practice or a legally imposed duty. This question is especially pertinent to a disease like HIV/AIDS, which is deeply private, socially stigmatizing, and medically incurable.

In truth, partner notification—whether applied to traditional STDs or to HIV/AIDS—is highly complex. Partner notification has deep roots in the historical, legal, and philosophical heritage of America. Why, then, does U.S. policy refrain from fully implementing one of the most well-established public health interventions in the HIV/AIDS epidemic?[13] To some, the failure to aggressively pursue partner notification shows that AIDS has attained an "exceptional" status[14] whereby civil liberties trump public health.[15] Yet this argument assumes that partner notification is effective and that syphilis and HIV/AIDS are truly analogous diseases.

Despite the use of partner notification in all of its forms, it has not been systematically examined from legal, ethical, empirical, and economic perspectives. This chapter discusses the three meanings of partner notification— governmental contact tracing, the duty of infected persons to disclose, and the duty of health care professionals to warn; provides an ethical analysis of partner notification, including competing claims of the right to privacy and the right to knowledge; presents an empirical analysis of partner notification, inquiring whether it is cost-effective; and offers an alternative to partner notification, namely, Social Network Analysis (SNA). The chapter concludes with some reflections on partner notification and its implications for privacy and protection of vulnerable people.

The Three Meanings of Partner Notification:
From Contact Tracing to the Duties to Disclose and Warn

Partner notification is a highly complex concept. Although it is often simplified to denote disclosure to persons who are at risk of becoming infected with a disease, partner notification has at least three distinct, at times overlapping, meanings: (1) *contact tracing*—public health agencies locate and inform partners who may have been exposed to infection, (2) *duty to disclose*—persons disclose their infection to their partners, and (3) *duty to warn*—health care professionals warn the partners of their infected patients.

These three meanings of partner notification evolved principally from syphilis control programs. The HIV/AIDS epidemic has presented challenges that are both similar to and different from conventional STDs. One obvious similarity between syphilis and AIDS is the societal response. Fear and stigmatization of persons affected prevailed during both epidemics. The societal response to gays and injection drug users (IDUs) living with HIV/AIDS ominously parallels the treatment of women, particularly sex workers, during the syphilis epidemic. In an earlier time, persons with syphilis were often categorized as either innocent or guilty. Wives, mothers, and children "innocently" infected with syphilis were treated with sympathy, whereas others were ostracized and punished.[16] STDs and HIV are similar in another important respect. Common STDs like syphilis, gonorrhea, chlamydia, and genital herpes are known to increase the risk of other STDs as well as HIV infection.[17] The epidemics of HIV and STDs are intertwined and, in many ways, inseparable.

Despite the similarities and interconnectedness of these two diseases, partner notification has never garnered the level of acceptance in the HIV/AIDS epidemic it has with other STDs. In the HIV/AIDS context, the notion of partner notification has angered gay rights organizations,[18] civil rights groups,[19] and even some public health officials.[20] Although some states have attempted to establish mandatory partner notification programs, most programs and state educational initiatives focus on individuals protecting themselves from infection.

Contact Tracing

Contact tracing is characteristically a governmental responsibility undertaken by public health authorities. The health department typically interviews an infected patient (index case) who voluntarily discloses the names and locations of past and present sex partners. Health authorities then locate (trace) the contacts, when possible, to notify them of their exposure to infection. In an attempt to preserve confidentiality, authorities do not inform those notified of the name of the index case. Moreover, health departments frequently offer medical treatment and personal counseling. For those persons found to be infected, the process is regenerated to determine additional contacts. The principal objective of contact tracing is to reduce disease transmission by locating and containing the spread of STDs, including HIV. It seeks to break the chain of transmission by identifying, counseling, and treating persons exposed to infection.

Contact tracing is primarily the responsibility of state health departments and is authorized or mandated under state law.[21] The differing needs of communities render contact tracing suitable to state and local, rather than federal, control.[22] Although there is no national system of partner notification, federal policy does exist. The Ryan White Comprehensive AIDS Resources Emergency Act of 1990 (CARE) authorizes the secretary of health and human services to provide grants to state public health departments to implement partner notification programs for persons living with HIV/AIDS.[23] The Ryan White CARE Reauthorization Act of 1996 conditioned the receipt of federal funds for state partner notification programs upon the implementation of good-faith efforts to notify spouses of index cases infected with HIV and offer them testing.[24]

Certain federal grants also require states and localities to implement partner notification programs according to CDC guidelines.[25] In 1997 the CDC issued parameters for partner notification, or what it called "partner notification support services."[26] The CDC requires federally funded contact tracing programs to provide a comprehensive set of supplemental services, including testing, medical treatment, and counseling, in addition to notification assistance. In 1998 the CDC issued new guidelines for partner counseling and referral services.[27] These guidelines recommend that services be client-centered, voluntary, confidential, and culturally appropriate. The CDC further recommends that these services be available throughout the client's lifetime. In 2003 the CDC announced that it would increase emphasis on partner notification and referral services by funding new models of early diagnosis and support for partners. This includes using rapid HIV testing, peer counseling, and treatment referral.[28]

In summary, contact tracing arose from governmental control of STDs. As one form of partner notification, contact tracing represents a traditional activity of the state to protect the public from epidemic diseases. A principal feature is voluntariness of participation. Similarly, maintaining the confidentiality of index patients encourages patients to cooperate with public health officials.

Duty of Infected Persons to Disclose

The second meaning of partner notification is the infected person's duty to disclose the risks to his or her partner. The partner's "right to know" emerged from the social hygiene movement of the early 1900s and was likely influenced by early principles of feminism. It developed under tort law, which held that a person has a duty of care toward his or her sex partner. This duty may entail an obligation to disclose HIV status to a sex partner or to reasonably protect the partner from avoidable health risks. Although the duty of infected persons to disclose shares characteristics with contact tracing, significant differences exist. These dissimilarities tend to confuse policy formation and impair society's understanding of contact tracing.

Statutes and courts have imposed duties on persons infected with HIV or other STDs to disclose the risk to their partners.[29] The duty to disclose represents a serious, obligatory side of partner notification, grounded in the responsibility to do no harm to others. It requires persons living with HIV/AIDS to inform their sex and needle-sharing partners of their infection.[30] Accordingly, spouses and other partners[31] can recover tort damages for breaches of this duty.[32]

A crucial issue is when the judiciary will impose the duty to inform a partner.[33] Certainly, courts have little difficulty imposing liability if the person knew, or reasonably should have known, that he was HIV-infected. Thus, courts may impose a duty to inform if an individual has some reasonable basis for knowledge such as a positive test result or persistent, noticeable symptoms. But the courts are reticent to impose a duty based solely on a person's sexual history.[34] For example, if an individual has had multiple sex partners, but has not been tested, the courts may not assume that he was aware of his HIV infection.

Duty of Health Care Workers to Warn

The third meaning of partner notification is derived from a related legal doctrine known as a "duty to warn." Through conversations with the infected patient, a physician or other health care worker (HCW) may conclude that certain persons are at risk of contracting the disease. Under the duty to warn, a physician treating a person living with HIV/AIDS has an obligation to inform foreseeable third parties, regardless of whether the patient consents to such notification or the patient's identity is protected.

The duty of HCWs to warn shares its origins with the same line of cases through which courts developed the duty of infected persons to disclose. *Tarasoff v. Regents of the University of California*, however, most famously recognized this duty.[35] In *Tarasoff*, the California Supreme Court held that mental health professionals have a duty to warn third parties of threats of violence by the professional's patients. "When a therapist determines, or pursuant to the standards of his profession should determine, that his patient presents a serious danger to another, he incurs an obligation to use reasonable care to protect the intended victim against such danger."[36] The *Tarasoff* decision has been widely accepted by courts in the United States.[37] It has been extended to include a duty of a HCW who is aware of a foreseeable danger posed by his or her patient to "instruct and advise" existing sex and needle-sharing partners.[38] The common law doctrine of the duty to warn has been codified in statutes in many states.[39] In practice, however, physicians tend to avoid an active role in partner notification. A national survey found that physicians instruct over 80 percent of patients who are newly diagnosed with HIV or another STD to inform their sex and needle-sharing partners themselves.[40]

An Ethical Analysis of Partner Notification

A systematic analysis of the justifications for partner notification, both theoretical and empirical, is helpful in assessing its continued usefulness. Partner notification creates a tension between the interests of persons living with HIV/AIDS (primarily the right to privacy) and their sex and needle-sharing partners (primarily the right to know). Because privacy and knowledge are incompatible interests, policymakers must sometimes choose one interest over the other.

Persons living with HIV/AIDS have strong reasons to maintain their privacy. Disclosure of a person's HIV status can cause embarrassment and stigma and result in discrimination. Society often stereotypes persons living with HIV/AIDS as homosexuals, drug users, or prostitutes and relegates them to a lesser social status. The resultant discrimination takes many forms, including refusal to provide medical treatment, adverse employment decisions, and refusals to contract (see Chapter 6).[41] Since most STDs are not transmissible through casual contact, discrimination in the form of barriers to access to employment, public accommodations, and services is especially egregious and morally unwarranted.[42]

Disclosure of HIV status also may result in emotional, economic, or physical abuse. Studies indicate that persons who participate in partner notification programs are disproportionately neglected, abandoned, and battered.[43] Once their partners find that they are HIV-infected, there is a potential for anger, betrayal, and retaliation. As a result, individuals with HIV who participate in contact tracing programs often fear the consequences should their identities be revealed. Moreover, they may forgo their duty to disclose out of concern that such information will circulate within the community. Therefore, adequate legal protection against discrimination and retaliation is critical to successful implementation of public health strategies. Such protections will likely have the added benefit of encouraging persons living with HIV/AIDS to participate in partner notification programs.

Balanced against the privacy claims of infected persons are the equally compelling claims of their partners to be informed of the risk. Sex partners understandably seek to know the unforeseen dangers of which their partners or associated health care professionals are aware.[44] Partners claim a "right" to know that they have been exposed to infection because knowledge (1) empowers individuals to avoid continuing risks, (2) facilitates access to early treatment, and (3) helps prevent further transmission.[45]

There is no sure way to resolve this dilemma ethically. Both claims—the right to privacy and the right to know—are based on autonomy. Persons living with HIV/AIDS can reasonably argue that they have the right to control highly personal information, particularly where unauthorized disclosure can be harmful. Their partners, however, may answer that absent full information, the freedom to make an autonomous choice is merely illusory. The level of risk of infection is highly relevant information when choosing to have sex or share needles. This is true despite the universal public health message that all people, irrespective of specific knowledge of HIV risk, should take precautions all of the time. Although theoretically wise, realistically, people will be more cautious if they are aware that their partners are HIV-infected. Moreover, the moral imperative of autonomous choice rests on every person's claim to have specific knowledge of his or her partner's HIV status. Given the equally strong normative claims, the best way to determine whether partner notification is a wise policy may be to examine its effectiveness empirically.

Efficacy of Partner Notification: An Empirical Analysis

Partner notification practices should also be evaluated with respect to their cost-effectiveness. To determine if partner notification should continue as a standard public health practice, it would be helpful to have demonstrably sound and scientifically verifiable evidence that it reduces the risk of infection. The central question is whether partner notification accomplishes the goal of reducing transmission and, if so, at what cost? Some studies suggest that partner notification is effective in limited environments involving high-risk populations. But evidence of the effectiveness of contact tracing as a widespread public health practice is inconclusive.[46]

Examining the objective data on partner notification is not a simple task.[47] There is no scientifically valid empirical standard. Rather, the consensus of opinion holds that "[a]ctive contact tracing programs have been effective (but costly) in controlling localized outbreaks of specific antibiotic resistant strains of sexually transmitted diseases with short latency periods and in targeting specific subgroups of the population."[48] Studies suggest that STDs such as syphilis,[49] gonorrhea,[50] and chlamydia[51] have been controlled among subgroups through contact tracing.

Studies of partner notification to prevent HIV/AIDS suggest that it is less effective than for other STDs.[52] The reasons proffered are the lack of a cure for AIDS and the long asymptomatic incubation period of the infection, which makes tracing among populations difficult. These observations, however, do not justify the failure to attempt to notify persons at risk of HIV infection. Although notifying former partners may be a difficult task, it can be useful in identifying individuals at an earlier stage of disease.[53] Clearly, "the key issue remains not whether sex and needle-sharing partners of HIV-infected individuals should be informed, but rather how this notification will occur."[54]

Public health studies suggest that HIV partner notification programs can be effective in locating and counseling the infected contacts of index cases[55] and reducing STD infection rates,[56] especially among at-risk groups.[57] Many of these studies emphasize the importance of voluntariness and confidentiality.[58] However, studies in Oregon[59] and North Carolina[60] involving syphilis and HIV respectively concluded that partner notification is less successful in containing disease where index cases have sex and drug partners too numerous to identify. Contact tracing is also less successful with STDs that have long latency periods such as syphilis and HIV. Canadian researchers who examined several partner notification studies found that evidence of effectiveness is inconclusive due to the paucity of well-designed studies.[61] Overall, the authors opined, "there is very little upon which to estimate the ultimate benefits and harms of partner notification for HIV infection," stating that "arguments for and against provider referral for HIV infection tend to be based more on convictions than on data."[62]

Alternative Models for Partner Notification

Despite the moral and legal claims supporting partner notification, impediments exist to its acceptance within affected communities. In addition to the difficulties of ensuring confidentiality, infected individuals often do not regard state-operated contact tracing programs as voluntary in light of the judicially enforced duties to disclose and to warn. In this sense, partner notification has a coercive component that discourages participation. These facts, coupled with the real-world potential of discrimination and physical harms, pose significant challenges for the future of partner notification. As a result, other public health measures should be examined to determine if they can be used to prevent HIV without the drawbacks of partner notification.

Social Network Analysis (SNA) offers public health professionals a viable alternative to explore.[63] Complex in practice, SNA attempts to measure the ways in which people relate to each other by examining determinants of their social structure or network. It transforms information obtained from individuals through interviews, surveys, or epidemiologic studies into data about their interaction within networks. Complementary approaches of network ascertainment and ethnography are combined to describe "a social process, such as the transmission of disease, and to contribute to disease control and program evaluation."[64] Instead of concentrating on information about partners as in traditional contact tracing, SNA attempts to identify persons in an infected individual's social setting and offer assistance (counseling, testing, and medical evaluations) to STD network members determined through ethnographic analysis. In this way, authorities can focus public health efforts on those who are calculated to be at risk of infection without invasion of individual privacy.

Among the benefits of SNA over traditional contact tracing are (1) the ability of public health authorities to focus efforts on a larger number of persons at risk, (2) the development of enhanced knowledge about existing transmission patterns within defined areas and subpopulations, (3) the nonnecessity to specifically inquire about partners of infected persons, (4) the provision of important information to at-risk individuals without breaching the confidentiality of sources, (5) the ability to identify and notify persons at risk who are not necessarily former or existing sex or IDU partners of infected persons, but may be in the future, and (6) the ability to develop more detailed information about at-risk behaviors to allow more effective interventions.

Of course, there are disadvantages to SNA as well: (1) SNA is dependent on information gathering and is thus labor-intensive, expensive, and time-consuming (this drawback is also true of contact tracing), (2) if the information is incomplete or incorrect, network behavioral calculations may be off-target; (3) SNA requires technologically advanced statistical calculations by knowledgeable experts to which smaller public health districts may lack adequate access; (4) network techniques may be incomparable for differing STDs and difficult to replicate in all communities; and (5) since SNA does not notify partners directly, participation by infected persons does not satisfy the legal duty to disclose.

Social Network Analysis thus needs rigorous evaluation. At present, its effectiveness is unclear. However, innovative strategies like SNA offer promising new methods for the prevention of infection with less adverse effects on individuals. In light of the benefits of SNA and the drawbacks of contact tracing, public health authorities should consider SNA in combination with contact tracing on a reduced scale, limited to those environments where contact tracing is most likely to be effective.

Conclusion

From its origins in the practice of reglementation to its development during the syphilis epidemic to its modern application in the HIV/AIDS epidemic, partner notification has been motivated by the moral imperative to notify and protect persons who are unaware of their risk to exposure. Few people question the underlying morality of open, honest information in relation to a "hidden epidemic." However, the consequences of partner notification are complex and not uniformly beneficial to infected persons, their partners, and the community. Even though it is defensible on normative grounds, partner notification has demonstrable flaws. Partner notification poses a cost to individuals in loss of privacy and discrimination. Particularly for women, it can result in abandonment, neglect, and abuse. And, just as importantly, research data do not convincingly demonstrate the effectiveness of partner notification. For these reasons, alternative strategies like Social Network Analysis should be considered to supplement partner notification. SNA, which involves focused education and notification of subpopulations at high risk, may change risk behaviors without infringing civil liberties.

As seen in the epidemics of syphilis and now HIV, STDs strike vulnerable populations and pose a complex dilemma between civil liberties and public health. One day HIV/AIDS will become a manageable disease, but its immediate lesson is clear: we must model our public health efforts within the social realities of the time. Contact tracing must conform to modern understandings of privacy, women's rights, and a rigorous determination of public health effectiveness.

Part of the reason for the advocacy community's opposition to partner notification is that it is perceived to have a coercive element. Although voluntary in theory, individuals interviewed by a state official may not fully appreciate the freedom they have to refuse to cooperate. There are, of course, public health powers that are explicitly coercive and the AIDS community has even more strenuously opposed them. The next chapter evaluates the most coercive public health interventions—isolation and quarantine, compulsory medical treatment, and criminal punishment.

Investigations by the Department of Human Services have revealed that you have been engaged in activities which are potentially harmful to the public health. You have been counseled as to the nature and risk of these activities. Nevertheless, there is evidence to suggest that you have continued to participate in these activities. Now, therefore, I, Commissioner of the Department of Human Services, order you, [name], to cease and desist from activities which are deemed to constitute a threat to public health, effective immediately. If you fail to honor this order, a court injunction may be sought to compel your compliance.
— **State of Maine, Department of Human Services** (1993)

Chapter 10

The Politics of AIDS

Compulsory State Powers, Public
Health, and Civil Liberties

Disease epidemics bring out the best and the worst in human beings. There are those who risk their own health to care for or treat others, befriend the ill, and advocate for services and rights. At the same time, the body politic often ostracizes and discriminates against persons with infectious disease. The history of epidemics tells the story of communities first fearing, then excluding, and finally punishing persons perceived as contagious. The community often regards persons with infectious disease as "the other," subjecting them to exclusion and separation from the wider society.

The use of compulsory public health powers can be a visible political symbol for controlling AIDS. Public opinion polls earlier in the epidemic consistently showed support for coercive action, with a significant proportion of respondents favoring "quarantine" of persons living with HIV/AIDS in "special

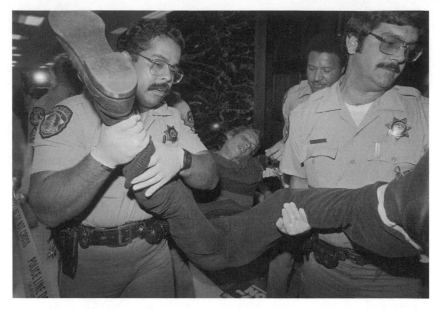

Latex-gloved police carry a demonstrator out of the governor's office in Sacramento, California, in 1986. The man was protesting job and housing discrimination against people who have AIDS. (© Bettmann/CORBIS)

places to keep them away from the general public."[1] The public similarly favored criminal penalties for persons who engage in risk behaviors such as sex, needle sharing, or donating blood while HIV-infected.[2]

Persons living with HIV/AIDS have, for the most part, been spared the indignity of systematic civil sanctions. Nevertheless, the community exhibited exaggerated fears of contagion and segregationist instincts during the first decades of the epidemic. Recall, for example, the burning of Ricky Ray's home when his mother insisted that he attend school.[3] Popular indignation was also evident in frequent proposals for punitive measures, such as branding with a tattoo,[4] confining,[5] and establishing special institutions.[6] More recently, there has been discussion of compulsory treatment or directly observed therapy for persons who are deemed "recalcitrant," particularly for pregnant women.[7]

Even though most forms of civil police powers were never systematically implemented, governments have resorted to criminal penalties against persons living with HIV/AIDS. Politicians have enacted a spate of laws ostensibly to deter individuals from engaging in HIV risk behaviors. Prosecutors have brought cases against persons living with HIV/AIDS for prostitution, assault with a deadly weapon ("mouth" and "teeth"), and attempted homicide. Similarly, they have brought charges under HIV-specific statutes for risking transmission of HIV. Persons living with HIV/AIDS have been charged and convicted for the full gamut of possible behaviors ranging from sex and needle sharing to biting, spitting, and donating blood.

Persons living with HIV/AIDS, particularly those associated with disfavored groups such as gays and injection drug users, have been blamed for their disease. They have been unfavorably compared with "innocent" "AIDS babies" and hemophiliacs.[8] The clear implication is that a person somehow is responsible for his disease if he engaged in volitional behavior such as sex or needle sharing, but not if HIV was contracted through a blood transfusion or perinatally. Indeed, AIDS earned its own sobriquet: AIDS phobia (often associated with homophobia).[9] In these ways, AIDS is much like the epidemics of the early twentieth century. During that period, *venereal insontium* referred to venereal disease of the innocent, and *phthisiophobia* referred to the fear of tuberculosis (TB).[10]

This chapter describes the history, politics, and law relating to compulsory powers exercised against persons living with HIV/AIDS. First, the chapter analyzes the major civil powers, including compulsory treatment, directly observed therapy, and isolation. Then it examines the use of criminal law as a tool in the HIV epidemic.

Police Powers: Compulsory Treatment and Civil Confinement

Public health authorities possess a variety of powers to restrict the autonomy or liberty of persons who pose a danger to the public. They can direct individuals to discontinue risk behaviors ("cease and desist" orders), compel them to submit to physical examination or treatment, and detain them temporarily or indefinitely. All of these powers are civil measures designed to prevent risks to the public. They are not intended to punish individuals for morally culpable behavior, as in the case of criminal prosecutions. Civil remedies, therefore, are forward-looking attempts to prevent harm and improve health, whereas criminal penalties are backward-looking attempts to punish wrongdoers. These civil powers would not appear to apply to persons living with HIV/AIDS because of the absence of airborne or casual transmission. Nevertheless, the public has sometimes called for coercive measures, and the government, on occasion, has obliged. For example, the notice to cease and desist risk behaviors in the epigraph at the beginning of the chapter was sent to a person living with HIV/AIDS who was deemed "recalcitrant."

Compulsory Medical Examination, Treatment, and Directly Observed Therapy

Public officials have taken a keen interest in the issue of medical treatment for HIV. Treatment benefits individuals by ameliorating symptoms and prolonging life. Treatment also benefits society by reducing infectiousness. Individuals are much less likely to transmit HIV infection if they are in treatment; therapy can dramatically reduce viral loads to undetectable levels.[11] These dual advantages of treatment, however, are placed at risk if individuals do not take the full course of their medication. Inconsistent treatment can result in drug resistance so that modern therapies become less effective. Indeed, antiretroviral resistance has become a major problem in the HIV epidemic.[12] Because of the benefits to individuals and the community, and the problem of drug resistance, public health authorities have an abiding interest in HIV treatment.

Surely, voluntary treatment with informed consent ought to be the preferred method of ensuring that everyone is treated for HIV. After all, the main barrier to treatment is not the individual's unwillingness, but rather the prohibitive cost. The most obvious solution, therefore, is to ensure culturally appropriate and affordable access to care. Compulsion is usually unnecessary in cases where the person benefits directly from treatment.

Some individuals, of course, may be unwilling or unable to participate in the arduous routine of an HIV treatment program. Highly active antiretroviral therapy (HAART) can produce unpleasant adverse effects.[13] The treatment regimen is also rigorous, requiring discipline to take medication at specific times each day over an indefinite period. Consequently, public officials have discussed the possibility of compulsory physical examination, mandatory treatment, or directly observed therapy.[14] Although these mandatory interventions may be superficially attractive and may even be constitutionally permissible, they raise serious questions of effectiveness and fairness.

The Supreme Court has ruled that health authorities may impose serious forms of treatment, such as antipsychotic medication, if the person poses a danger to himself or others.[15] The treatment must be medically appropriate so that the person benefits. Lower courts, using a similar harm prevention theory, have upheld compulsory physical examinations,[16] compulsory treatment, and directly observed therapy.[17]

Despite the attractions of mandatory HIV treatment, it would be counterproductive. In the past, compulsion has been used in the treatment of persons with sexually transmitted diseases (STDs) or TB.[18] Compulsory treatment for these health conditions is based on the fact that TB is transmitted casually through the air, and most STDs can be treated and cured with relatively short, uncomplicated regimens. But treatment of HIV is much more complex and burdensome. HIV is not casually transmitted, so the primary justification for compulsion does not exist. If a person does not engage in high-risk behavior, the probability of HIV transmission is exceedingly low. Therefore, there is no justification for the use of compulsion in cases where the person does not pose a significant risk to the public.

The HIV treatment regimen is exceedingly difficult to follow and lasts for a lifetime. This means that compliance cannot easily be enforced because persons living with HIV/AIDS would have to be supervised intrusively, systematically, and indefinitely. Thus, the human rights burdens would be so high that it would not be worth the benefits. Moreover, if government attempted to compel such arduous, and long-term, forms of treatment compliance, it is possible that persons living with HIV/AIDS would not come forward for testing, counseling, and treatment. Rather than promote the population's health, the exercise of compulsion could actually undermine clinical and public health objectives.

Quarantine, Isolation, and Civil Commitment

Public health authorities have used isolation and quarantine throughout history to contain infectious diseases.[19] It is thus not surprising that the idea of confining persons living with HIV/AIDS surfaced early and often in the epidemic.[20] Although the terms "isolation" and "quarantine" are often used interchangeably, both in public health statutes and in common parlance, there is a technical distinction between them. The modern definition of quarantine is the restriction of the activities of *healthy* persons who have been exposed to a communicable disease during its period of communicability to prevent disease transmission during the incubation period if infection should occur. In contrast, isolation is the separation, for the period of communicability, of *known* infected persons in such places and under such conditions as to prevent or limit the transmission of the infectious agent.[21] Since HIV can be readily identified through testing, the term "isolation" is most appropriate.

Two different kinds of proposals for isolation have been made: one authorizes confinement on the basis of HIV status alone ("status-based" isolation), and the other authorizes confinement of HIV-infected persons who engage in dangerous behavior ("behavior-based" isolation). The distinction between status-based and behavior-based isolation is pivotal, because one is concerned with an immutable health status, while the other is targeted directly to those who engage in risk behaviors. Clearly a status-based isolation would be grossly unfair and impractical. It would be inequitable since many people who do not engage in risk behaviors would lose their liberty unnecessarily. It would also be impracticable since it would potentially include the entire population of people living with HIV/AIDS, estimated at 900,000 in the United States.[22]

Behavior-based isolation would perhaps be more practicable and politically acceptable, but it would also be ineffective and unjust. It would require a finding that the person is unable or unwilling to control his risk behavior. Predictions of future dangerousness are notoriously unreliable.[23] Consequently, people would lose their liberty based on subjective opinions about their future sex or needle-sharing behavior.

Isolation, whether disease-based or behavior-based, is a uniquely serious form of deprivation of liberty because it can be utilized against competent and unwilling persons, even in the absence of a criminal conviction.[24] It restricts the personal liberty of rational adults, not out of concern for their welfare, but out of concern for the safety of others. Furthermore, it is a form of preventive confinement based on what a person *might* do rather than what he or she has already done. The law is usually loath to confine individuals for acts they have yet to commit. Even more telling is the fact that isolation has no temporal limitation; indeed, inasmuch as persons living with HIV/AIDS are presumed to be infectious for the rest of their lives, isolation amounts to a civil life sentence. Unlike a criminal sentence, however, the duration of isolation is not necessarily proportionate to the gravity of the behavior. Rather, consensual sexual behavior (or even acts such as spitting or biting) could result in lifelong confinement. In short, AIDS does not display the paradigmatic conditions that call for isolation. HIV is not transmitted by casual contact, the person is presumed infectious for an indefinite period of time, and there is no known cure.

If persons living with HIV/AIDS were subjected to isolation based on their health status or behavior, it would still be necessary to ensure that they received a fair and impartial judicial hearing. Persons subject to detention are entitled to procedural due process. As the Supreme Court recognized, "There can be no doubt that involuntary commitment to a mental hospital, like involuntary confinement of an individual for any reason, is a deprivation of liberty which the State cannot accomplish without due process of law."[25]

In *Greene v. Edwards*, the West Virginia Supreme Court reasoned that there is little difference between loss of liberty on mental health grounds and loss of liberty on public health grounds.[26] Persons with an infectious disease, therefore, are entitled to similar procedural protections as persons with mental illness facing civil commitment. These procedural safeguards include the right to counsel, a hearing, and an appeal. Such rigorous procedural protections are justified by the fundamental invasion of liberty occasioned by long-term detention, the serious implications of erroneously finding a person dangerous, and the value of procedures in accurately determining complex facts that help predict future dangerous behavior.

The Criminal Law: Knowing or Willful Exposure to Infection

In 1997 public health authorities in Chautauqua County, New York, discovered that a man infected with HIV had sexual intercourse with between fifty and seventy-five women over a two-year period. Authorities further learned that he had infected thirteen women, and they, in turn, infected others.[27] Similar cases have been documented in Tennessee,[28] Missouri,[29] Pennsylvania,[30] and other states.[31] Countless additional detected and undetected cases of knowing or willful exposure to HIV infection likely exist.[32] Research suggests that a substantial minority of persons infected with HIV engage in sex or needle sharing without disclosing the risk to their partners;[33] in many cases the individual does not use a condom or sterile drug-injection equipment.[34]

There is a powerful appeal in using the criminal law in response to willful or knowing exposure. The public views individuals who engage in this behavior as morally blameworthy[35] and supports criminal sanctions for aberrant and irresponsible conduct.[36] The criminal law deters risk behavior and sets a clear standard for behaviors that society will not tolerate. According to the presidential commission on the HIV epidemic, criminal liability is "consistent with society's obligation to prevent harm to others and the criminal law's concern with punishing those whose behavior results in harmful acts."[37]

The attraction of the criminal law as a public health measure is also based on its clarity, objectivity, and safeguards.[38] Whereas civil confinement (e.g., isolation or quarantine) often uses broad standards such as "dangerousness," the criminal law must specify the behavior that is prohibited. If its language is vague, a criminal statute fails to forewarn and is for that reason unconstitutional.[39] Whereas civil confinement authorizes detention based on predictions of the future, the criminal law focuses on behavior that has already occurred. Whereas "dangerousness" need only be proved by clear and convincing evidence, each element of a crime must be proved beyond a reasonable doubt. And whereas the period of civil confinement is indefinite, the period of criminal confinement is usually finite and proportionate to the gravity of the offense.

Despite its social and political appeal, the use of the criminal law against persons living with HIV/AIDS is highly complex, raising fundamental issues of fairness and effectiveness as a public health measure. This discussion first examines criminal law theory. Next it surveys the two main approaches: (1) traditional crimes of violence and (2) public health offenses (particularly HIV-specific offenses).[40] Finally, it evaluates the criminal law as a tool of public health.

Criminal Law Theory

The legal definition of a crime is an act performed in violation of duties that an individual owes to the community.[41] It includes both harmful conduct (*actus reus*) and a culpable state of mind (*mens rea*). This discussion covers criminal offenses involving the transmission of HIV infection; the underlying assumption is that persons living with HIV/AIDS owe a public duty to avoid transmission of the infection. These offenses, however, are far more complex and varied than they first appear because they incorporate a wide variety of behaviors and culpable states of mind.

Individuals living with HIV/AIDS have been prosecuted for acts that range from the trivial to the highly dangerous and from the common to the rare.[42] At one end of the spectrum are acts that are common and not usually dangerous, such as donating blood. However, if the blood donor is infected with HIV, the act carries risk, though the probability of the risk is quite low because the blood supply is screened for HIV. Persons living with HIV/AIDS are also prosecuted for assaults such as biting, spitting, and splattering of blood. Although these acts can be harmful in themselves, they often do not pose significant risks of transmission of infection. Finally, some acts are generally benign but become harmful if persons with an infectious disease engage in those acts. For example, having unprotected sex and sharing drug-injection equipment become potentially harmful acts if one person has the HIV infection.

Harmful acts in and of themselves do not constitute an offense. The individual also must have a culpable state of mind. States of mind in the criminal law are highly complex, but, generally speaking, persons may act purposefully, knowingly, or recklessly.[43] Persons act *purposefully* when they intend to cause a harmful result—they desire the consequences of their act. A person who actually seeks to transmit an infection acts purposefully.

Persons act *knowingly* when they are aware that their conduct will cause harm. For example, a person who tests positive for HIV and understands the modes of transmission acts with knowledge. Persons can also act with constructive knowledge when they reasonably *should* know that their behavior poses an unreasonable risk. For example, a person who has had a long-term relationship with an infected person and has symptoms may be assumed to know his sero-logic status even though he has never been tested. Persons who act with knowl-edge, or constructive knowledge, are deemed blameworthy because they un-derstand the consequences of their harmful behavior.

Persons act *recklessly* when they consciously disregard a substantial and un-justifiable risk. Individuals who blatantly disregard risks to others deviate from the standard of conduct to which reasonable, law-abiding persons placed in similar situations would adhere. For example, a person living with HIV/AIDS who has unprotected sex with numerous partners and fails to disclose the risk grossly deviates from acceptable conduct and may be thought of as criminally reckless.

In summary, persons living with HIV/AIDS are subject to prosecution for a wide range of behaviors and states of mind. Behaviors range from blood do-nations and simple batteries (e.g., spitting or biting) to sexual intercourse and sharing drug-injection equipment. It is obvious that each of these behaviors carries very different probabilities of transmission. Individuals may also en-gage in these behaviors with varying states of mind (i.e., purposeful, knowing, or reckless), each with its own degree of culpability.

To understand the complexity of the criminal law, consider a hypothetical situation involving persons living with HIV/AIDS who engage in the same be-havior (i.e., sexual intercourse) but with different states of mind: one woman is a prostitute who is paid for sex, another is a victim in a physically abusive re-lationship, and a third seeks revenge. Now consider a hypothetical involving the same state of mind (i.e., intent to kill) but different behaviors: one man jabs his victim with a contaminated needle, one has sex with her, and a third spits in her face. Each of these cases poses different risks of harm and different de-grees of culpability. Ideally, the criminal law would be able to identify the truly harmful and blameworthy cases, but, as we will see, this is a difficult distinction.

Traditional Crimes of Violence

The traditional crimes of violence that can be read to apply to the transmission of HIV are homicide (actual and attempted) and assault.[44]

Homicide

Murder prosecutions resulting from transmission of HIV infection are rare be-cause they require the death of the victim. HIV does not always result in death, and, if it does, the length of time from infection to death usually precludes prosecution; either the defendant has already died from the infection or there is a statutory requirement that death must occur within one year of the act. Additionally, homicide requires proof of causation, and it may be difficult to demonstrate that the decedent contracted the infection from the defendant.

Attempted Homicide

Prosecutions for attempted murder are also rare and difficult to prove. As Kathleen Sullivan and Martha Field observe, "Having sex or sharing needles is a highly indirect modus operandi for the person whose purpose is to kill."[45] Nevertheless, attempted homicide charges have been brought for a broad range of conduct, but with mixed results. The Maryland Supreme Court held that, even in the context of a rape by a person with HIV infection, intent to kill could not be inferred.[46] But an Oregon court convicted a man of ten counts of attempted murder for having consensual unprotected sex with multiple women after he had been counseled to refrain from sex or, minimally, to use a condom.[47] An Ohio court also upheld an attempted aggravated murder conviction of a man who was aware that he had AIDS and intended to kill his eight-year-old rape victim.[48]

The criminal law uses a subjective standard for criminal attempts: if the facts are as the person believes them to be, it is an offense.[49] This is important in the field of AIDS because a person could be convicted of attempted murder if his intent was to kill, regardless of whether the method used posed a significant risk of transmission. Indeed, courts have determined that if the defendant believed his actions could transmit a lethal infection, it was irrelevant if the actual risk was negligible. Under this theory, persons with HIV infection have been convicted of attempted murder for conduct that has exceedingly low risks: biting,[50] spitting,[51] and splattering of blood.[52]

If a person living with HIV/AIDS plans to kill for revenge or greed and uses a primary mode of transmission, that person should bear full criminal responsibility. Consider the case of a father who injected his child with an HIV-contaminated needle hoping to avoid making child support payments,[53] or a physician who exacted revenge on his ex-lover by injecting her with HIV and hepatitis C.[54] But would it be contrary to public policy to punish nondangerous behavior? Think about an inmate who spit at a prison guard hoping to harm him. Should he be subject to prosecution for attempted murder because of his mistaken belief that his saliva could kill? Finally, what is the preferred public policy if a person acts in ways that appear to be more of a cry for help than a malicious attempt to kill? In *State v. Haines*, an HIV-infected defendant attempted suicide by slashing his wrists. When police and emergency workers came, he pleaded with them, "Let me die I have AIDS." When they continued to intervene, he splattered his blood on the officers. Mr. Haines was convicted of attempted murder.[55]

Assault and Aggravated Assault

A simple assault is a purposeful, knowing, or reckless causing of bodily injury.[56] Defendants with HIV infection who engage in harmful behavior, such as biting,[57] spiting,[58] or throwing "body waste,"[59] have been convicted of assault instead of attempted murder. The crime becomes aggravated assault if the person causes a "serious" bodily injury or uses a "deadly weapon."[60] Two federal courts of appeal have convicted inmates of aggravated assault, holding that teeth, under certain circumstances, can constitute a deadly weapon.[61] In Virginia, a man was charged with "infected sexual battery" for infecting his wife via sexual contact.[62] Certainly, persons who engage in assaultive behavior deserve criminal punishment. However, should individuals be convicted of more serious offenses (e.g., assault with a deadly weapon) *because* of their infectious state? From a public health perspective, the answer would be no because criminal punishment leads to prevention of only negligible risks of disease transmission.

Despite the prosecutions for traditional crimes of violence, the mental elements of "purpose" or "knowledge" can be difficult to prove. A person acts with purpose only if she actually desires to transmit the infection. A person acts knowingly only if she is "practically certain" that her conduct will cause harm.[63] Since risks of disease transmission are highly variable, and frequently low, a person cannot realistically know that any single act will transmit the infection. Consider the most common behavior that is subject to prosecution—sexual intercourse. Sexuality is a highly complex behavior involving many different passions, desires, and fears. Usually, neither partner wants to harm the other but is willing to take risks. To establish beyond a reasonable doubt what the person knew or whether he acted with intent, it may be necessary to discover what went on and what was said in the privacy of a sexual encounter. Did the person know he was infected? Did he inform his sex partner? Did he use a condom? Did the partner assume the risk? The answers to these questions are difficult to ascertain, and, even if they could be known, police surveillance of intimate behaviors may be so intrusive that it would not be worth the cost.

Partly in frustration with proving intentionality or knowledge, and partly in response to political pressure, legislatures have sought other avenues to criminalize the risk of transmission. Infectious disease statutes create public health offenses that vary from state to state. A few states have broad provisions that punish behavior that risks transmission of *any* contagious disease.[64] Most statutes, however, create "disease-specific" offenses that were often enacted in waves in response to public misapprehensions about epidemics of the day. In the early twentieth century states enacted statutes directed at TB,[65] followed by STDs,[66] and, in the latter part of the century, HIV/AIDS. In each case, politicians vilified persons who had the disease, both blaming them for their own affliction and holding them morally accountable for placing the public at risk.

Most public health statutes do not define HIV/AIDS as a sexually transmitted or venereal disease so that the statutory offense of transmitting an STD does not apply.[67] The highest court in New York, for example, upheld the commissioner's determination not to add HIV to the list of STDs.[68] Although a few states have explicitly defined "venereal disease" to include HIV,[69] most have enacted HIV-specific statutes modeled on older STD offenses.[70] The federal government has enacted an HIV-specific offense relating to blood and tissue donation[71] and conditioned receipt of AIDS-related funding based on state certification that the state's criminal laws are adequate to prosecute persons who risk transmission of HIV.[72]

At the beginning of 2002, twenty-eight states had at least one law criminalizing behavior that risks transmission of HIV infection. Fifteen of these states had more than one such law (see Map 10-1).

State HIV-specific criminal statutes vary widely. The most common form criminalizes an act where (1) the person knows he is HIV-infected (e.g., tests positive for HIV), (2) engages in specified risk behavior (not always limited to sexual behavior), and (3) fails to inform his partner of the risk (see Table 10-1).[73]

HIV-specific criminal statutes vary according to (1) the behavior needed to commit the offense, (2) the degree of intent needed, (3) the result of the behavior (exposure or actual transmission of HIV), (4) whether consent of the partner is a defense, and (5) the penalty for a violation of the law (see Table 10-2).

The Behavior Criminalized

Many states criminalize the behavior of exposing another person to HIV without specifying any particular act. These laws may be regarded as wide-ranging and possibly unconstitutionally vague, because the person is not apprised in

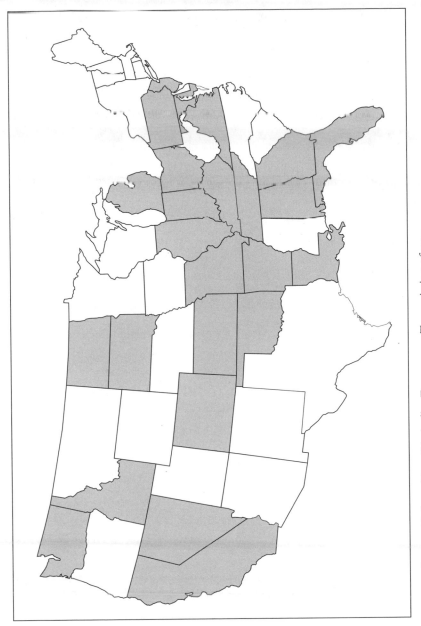

MAP 10-1. States with Laws That Criminalize Exposure or Transmission of HIV

TABLE 10-1. Standard Elements of HIV-Specific Offenses

1. Knowledge of serologic status

2. Behavior risking transmission—e.g., sex, needle sharing, blood donation

3. Failure to inform

advance which behaviors are criminal and which are not. Some states criminalize only "sexual contact," although this term may not be clearly defined. These statutes often do not distinguish between "safe" and "unsafe" sex, so a person would be equally culpable if he had sexual intercourse with, or without, a condom.[74] In addition to specifying sexual conduct, many states criminalize multiperson use of drug-injection equipment or donation of blood, semen, breast milk, or other tissue. Still other states specifically criminalize low-risk activities such as spiting, biting, or general "exposure to bodily fluids."

Degree of Intent Required

The majority of HIV-specific statutes lack a specific intent requirement. It is sufficient if a person has knowledge or constructive knowledge of his HIV infection and engages in the prohibited conduct. Thus, the person commits the offense if he knows (e.g., tested positive for HIV) or should know (e.g., his partner is dying of AIDS) he is infected, makes no disclosure, and engages in risk behavior. It does not matter that the person living with HIV/AIDS has no specific desire to harm his partner.

The Result of the Behavior

Almost all HIV-specific statutes make it a criminal offense to expose another person to HIV. It does not matter if the infection is actually transmitted. Only two states, Alabama and Indiana, require that the victim contract HIV infection for the purposes of prosecution.

Disclosure of HIV Infection (Consent as a Defense)

Since most statutes specify that a "failure to inform" is an element of the offense, informed consent is usually a defense. Indeed, several laws explicitly make consent of the partner an affirmative defense. As explained above, under a strict reading of the statutes, use of a condom would not excuse the failure to inform. HIV-specific offenses, therefore, undermine the "safer sex" ethic held by many in the gay community that people are not required to disclose their HIV status as long as they use a condom.[75] Those adhering to this ethic

TABLE 10-2. State HIV-Specific Criminal Statutes

	States That Make HIV Transmission a Criminal Offense
Behavior Criminalized	28
Without specifying prohibited behaviors	9
Risking transmission by needles, syringes, or injection equipment	10
Risking transmission by biting, spitting, or exposure to bodily fluids	7
Risking transmission by sexual contact	16
Laws that define prohibited sexual behaviors	11
Laws that distinguish between safe and unsafe sex	2
Degree of Intent Required	
States that require intent to infect as an element of the crime for people who engage in prohibited conduct:	
While engaging in sexual behavior	5
While engaging in drug use	4
Result of the Behavior	
States that require actual infection for prosecution	2
Disclosure (Consent as a Defense)	
States in which failure to inform partner of the risk is an element of the crime for people who engage in prohibited conduct:	
While engaging in sexual activity	10
While engaging in drug use	4
States that make consent of the other person an affirmative defense	11
Penalty	
States in which violations of the law are felonies	22
States in which violations of the law are misdemeanors	4

Source: Zita Lazzarini, Sarah Bray, and Scott Burris, "Evaluating the Impact of Criminal Laws on HIV Risk Behavior," Journal of Law, Medicine, and Ethics 30 (Summer 2002): 239–53.

would be liable to prosecution since many persons living with HIV/AIDS have sex without disclosing their serologic status.

The Penalty

HIV-specific statutes are often modeled after STD laws enacted in the mid-twentieth century in response to epidemics of syphilis, gonorrhea, and herpes. It is important to emphasize, however, that whereas STD statutes tend to impose mild "public health" sanctions (e.g., misdemeanors), HIV-specific statutes often pose harsher sentences (e.g., felonies). In one case, a court sentenced a person to between seven and fifteen years in prison for "transferring bodily fluids that may contain HIV."[76]

Prosecutions

Compared with prosecutions for other sexually related offenses such as rape or prostitution, HIV-specific criminal charges are rarely brought. Zita Lazzarini and colleagues identified 316 such prosecutions between 1986 and 2001: 67 percent for sexual exposure; 23.4 percent for biting, spitting, or scratching; 5.4 percent for selling blood, sharing needles, or threats involving a syringe; and 4.7 percent for an unknown, or no apparent, mode of transmission.[77]

One possible reason for the relatively small number of prosecutions is that police are unaware of a person's HIV status. The number of prosecutions would probably increase if public health departments shared HIV data with law enforcement. In 2003 South Dakota passed a law authorizing the Department of Health to release a person's medical information to law enforcement officials if the department suspects that the person has violated the state's law that criminalizes HIV-risk behavior.[78] This is a worrying precedent because it threatens the privacy rights of persons living with HIV/AIDS and will facilitate a punitive approach to the epidemic.

Constitutionality

Courts have upheld the constitutionality of HIV-specific statutes against challenges based on vagueness,[79] overbreadth,[80] and the absence of a mens rea or specific intent requirement.[81] In particular, courts have found that HIV statutes are not impermissibly vague as applied to persons who engage in unprotected sexual intercourse, especially after being counseled about safe sex.[82] It is certainly possible, however, that HIV statutes would be invalidated on grounds of vagueness if used to charge people with "exposure" for engaging in low-risk behavior. This kind of language appears highly ambiguous and does not forewarn individuals of the behaviors that are prohibited.

Evaluating HIV-Specific Offenses

HIV-specific offenses have advantages over traditional crimes of violence. If each of the elements is present, prosecutors need not prove specific intent or knowledge to harm. If narrowly written, they also can be more precise than the traditional criminal law: individuals are forewarned of the prohibited behaviors, and prosecutors are vested with less discretion. Finally, HIV-specific offenses declare a public interest in responsible behavior and encourage disclosure to persons at risk of infection.

Despite these benefits, HIV-specific offenses may not actually improve the public's health and, conversely, may be detrimental. First, because these statutes often apply to low-risk behavior, any deterrent value may be misplaced. Public health authorities must prioritize prevention activities; public resources devoted to conduct that poses little or no risk of transmission represents an opportunity cost. Second, to the extent that laws create incentives of any kind, they may create the *wrong* incentives. Persons at risk may be better off not knowing their serologic status because only those who are aware of their status can be prosecuted. Similarly, while HIV-specific offenses encourage people to disclose their status, the disclosure must take place prior to the first sexual encounter. If an infected person fails to disclose in the beginning, he will have no incentive to inform his partner thereafter. As a matter of public health, of course, late disclosure is preferable to no disclosure at all. Finally, by creating a specific offense legislatures implicitly invite the interest of police, prosecutors, and the apparatus of the criminal justice system. This, in turn, engenders concerns about intrusive surveillance, selective enforcement, and loss of privacy, undermining the public education approach to disease prevention.

It is important to recall that, even though relatively few cases are actually prosecuted, HIV-specific offenses criminalize a wide range of quite ordinary behavior. The fact that a substantial proportion of persons living with HIV/AIDS engage in behaviors that are criminally prohibited has profound implications. First, it places a large number of otherwise law-abiding citizens into the category of criminals. Second, persons living with HIV/AIDS may not be aware that behaviors they believe are relatively safe (e.g., sex with a condom) are criminally proscribed. Indeed, due to the variability of state laws, an identical act with the same partner could be unlawful in one state but lawful in another. Finally, some jurisdictions neither make informed consent an affirmative defense nor specify nondisclosure as an element of the offense. In these states, the law could be construed to criminalize all sex by persons living with HIV/AIDS. As Lazzarini and her colleagues have observed, "Such a lifetime ban on sexual activity is unreasonable and unnecessary given the possibility for responsible sexual activity by persons with HIV."[83]

Evaluating the Criminal Law as a Tool of Public Health

Incarceration does not prevent a person from spreading the virus, nor is it likely to rehabilitate complex human behavior around sexual activity and drug use; criminal sanctions for

HIV transmission cannot be justified on the basis of retribution, because this approach is not related to the primary objective of preventing new infections and it reinforces harmful social stigma; and laws criminalizing intentional transmission of HIV are likely to scare people away from testing, rather than deter them from high-risk behaviors.—Richard Elliott and Miriam Maluwa, UNAIDS (June 2002)

In thinking about the value of the criminal law in the context of the HIV epidemic, it is helpful to inquire whether prosecution would achieve any of its traditional goals: deterrence, retribution, incapacitation, and rehabilitation.[84] The answer is not simple; rather, it depends on the severity of the case. Most everyone would agree with prosecuting a person who truly intends to kill and who uses a means reasonably calculated to achieve that end (e.g., the father who injects his son with a contaminated needle to avoid paying child support). So, too, would most people agree with prosecuting a person who, knowing that he has a serious infection, exposes many people (e.g., the person in Chautauqua County who hid his HIV status from multiple sex partners). In these cases, society legitimately holds persons living with HIV/AIDS criminally accountable for the same reasons it would hold anyone accountable: the person has a culpable state of mind and poses a significant risk that is outside the socially acceptable range of conduct. In these cases, prosecution achieves several objectives of the criminal law—deterrence of high-risk behavior, punishment of morally blameworthy individuals, and incapacitation and rehabilitation of dangerous persons.

It is much more difficult to judge the utility of prosecutions in the majority of cases that involve minimal risks and behaviors that are common in society. After all, many prosecuted cases involve epidemiologically low risks such as biting, spiting, or donating blood; and defendants, in fact, rarely transmit infection. The criminal justice system does not achieve its goals if the behavior deterred involves negligible risk and the effect is to incapacitate and rehabilitate a minimally dangerous person.

A related problem is that many of the behaviors are common and resistant to change. Most adults engage in sexual behavior, and persons living with HIV/AIDS often have sex without disclosing the risk. The result is that persons who engage in socially common behaviors are subject to serious criminal sanctions. Arguably, it is not in society's interest to seek retribution against persons who behave like many other people and who, in any event, are suffering from a serious, sometimes life-threatening, disease.

Suppose that policymakers want to use the criminal law as a tool of prevention rather than retribution. They might reason that criminal sanctions will promote the public's health by deterring individuals from risk behavior. Although there is little empirical evidence to draw on, it is conceivable that criminal law is actually antithetical to public health.

For an array of psychological and practical reasons, the criminal law may not deter HIV risk behavior. Few persons living with HIV/AIDS are aware of criminal law's prohibitions, so the law is unlikely to affect their behavior. Moreover, sexuality, needle sharing, and other risk behaviors are not rationally motivated, but rather are highly complex behaviors. It is unclear whether persons would alter their behavior even if they were aware of the criminal sanctions against it.[85]

The criminal law may actually discourage individuals from being tested, providing accurate information to health professionals, and participating in clinical and public health programs. As explained earlier, criminal sanctions provide an incentive not to be tested because, legally, it is better not to discover one's serologic status. If individuals are not tested, they may be more likely to engage in risk behavior. Similarly, if having sex while infected is a crime, individuals may be less likely to reliably disclose their symptoms and behavior or to seek access to services. Failure to disclose impedes counseling and education. Moreover, if fewer people receive clinical treatment, the risk to the public increases. Highly active therapy for persons living with HIV/AIDS significantly reduces their infectiousness. Finally, if persons believe that discussions with public health authorities place themselves and/or their partners at risk of criminal prosecution, they may not cooperate. For example, persons may not participate freely in partner notification services for fear that their partners will be implicated in a crime. The criminal law, therefore, breaks down the trust that is vital to the success of clinical and public health programs.

Even if the criminal law could effectively deter risk behavior, it may be overly intrusive and unfair. Once statutes make intimate behavior unlawful, they legitimize police surveillance of deeply private activities. Further, law enforcers and prosecutors may selectively enforce the law by targeting vulnerable, and visible, populations such as prostitutes, homosexuals, the poor, and minorities. Indeed, since the targeted behavior is so common, it opens the door to discrimination in enforcement—for example, white, middle-class individuals who have sex without disclosing the risk are seldom prosecuted, whereas those from lower socioeconomic classes and racial or sexual minorities are prosecuted for the same behavior.[86]

The criminal law allows society to place a boundary around behavior that it will and will not tolerate, and to express its moral outrage at egregious conduct. The criminal law is justifiably applied to cases involving truly dangerous behavior and culpable states of mind. Yet the generalized use of the criminal law is unlikely to become an effective tool for public health. It discourages exactly those behaviors necessary for the collective good—testing, disclosure, and participation in clinical and public health programs. The criminal law also invites intrusive surveillance, selective enforcement, and discrimination.

Conclusion

This chapter has demonstrated that compulsory state powers are seldom justified as a response to HIV/AIDS. Even if coercion was appropriate in past epidemics (and it is far from clear that it was), there are persuasive reasons why HIV/AIDS is different. HIV cannot be transmitted casually, treatment is long-term, there is no currently known cure, and the social and political environment in America has shifted toward a renewed respect for civil liberties. It is true that personal entitlements should not necessarily trump public health. But it is equally true, and AIDS advocates have made this point powerfully, that coercion often undermines public health goals, driving the epidemic underground. Consequently, there are good reasons, based on civil liberties and public health, to reject the use of compulsion in the HIV/AIDS epidemic.

Part III of this book has assessed some of the most socially and politically charged issues in the HIV/AIDS epidemic: screening, reporting, partner notification, and personal control measures. The next part explores four special populations that have been much discussed by government and in the media: survivors of sexual assaults, health care workers, pregnant women, and injection drug users.

Part 4 Special Populations

We are not adequately giving information to victims about testing and about exposure. Only about 16% of victims actually report that they have been assaulted. Some sexual assaults happen in marriage and those people are chronic sexual assault victims. How do we deal with that?—**Susan L. Higgenbotham,** executive director of the South Carolina Coalition against Domestic Violence (1997)

Chapter 11

Testing, Counseling, and Treatment after Sexual Assault

Little attention has been devoted to the risk of HIV infection for survivors of sexual assault. This may be due in part to society's conflicting attitudes and beliefs concerning sexually transmitted diseases (STDs) in general and AIDS and rape in particular. Historically, powerful cultural and social constructs have shaped the meaning of STDs. Society often views these diseases as the result of socially unacceptable sexuality, as a morally based failure of impulse control by individuals, and as fair punishment for the transgression of social norms.[1] Similar moralistic reasoning often underlies the conventional wisdom concerning rape and AIDS. Rape, a violent crime where sex is used to intimidate and harm, is often seen as the result of inappropriate seductive behavior or a sudden change of heart on the part of the victim who initially had consented to a sexual encounter.[2] Similarly, some view AIDS as a just consequence for the "sins" of homosexuality, promiscuity, and substance abuse.[3]

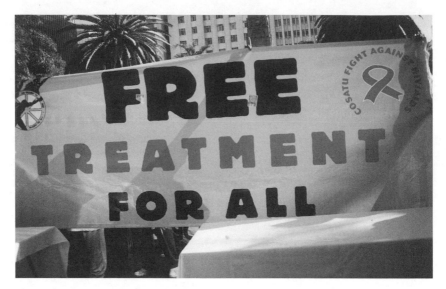

The Treatment Action Campaign, based in South Africa, is among the organizations fighting to ensure access to quality treatment for all. Many survivors of sexual assault do not access counseling and health care.

Those who hold less judgmental and culturally determined views concerning STDs, AIDS, and rape may argue that the potential for HIV infection in sexual assault has garnered less attention because of the relatively low risk of transmission during any individual encounter.[4] But this argument fails to consider other low-risk situations that nevertheless have received substantial attention during the AIDS epidemic—most notably, HIV transmission between health care workers (HCWs) and patients in the course of invasive procedures (see Chapter 12). Health authorities have instituted detailed policies and procedures to further reduce these minimal risks.[5] In contrast, few policies and protocols exist to minimize the risk of HIV infection for survivors of sexual assault and the concomitant psychological burdens imposed on them.

This chapter considers proposals from the Working Group on HIV Testing, Counseling, and Prophylaxis after Sexual Assault for the development of policies and principles of clinical intervention in the postassault care of survivors. The recommendations are intended to guide health care providers, sexual assault counselors, and allied service professionals in providing compassionate and effective counseling, testing, and treatment to survivors of sexual assault. The chapter also examines the ethical, public health, and legal justifications for a policy of limited compulsory testing of persons accused of sexual assault.

Assessment of Risk

Rape is a crime that is often hidden, underrecognized, underreported, and underdocumented.[6] The U.S. Department of Justice reported that there were 225,320 forcible rapes of adult women in 2001; 30 percent of rapes were by strangers, and 39 percent were reported to the police.[7] Significant numbers of adolescents and children are the victims of sexual assault, often involving multiple encounters.[8] The Department of Justice estimated that there were 22,930 sexual assaults of males ages twelve and over in 2001.[9]

The level of risk of contracting HIV infection for a survivor depends on the serologic and clinical status of the assailant, the type of sexual assault, and the frequency of assaults. Although persons with HIV infection who have committed sexual assaults have been documented in medical literature,[10] the seroprevalence in relevant populations is difficult to assess. High variability in infection rates of the same risk groups at different geographic sites has been reported.[11] In 2000 the overall rate of AIDS was approximately four times higher in state and federal correctional systems (0.52 percent) than in the U.S. population (0.13 percent).[12] However, there are insufficient data to determine whether sex offenders have different rates of HIV than other offenders.

The type of sexual exposure (genital, anal, or oral), the associated physical trauma, the presence of other STDs, and the exposure to sexual secretions and/or blood are relevant in assessing the risk of HIV transmission.[13] HIV is transmitted less often through sexual intercourse than other STDs such as gonorrhea,[14] syphilis,[15] or hepatitis B,[16] which may have per-contact infectivity rates as high as 25 percent. The per-contact HIV infectivity rate from consensual male-to-female penile-vaginal intercourse is estimated at less than two per thousand.[17] The per-contact infectivity rate for consensual receptive anal intercourse between homosexual partners is estimated at between one and thirty per thousand.[18] Receptive oral exposure to ejaculate has also been associated with HIV seroconversion in rare cases.[19] The presence of lesions or blood from violent assaults may significantly increase the probability of transmission.[20] The estimates of per-contact risk for transmission of HIV and other STDs are confounded by the retrospective and aggregate nature of the data collected in most studies.

The risk of HIV transmission is highly variable, with some individuals infected after the first encounter; others remain uninfected after hundreds of unprotected sexual contacts.[21] In some cases, high efficiency HIV transmitters have been identified.[22] The infectiousness of an assailant is affected by the clinical stage of HIV infection, with recently infected individuals and those at late stages being the most infectious to their partners.[23] Persons with untreated HIV disease are likely to have higher viral loads than those in treatment, thereby increasing their contagiousness.[24] Moreover, it may reasonably be hypothesized that persons who engage in violent criminal behavior are less likely to be in treatment. Genital ulcerative STDs have also been associated with increased infectiousness, as well as susceptibility to HIV.[25] Another salient variable is the virulence of the viral strain,[26] but the ability to measure this parameter and correlate it with infectiousness is still rudimentary.

Given the multiplicity of factors, the risk of HIV transmission from a sexual assault involving anal or vaginal penetration and exposure to ejaculate from an HIV-infected assailant is conservatively estimated to be in the same range as that for receptive anal and penile-vaginal intercourse—greater than two per thousand assaults. The actual per-contact risk will be higher with the existence of other factors such as violence producing trauma and blood exposure or the presence of inflammatory or ulcerative STDs.

Psychological Burdens of Sexual Assault

Extensive clinical observation and research show that sexual assault causes grave consequences for its survivors. Among them are persistent fear, loss of self-esteem, sexual dysfunction, and problems with social adjustment and relationships. Psychiatric symptoms can include depression, social phobia, obsessive-compulsive behavior, and anxiety.[27] The chronic psychological effects of sexual assault were initially described as the Rape Trauma Syndrome[28] and are now accepted as a special example of post-traumatic stress disorder (PTSD).[29]

Survivors frequently worry about contracting an STD from their assailants.[30] The fear of contracting an STD, particularly HIV infection, following rape appears to be an additional and significant stressor adding to the incidence, prevalence, and severity of psychiatric morbidity in rape survivors. The emotional trauma of sexual assault, including the fear of STDs, is often also experienced by persons closest to the survivor, particularly sex partners.[31]

Counseling, Testing, and Prophylaxis for Survivors

There are approximately 10,000 victim service programs in the United States based in police departments, prosecutors' offices, correctional settings, schools, community-based organizations, hospitals, domestic violence shelters, and rape crisis centers.[32] In practice, however, not all survivors of sexual assault receive information regarding HIV from a victim service program. The National Women's Study in 1992 found that fewer than 20 percent of survivors had a medical exam following their assault and, of those who were examined, 73 percent did not receive information about HIV infection in conjunction with the exam.[33] More recent data on postassault medical examination and HIV counseling were not available as of this writing.

In most programs, victim service professionals should give survivors information concerning HIV infection as soon as possible so that they can make the best use of the information.[34] One hospital rape crisis intervention program reported that about two-thirds of patients never returned for follow-up, thus losing important opportunities to receive information and counseling about HIV infection.[35]

Information and counseling should be provided in a nondirective manner, offering the survivor the opportunity for an open-ended discussion of his or her questions in a nonjudgmental manner. The information and counseling given should cover the risks of HIV infection, the meaning of HIV antibody tests as well as their advantages and disadvantages, and the limited data on the efficacy of chemoprophylaxis for HIV infection.

Different ethnic and cultural groups view rape and AIDS in ways that are not necessarily represented in the dominant culture. For example, conceptions of sexual behavior as being intensely private in some communities can pose challenges to open and constructive counseling.

Some service situations may not present an appropriate environment in which to raise the possibility of HIV infection. Rape crisis hotlines or other settings without face-to-face contact may not allow the service provider to adequately evaluate the physical and psychological needs of the survivor or to offer immediate follow-up. Sexual assault service providers must work to initiate discussions regarding the risk of HIV infection whenever possible. Survivors should be offered referrals to agencies that provide information and counseling about HIV/AIDS. In settings where provider and survivor are face-to-face, HIV-related issues should be addressed as soon as clinically appropriate. This may be delayed, for instance, when the provider must give priority to the acute physical and psychological needs of the survivor who is gravely injured, unconscious, or so psychologically traumatized that he or she cannot assimilate the information.

A study of a British Columbia emergency room program that offered HIV prophylaxis to victims of sexual assault revealed the limitations of treatment directed to all sexual assault victims regardless of their risk of HIV infection.[36]

The study found that few sexual assault victims completed and complied with the prescribed treatment: 71 out of 258 clients accepted the offer of HIV post-exposure prophylaxis; only 29 continued the treatment after five days; and only 8 completed the full four-week regimen and returned for their final follow-up visit. However, many of the victims who did not complete the treatment were at low risk of contracting HIV either because of the type of assault or because the assailant was not known to have HIV. Further, health care providers had difficulty explaining the treatment because the victims were generally too traumatized to understand the complex regimen. After the study, the hospital modified its program to offer prophylaxis only to victims at high risk of contracting HIV.

It may be argued that discussion of HIV infection following sexual assaults could introduce ideas and anxieties where none existed or exacerbate existing fears. Moreover, feelings of shame or a reluctance to talk about sexuality may keep survivors from asking questions they have about HIV. After careful consideration of all of these factors, respectful and nonthreatening inquiry may assist survivors in discussing their concerns.

Testing of Survivors

Survivors of sexual assaults need careful diagnosis and follow-up for a multiplicity of clinical conditions, including screening for STDs.[37] Voluntary HIV testing, with confidentiality protections, should be provided only after obtaining individual informed consent. Professional counseling, education, and avoidance of high-risk behaviors are essential.

It usually takes at least two weeks after exposure to HIV before standard tests reveal antibodies.[38] The vast majority of individuals infected with HIV have detectable antibodies within three to six months,[39] though in rare cases it may be longer.[40] Advanced diagnostic technologies, such as the polymerase chain reaction technique, narrow "the window period" in which persons may be newly HIV-infected, but antibody negative.[41] These tests are expensive and therefore not routinely available in many settings. Periodic testing for HIV infection beginning within six weeks after the sexual assault can provide a number of potential benefits to the survivor. It can ease the psychological burden of wondering whether he or she has contracted HIV. Knowledge of test results can also enable survivors to make educated decisions regarding their health, sexual or needle-sharing behavior, reproduction, breast-feeding, and parenting.

Immediate postassault testing is of limited import for medical or psychological purposes primarily because it will not indicate whether survivors have been exposed during the assault or whether they are likely to become infected. If survivors wish to demonstrate in subsequent criminal or civil proceedings that they contracted HIV infection from the assailant, they should be offered initial (baseline) testing soon after the assault. A successful prosecution or civil suit would need to show that the survivor's seroconversion was due to the assault, not other risk behaviors. In attempting to prove that seroconversion was due to the assault, a survivor might find that his or her sexual history was not protected by rape shield laws and thus might have to testify regarding past and present sexual activity.

A significant problem that arises from HIV counseling and testing in some states is that the alleged assailant may have a right to the survivor's medical and psychological service records. The Supreme Court has held that, although a defendant does not have free access to a victim's records, due process requires that a trial judge review the information and determine whether to authorize its release.[42] Accordingly, some states allow a breach of the therapist-client confidentiality in various situations.[43] In Massachusetts, the victim's medical and psychological records may be released if the defense meets certain requirements. Specifically, the judge will undertake an in-camera review of the victim's otherwise privileged rape counseling records if the defendant has demonstrated a "good faith, specific, and reasonable basis" to believe the records contain evidence that is relevant and material to the issue of guilt.[44] If, after review, the judge believes the records do contain relevant information, both the defense and the prosecutor may have access to the records.[45] Victim records may include information from psychiatrists, psychologists, and other health care and victim service professionals.[46] To avoid documentation of the test results in the medical record, some survivors may prefer anonymous testing at an alternative test site.

Postexposure Prophylaxis for HIV Infection

Survivors, advocates, and victim service professionals debate whether survivors of sexual assault should receive counseling and be offered antiviral treatment as a prophylaxis for HIV infection. The effectiveness of antiretroviral therapy in inhibiting HIV replication led to clinical interest in whether drugs like zidovudine (AZT) could prevent HIV transmission after exposure.[47] Studies have shown that use of antiretroviral agents by health care workers after occupational exposure to HIV reduces their infection rate by 80 percent.[48] Other studies provide evidence that treatment of a mother and her newborn helps prevent perinatal transmission of HIV.[49] Together these studies indicate that postexposure prophylaxis of sexual assault victims might significantly reduce the risk of HIV infection[50] at a reasonable cost.[51]

The decision to take antiretroviral agents following a sexual assault should be based on a risk assessment of the exposure. The risk assessment must consider the serologic status of the assailant, the type of exposure (anal, vaginal, or oral penetration and ejaculation), the nature of the physical injuries, and the number of assaults. Individual assessment of the exposed individual must also be considered, including his or her reproductive health status and ability to tolerate potential side effects. The initiation of high-dose chemoprophylaxis may have many uncomfortable associated side effects (e.g., anemia, sleep disturbances, gastrointestinal complaints, myalgia, and headache) and occasionally more serious adverse effects (e.g., diabetes mellitus, pancreatitis, and severe drug interactions). For example, data indicate that nearly 50 percent of health care workers report adverse events while taking antiretroviral drugs prophylactically.[52] Further, as indicated above, a substantial number of sexual assault survivors who begin prophylaxis do not complete the full course of medication.

An equally significant obstacle to the potentially effective use of chemoprophylaxis is the short window of time for initiation of effective therapy. Even a potentially efficacious intervention may not work after the virus is well integrated into deeper tissue cells. The CDC recommends that therapy begin within hours of occupational exposure and continue for four weeks.[53] Initiation of treatment is still recommended thirty-six hours after exposure because the window of efficacy in humans is undetermined. When the risk of transmission is high, treatment is recommended even if initiation begins one to two weeks later, because early treatment of HIV infection has been shown to be beneficial. It is unknown whether there might be differences for infections that are transmitted sexually rather than by parenteral inoculation.

Victim service professionals face significant dilemmas when addressing prophylaxis. Information about an unsubstantiated prevention, in an already low-risk situation, may simply exacerbate anxiety and create false hope. However, the survivor has the right to evaluate the information and make a decision. In fact, U.S. foreign policy favors postexposure prophylaxis. In the Global AIDS and Tuberculosis Relief Act of 2000, Congress specifically supported measures for providing postexposure prophylaxis to victims of rape and sexual assault in other countries.[54]

Testing the Accused for HIV Infection

Some survivors claim the right to know their assailant's HIV status and may want to pursue having him tested. Testing the accused for HIV infection is feasible only where the assailant has been identified and apprehended. Statistics indicate that only a small proportion of survivors have this option. In 2000 only 30 percent of the rapes reported to the police resulted in an arrest of at least one suspect.[55] The average time between arrest and conviction was 289 days.[56] Informing the survivor about the small proportion of assailants who are arrested and convicted, and the extended time between assault, arrest, and conviction, could affect the survivor's expectations for testing the assailant and his or her own decisions regarding testing and prophylaxis.

Current Status of the Law

The Ryan White CARE Act requires states to authorize or mandate HIV testing of the assailant at the request of the survivor.[57] The person tested must be either charged or convicted of a sexual offense. As of 2001, all states except Alabama, Massachusetts, Nebraska, Vermont, Washington, and West Virginia had complied.[58] Additionally, the 1990 Martin Amendment to the Comprehensive Crime Control Act directed states to test convicted sex offenders for HIV and made funding from the Bureau of Justice conditional on state compliance. Under the Martin Amendment, the state must pay for one test for the survivor and reveal the results to victims and defendants.[59]

As of 2001, forty-five states authorized compulsory HIV testing of sex offenders.[60] The terms of the state laws vary significantly, particularly as to whether they apply to persons who are simply accused or those who are actually convicted of an offense. Two states (Tennessee and Nevada) allow HIV testing of a suspect merely upon arrest. Thirty-one states allow testing of a defendant after being charged but before being convicted of a crime. Thirteen states allow testing only after conviction.

State laws addressing compulsory HIV testing of sex offenders either permit or mandate testing. Of the thirty-one states that allow testing prior to conviction, eight states mandate testing. In Tennessee and Nevada, testing is mandatory upon arrest. The other twenty-three states that allow testing prior to conviction do not mandate it. Eight states allow the court to order HIV testing of the accused without the victim's request but require that the court make a finding based on the facts of the case that transmission could have occurred.

Nine states require both the victim's request and a court finding that transmission could have occurred before a court is permitted to order HIV testing of a defendant.

State HIV testing statutes also outline who is required to pay for the tests. Most states require either the defendant (if convicted) or the health department to pay for them. A smaller number of states place the burden of payment on the survivor or the county where the defendant is being held. States have identified different exceptions to the rule of confidentiality. In all states, both the defendant and survivor have access to the test results. Some states allow further disclosure to the judge, attorneys, or the survivor's family or sex partners. Most states also allow disclosure of the test results to the state or county health department.

Finally, thirty-one jurisdictions provide counseling for the survivor regardless of the defendant's HIV status. Eight states offer counseling only if the defendant is HIV positive. One state (Louisiana) provides counseling for the survivor only when the survivor is found to be HIV positive. Thirteen states and Washington, D.C., give counseling to the defendant as well.

The spectrum of state laws pertaining to the confidentiality, counseling, and funding for HIV tests demonstrates the different approaches to balancing the survivor's rights against those of the defendant.

The Case for Limited Compulsory HIV Testing

Testing the accused will not benefit most survivors because of the small percentage of assailants who are arrested and convicted in a timely manner. Meeting the needs of survivors therefore requires that states first establish comprehensive systems of counseling, treatment, and anonymous or confidential testing of the survivor. These programs should allow the survivor to come to terms with the assault and take measures to protect his or her health, as well as the health of family and loved ones.

States that wish to go further and permit survivors to learn the HIV status of their assailants have at least four alternatives, all of which are imperfect: (1) relying on counseling and testing of the survivor alone, (2) seeking the consent of the accused to testing, (3) testing the accused without consent (compulsory testing) but only after conviction, and (4) compulsory testing, before conviction, with procedural safeguards.

For the reasons given below, the policy alternative that may produce the greatest benefit for the largest number of survivors may be to allow preconviction testing of the accused at the request of the survivor. Adequate procedural safeguards would need to be in place to reduce the likelihood of testing persons wrongly accused, to limit disclosure of the results, and to prevent punitive use of the information.

A policy designed for this purpose would (1) authorize preconviction testing, initiated at the survivor's request; (2) require the prosecution to demonstrate probable cause to believe that an assault was committed, that the accused committed the assault, and that the assault was of a type that could transmit HIV infection; (3) authorize retesting of the accused six months after the assault, if the initial test was negative, unless the accused had already been acquitted, (4) disclose the test results only to the survivor and the accused, but allow the accused to exercise a prerogative not to be informed of his serostatus; (5) protect the confidentiality of the test results, except as required to inform the survivor, with civil penalties for unauthorized disclosure to other parties; and (6) limit the use of information obtained by compelled testing by making test results generally inadmissible as evidence in the criminal or subsequent civil proceedings.

The particular characteristics of sexual assault distinguish it from other situations involving potential exposure to HIV infection. A proposal for compulsory testing, therefore, must be analyzed under fundamentally different standards. Survivors of sexual assault did not consent to the behavior that caused the potential exposure. Assault, by definition, is coerced; it is both a violation of dignity and a harm to the survivor. Its nonconsensual nature sharply differentiates sexual assault from many other potential exposures to HIV, including consensual sexual intercourse or needle sharing and voluntary employment in a setting where occupational exposure may occur. Because the survivor's exposure starts with a wrong, the assailant owes the survivor a duty to limit the harm caused by the assault. The duty the assailant owes the survivor neither ends nor is expunged after the completion of the assault. Sexual assault causes ongoing harms, including a continued fear of HIV infection that can postpone or limit recovery. The dynamic and ongoing nature of the harm suggests that public policy must do everything possible to limit future harm and preserve the health of survivors and their partners and children.

Even if policymakers conclude that the survivor has a legitimate claim for compelled testing, they face a dilemma when choosing the point in time to impose the test. The dilemma arises from the changing relationship over time between the usefulness of the information to the survivor and the strength of the privacy interests of the accused. In most cases the survivor's strongest claim to a benefit from testing the accused comes from knowing the results of the test as early as possible. Testing the accused late in the criminal process fails to assist survivors because they have already borne the burden of worrying about contracting HIV infection. At the same time, the accused has the strongest claim to protection early in the criminal process. The problem with testing the accused before conviction is that the accused sustains a significant invasion of his autonomy and privacy before a trial has established his guilt or innocence. Therefore, any solution results in either a diminution of the usefulness of the information to the survivor or an infringement on the legitimate interests of the accused.

Due to the serious nature of the invasions of the accused's interests caused by compulsory preconviction testing (autonomy, privacy, and procedural fairness), it is justified only where there are compelling reasons. There are four possible justifications for testing the accused, each of which, if achieved, could reduce some facets of the harm of sexual assault: (1) the clinical benefit of the survivor, (2) a public health benefit, (3) the psychological benefit of the survivor, and (4) use of the results as evidence in legal proceedings.

Clinical Benefit of the Survivor

Early knowledge of HIV infection that allows the survivor to receive beneficial treatment provides a powerful justification for preconviction testing. The efficacy of prophylaxis against HIV is proven, and early initiation is recommended. Even in the rare event that the assailant is apprehended immediately, rapid testing would require elimination of all but the most cursory procedural protections for the accused, as well as reliance on the most rapid test procedures and no confirmation of positive test results. Despite these significant limitations, preconviction testing can permit the survivor to begin antiviral therapy. If the survivor learns that the accused has tested negative, he or she can discontinue the prophylaxis and avoid the potential side effects of continued treatment with antiviral drugs. Of course, the survivor cannot rely on a single negative test to completely eliminate the risk of a false negative result.

The clinical benefits from timely treatment with antiretrovirals[61] and prophylaxis for opportunistic infections[62] are generally accepted by medical practitioners. In addition, because early initiation of therapy has been shown to be more effective in preventing HIV infection, testing the accused soon after the assault can assist the survivor in determining whether or not to begin treatment.

Public Health Benefit

A better case for imposed testing rests on the public health benefits it may offer. Survivors of sexual assault do not exist in a vacuum. They may be involved in sexual relationships, and they often return to those relationships soon after the assault. One study found that 37 percent of survivors had voluntary sexual intercourse one day to five months after the assault.[63] Survivors may be pregnant or contemplating starting a family. Therefore, an objective of testing the accused is to alert the survivor to the possibility of infection and allow him or her to take precautions to prevent further transmission.

Certainly, testing the accused will not give the survivor definitive guidance. However, it can provide some reassurance, or caution, about whether she should continue to take precautions before her own serostatus is detectable. Nor is testing the accused absolutely necessary to protect the health of others. The survivor has alternatives that are less intrusive for the accused, but more burdensome for her. The survivor can protect sex partners by abstaining from intercourse or using condoms; she can also protect offspring by delaying pregnancy or avoiding breast-feeding. However, these preventive measures entail substantial behavioral changes, some risk to others (HIV transmission and pregnancy from improper use of condoms), and costs (both personal and financial) including alteration of life plans (delaying parenthood, marriage, or sexual relationships). Fairness dictates that the burden of limiting future harm should not rest solely with the survivor.

Psychological Benefit of the Survivor

The case for imposed testing may also rest on the psychological benefits it may offer the survivor. The psychological well-being of survivors of sexual assault is a crucial part of their overall health. The psychological harm from sexual assault includes not only the trauma of the original assault, but also the rational fear of HIV infection. Moreover, the burden of anxiety persists for a substantial period of time. Without testing the accused, the survivor cannot rule out HIV infection for up to twelve months after the assault.

Policies authorizing early testing of the accused could help relieve this concern in many cases. Despite the small possibility of false positive or negative test results, the news would provide substantial reassurance to the survivor. Of course, where testing reveals that the accused is infected, the survivor can experience additional psychological stress. This burden, while heavy, would fall on far fewer survivors than those who currently worry about infection. Knowledge of exposure might even allow survivors to begin psychological preparation for the results of their own testing.

Use of the Results as Evidence in Legal Proceedings

Some survivors may seek testing of the accused to use the information in criminal or civil litigation. Thirty-one states have specific criminal penalties for

knowingly exposing others to HIV infection (see Chapter 10).[64] Several courts
have awarded significant damages to individuals who were exposed to, but not
infected with, HIV (see Chapter 3).

In most jurisdictions, a court cannot find the accused guilty or liable based
solely on HIV status. In criminal cases, the state of mind of the accused is relevant—usually intentional or knowing transmission of infection is required. In
civil cases the plaintiff must demonstrate that the assailant knew he was HIV-infected and the intercourse was nonconsensual or that the assailant's HIV status
was not disclosed. To prove that transmission occurred as a result of the assault, the survivor would have to consent to baseline testing and demonstrate
that subsequent seroconversion was not due to other risk behaviors.

Constitutional Rights of Accused Persons

Defendants in criminal cases involving sexual assault have challenged compulsory HIV testing on a number of constitutional grounds, notably the Fourth
Amendment right to be free from unreasonable searches and seizures. Evolving Fourth Amendment case law indicates that a carefully crafted testing program would probably be held constitutional. Such a program would require a
probable cause hearing prior to compelled testing, protect confidentiality, and
place limitations on the use of test results.

The Fourth Amendment guarantees individuals the right to be "secure in
their persons . . . against unreasonable searches and seizures."[65] Supporting this
guarantee is the amendment's requirement that all search warrants be supported by probable cause that the person committed the offense. The Supreme
Court has long held that an invasion of the body such as through compelled
testing of blood, urine, or "deep lung" breath is a search and seizure within the
meaning of the Fourth Amendment (see Chapter 7).[66]

When the information obtained is to be used as evidence in a criminal trial,
the Supreme Court normally requires a judicial warrant issued on probable cause
before a search. However, in exceptional cases (e.g., under exigent circumstances, such as when the evidence may be evanescent[67] or there is an imminent risk to life),[68] a warrantless search may be constitutional as long as the
search is "reasonable" under the circumstances. Testing for HIV infection for
use in a criminal trial[69] will likely require a warrant because HIV infection, unlike blood alcohol or drug metabolite level, will not disappear if the test is delayed. Nor would there be an immediate threat to the health or life of the survivor. If there is no demonstration that the infection is probable and relevant
to proof of the crime, a warrant for HIV testing for use as evidence in a crim-

inal trial could conceivably represent an unconstitutional infringement of a defendant's rights.[70]

A court would probably examine the policy for proposed compulsory testing under the Supreme Court's "special needs" doctrine. The Court developed the special needs standard in two companion cases involving the constitutional authority of the government to test individuals for illicit drug use.[71] The standard applies "when special needs, beyond the normal need for law enforcement, make the warrant and probable cause requirement impracticable."[72] If the HIV test results may not be used in a criminal prosecution without the consent of the accused, and the purposes of testing are to promote the health and well-being of the survivor, the program should be held constitutional if it is reasonable.

A number of court decisions following the drug testing cases suggest that when the government is trying to achieve an important public purpose and the intrusion on privacy is not substantial, the testing program will be upheld.[73] Alternatively, if the invasion of privacy is serious and the results may be used for arrest or conviction, testing may be held unconstitutional. In *Ferguson v. City of Charleston*, the Supreme Court ruled that hospitals may not test pregnant women for drugs and share the results with police: "While the ultimate goal of the [drug testing] program may well have been to get women into substance abuse treatment and off drugs, the immediate objective of the searchers was to generate evidence for law enforcement purposes to reach that goal. . . . In our opinion, this distinction is critical."[74]

In the case of HIV testing of persons charged with sexual assault, the government has a compelling interest in obtaining information that directly affects the physical and mental well-being of survivors.[75] The exchange of semen poses a real, albeit low, risk of transmission of HIV infection. It is, therefore, distinguishable from those cases, such as a bite or nonsexual assault where the risk is "minuscule, trivial . . . approaching zero."[76] Moreover, preconviction testing of defendants, though not perfect, is essential if the purposes of the testing are to be achieved.[77]

Although the Supreme Court perceives government-imposed blood tests as "commonplace" and not unduly intrusive,[78] preconviction HIV testing ought to be acknowledged as much more intrusive than most tests. The personal interest of the accused is not merely the drawing of blood without consent, but the intimate information obtained that could result in a deep invasion of privacy and discrimination. The proposed policy, however, reduces the intrusion on the individual by seeking to ensure confidentiality, protecting against forced disclosure of the test results to the accused, and prohibiting use of the information against him in judicial proceedings. Thus, the constitutionality of the policy proposed here, though not assured, is likely to be affirmed by the judiciary.

Conclusion

This analysis of compulsory testing emphasizes the particular usefulness of knowing the accused's serostatus in mitigating any ongoing harm to the survivor of sexual assault. This information is especially significant for the psychological well-being of survivors and the potential protection of their partners and children. The reassurance provided by early testing of the accused could further assist survivors and their families in their adjustment to the traumatic experience and their reintegration into productive lives.

The needs and rights of sexual assault survivors have not been discussed in the media and at the highest levels of government. That certainly is not true for another population that faces an even lower risk of contracting HIV infection —patients in health care settings. The next chapter explores the controversial issue of health care workers living with HIV/AIDS.

As health care professionals, we may sometimes feel overwhelmed by the massive gaps between what is needed and what is available to help communities fight HIV. We know, however, that we have no choice but to respond to the millions of individuals whose lives are
destroyed or severely compromised each year by this virus, and the tens of millions more
whose standards of living are put in danger.—**Gro Harlem Brundtland,** director general,
World Health Organization (2001)

Chapter 12

Rights and Duties of Health Care
Workers Living with HIV/AIDS

More than a decade ago the Centers for Disease Control and Prevention (CDC)
reported a cluster of six cases of transmission of human immunodeficiency
virus (HIV) infection from a Florida dentist to his patients.[1] These cases, in
which the mode of transmission was never determined, had a direct effect on
federal and state policy. In 1991, after a year-long national debate, the CDC recommended that health care workers (HCWs) infected with HIV or hepatitis B
virus (HBV) (HbeAg positive) should be reviewed by an expert panel and should
inform patients of their serologic status before engaging in exposure-prone
procedures. Later in 1991 Congress mandated states to adopt the CDC guidelines or their equivalent.

Public health authorities, in the face of scientific uncertainty, took the path
of caution.[2] Yet, considerable evidence has emerged since 1991 suggesting that
Congress and the CDC should reform national policy. Data demonstrate that

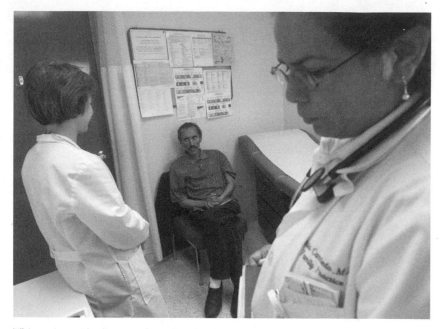

This patient, who lives on the U.S. side of the border, is regularly evaluated at an HIV clinic in San Ysidro, California. On this visit in 2002, he received care from two doctors, attending physician Ronell Campbell (left) and resident Maria Carriendo Ceniceros. Data demonstrate that the risk of blood-borne pathogen transmission in the health care setting is remote. (Reprinted with the permission of the *San Francisco Chronicle*)

the risk of blood-borne pathogen transmission in the health care setting is exceedingly low.[3] Current policy, moreover, does not improve patient safety. At the same time, implementation of CDC policy places significant human rights burdens on HCWs. Consequently, national policy should no longer include professional practice restrictions or require disclosure of an HCW's HIV or HBV infection status to patients.

After describing current CDC guidelines, this chapter presents evidence from the fields of epidemiology and law to demonstrate why revision of national policy is desirable. Although the focus is on HIV infection, much of the analysis is relevant to other blood-borne infections such as HBV and hepatitis C virus (HCV). The chapter concludes by proposing a new national policy that emphasizes patient safety by ensuring that infection control procedures are systematically implemented in health care settings. The policy, therefore, focuses on safer systems of practice rather than on excluding and stigmatizing infected HCWs.

Current National Policy for Protecting Patients from Blood-borne Pathogens

In 1991 the CDC recommended that HCWs infected with HIV or HBV (HbeAg positive) should not perform exposure-prone procedures unless they have "sought counsel from an expert review panel and been advised under what circumstances, if any, they may continue to perform these procedures."[4] Even if panels permit them to practice, HCWs must still disclose their serologic status to patients. The CDC defined an exposure-prone procedure to include "digital palpitation of a needle tip in a body cavity or the simultaneous presence of the health care worker's fingers and a needle or other sharp instrument or object in a poorly visualized anatomic site." The CDC sought help in clarifying the definition of exposure-prone procedures, but professional medical and dental associations declined to offer assistance.[5]

In October 1991 Congress enacted a statute requiring each state, as a condition of receiving U.S. Public Health Service funds, to certify that CDC guidelines "or their equivalent" had been instituted.[6] During the following year, the CDC notified states that "the agency would be flexible in accepting the certifications of equivalency." States could determine exposure-prone procedures "on a case-by-case basis, taking into consideration the specific procedure as well as the skill, technique, and possible impairment of the infected HCW."[7] As a result, variability exists in state law and practice. Significantly, many states do not require disclosure to patients even though this is currently recommended by the CDC.[8]

In December 1995 the Presidential Advisory Council on HIV/AIDS asked President Clinton to "instruct the CDC to review its guidelines that arbitrarily restrict HIV-infected HCWs and lead to discrimination." Later, professional organizations recommended a change in policy so that HCWs would not be required to be tested, hospitals would not be required to notify patients, and infected HCWs would not be excluded from practice.[9] The CDC, although it has the legal power to do so, has not changed its policy about testing and exclusion of HIV-infected HCWs.

The CDC held expert committee meetings in the late 1990s to reform existing policy about the testing and exclusion of HIV-infected HCWs. Despite almost unanimous consensus among the experts, the agency did not alter its policy. This may be explained not by science, but by politics. The issue of HIV-infected HCWs is still politically charged, and any CDC recommendations would be subject to intense scrutiny by the White House and Congress.

If the CDC were to change its guidelines, it would significantly affect national policy for two reasons. First, because current federal legislation requires states to adopt CDC guidelines or their equivalent, changes in CDC guidelines should result in statewide reforms. Second, under state tort law, courts usually measure professional and hospital practices against a national standard of care. CDC guidelines do not necessarily set that standard, but they are highly influential in judicial cases.[10]

Other branches of government may not necessarily agree with revised federal agency guidelines. The issue of infected HCWs is controversial, and Congress holds the ultimate power to set policy.[11] Congress, therefore, could enact new legislation reinstating an exclusionary policy with respect to infected HCWs. Further, the courts are not bound by CDC guidelines. Since judges retain discretion in applying tort law and disability discrimination law, the courts could continue to decide cases against the interests of infected HCWs. As a result, hospitals—due to their fear of liability—might still insist that infected HCWs inform patients or refrain from practice. Despite these concerns, reform of CDC guidelines could have significant positive effects on the lives of HCWs and their patients.

New Scientific Evidence

Published data suggest that the risk to patients of contracting HIV in a health care setting is exceedingly remote. Transmission of HBV and HCV to patients appears to be rare. The risks of blood-borne disease transmission, moreover, are significantly lower than other risks faced by patients in hospitals, such as the possibility of adverse outcomes from medical error.[12] Risks can be minimized if HCWs take recommended precautions. Further, if all transmissions from HCWs to patients were entirely prevented, the public health burden resulting from the HIV epidemic would only be reduced infinitesimally.[13]

Health Care Worker-to-Patient Transmission of HIV

At the time of the 1991 guidelines, there was little evidence from which to assess the risk of HIV transmission in the health care system. Since then, data from reported cases, retrospective investigations, and national HIV/AIDS surveillance have shown that the risk is extremely low. Since the beginning of the HIV epidemic more than two decades ago, more than 23,000 HCWs have been diagnosed with AIDS. Yet as of December 2001, the CDC reported only 57 documented cases where HCWs were infected with HIV following an occupational exposure, although an additional 138 cases were considered possibly attribut-able to an occupational exposure.[14] The risk to patients was even lower: fewer than 10 episodes of HIV transmission from HCWs to patients have been docu-mented. Since the 6 infected patients in the Florida dental cluster, there have been no other reported cases of HCW-to-patient transmission of HIV in the United States. A single case was reported in 1997 involving an orthopedic sur-geon in France with advanced symptomatic, but undiagnosed, HIV disease.[15] A further possible case of nurse-to-patient transmission in France was reported in 2000.[16]

Comprehensive retrospective investigations, particularly among physicians engaged in invasive procedures, identified no additional cases.[17] The CDC has analyzed HIV test results for more than 22,000 patients of 63 HIV-infected HCWs, and no documented case of transmission has occurred.[18] Similarly, in 1997, 1,180 surgical patients of an HIV-infected physician in obstetrics and gy-necology were tested in the United Kingdom; no patient was found to be pos-itive.[19] Finally, state health department follow-up of reported cases of HIV or AIDS has failed to confirm additional cases of HCW-to-patient transmission.

In addition to the epidemiological data, there are theoretical reasons to be-lieve that the risk of transmission to patients is exceedingly remote. New ther-apies can reduce the HIV viral load in plasma to very low levels.[20] Consequently, if HIV-infected HCWs are in treatment, it ought to be possible to monitor their health status and ensure low viral loads,[21] thus reducing risks to patients even further.[22]

Health Care Worker-to-Patient Transmission of Hepatitis B

The likelihood of transmission of HBV is significantly greater than the trans-mission of HIV. Model-based calculations estimate that the risk of surgeon-to-patient transmission of HBV is 0.24 percent during a single procedure as com-pared to a 0.0024 percent risk of HIV transmission from surgeon to patient.[23] Despite the elevated risk, HCW-to-patient transmission of HBV has also been rare since the early 1990s. In 1992 a cluster of nineteen cases of transmission occurred from a HbeAg-positive cardiothoracic surgeon in California who did not double-glove even after infection was diagnosed.[24] Transmission has also been documented in the United Kingdom[25] and Canada.[26] A cluster of HBV in-fections did occur in the United States between December 1995 and May 1996 among chronic hemodialysis patients, but the apparent mode of transmission was through the use of medical equipment shared by infected and uninfected patients.[27]

The 1991 guidelines did not address HCV because it had only recently been discovered, and data to support such guidelines did not exist. In 1998 the CDC found the risk of HCV transmission to be "very low."[28] There is a documented cluster of cases of HCV transmission from a cardiothoracic surgeon in Spain to five patients between 1988 and 1993, but investigation of those cases did not identify factors that might have contributed to transmission.[29] In 1998 an anesthesiology assistant in Germany transmitted HCV virus to five patients.[30] The anesthesiology assistant was himself infected through occupational exposure to a patient with HCV. Investigation revealed that the HCW never wore gloves and, at the time he treated all six patients, had a weeping wound on his right hand. Reports of the incident noted that the infections most likely could have been prevented by the use of universal precautions. Likewise, a Spanish anesthetist, who was addicted to morphine, reportedly infected over two hundred patients.[31] When giving patients postoperative painkillers, the anesthetist would often inject himself with part of the syringe contents and then inject the remaining painkiller into the patients using the same syringe. Apart from these exceptional cases, reported transmission of HCV from HCWs to patients has been rare.[32] Model-based calculations similarly suggest a low rate of HCV transmission of about 0.014 percent from surgical staff to patients.[33] This risk is approximately the same as a patient's risk of anesthesia-associated mortality.

Currently, no federal policy exists regarding management of HCWs with HCV. However, the American College of Surgeons states, "There is no indication for surgeons to take special measures to protect their patients except during acute, symptomatic illness with hepatitis C."[34] The level of risk entailed in HCV transmission in the health care setting appears to be comparable to that of other blood-borne infections. Consequently, national policy should include strategies for the management of HCV as well as HIV and HBV.

Prevention Techniques Minimize the Risk of Health Care Worker-to-Patient Transmission

Preventive measures greatly reduce the risk of HCW-to-patient transmission of blood-borne pathogens. The CDC has long recommended the use of universal precautions to reduce blood-to-blood contact between HCWs and patients.[35] The Occupational Safety and Health Administration's (OSHA) blood-borne pathogen standard also requires such precautions.[36] Some clusters of HCW-to-patient transmission of blood-borne pathogens could have been prevented entirely if the HCW had taken these universal precautions. Moreover, by adopting precautions HCWs can reduce the probability of percutaneous injuries during invasive procedures. For example, double-gloving protects both the patient and the provider against blood-to-blood exposure more effectively than single-gloving.[37]

Experts encourage surgeons and other HCWs to manage intraoperative injuries in the same way as other occupational injuries. Surgeons should avoid recontact between a contaminated instrument and the patient. The CDC recommends postexposure prophylaxis for HCWs occupationally exposed to HIV- or HBV-infected blood to prevent these HCWs from developing HIV.[38] Patients exposed to an infected HCW's blood can receive postexposure prophylaxis if exposure is promptly recognized and reported.[39]

Over the last decade scientists have made great strides in developing safer medical technology. In fact, the CDC has estimated that 177,000 injuries in hospital settings can be prevented each year through the use of needles with safety devices, needleless technologies, and safer work practices.[40] In response to the availability of safer needles, Congress passed the Needlestick Safety and Prevention Act in November 2000 amending OSHA's blood-borne pathogens standard to require health care employers to develop plans for the use of safe technology where possible.[41]

Human Rights Burdens

Sanctions against HIV-infected HCWs would be ethically permissible if they were necessary to avert a serious risk to patients or if the limitations on human rights were trivial. At present, however, the risks to patients are negligible, especially when appropriate preventive measures are taken, while the burdens on HIV-infected HCWs are disproportionately high. Qualified and experienced professionals face discrimination, invasion of privacy, and potential liability. An unintended consequence of the CDC guidelines is that health care organizations and the courts have used them to justify adverse treatment of infected HCWs.[42]

Discrimination

The Americans with Disabilities Act (ADA), and similar state statutes,[43] proscribe employment discrimination against "qualified" persons with a disability. (For further explanation of the ADA, see Chapter 6). Notably, "qualification" standards include a requirement that a person does not pose a "direct threat" to the health or safety of himself or others.[44] The ADA, however, requires an employer to provide reasonable accommodations that would enable persons with disabilities to perform their job effectively and safely (i.e., without posing a significant risk).[45] Thus, if reasonable accommodations could help HCWs practice safely, health care organizations must provide them.[46]

The critical questions, therefore, are whether HIV-infected HCWs pose a significant risk to patients and, if so, whether there are reasonable accommodations to reduce that risk.[47] The Supreme Court assesses "significant risk" by its nature (the mode of transmission), probability (the likelihood of transmission), severity (the magnitude of the harm should the infection be transmitted), and duration (the length of time the person would remain infectious).[48] The Equal Employment Opportunity Commission, moreover, maintains that "an employer . . . is not permitted to deny an employment opportunity to a person with a disability merely because of a slightly increased risk."[49]

Despite this clear language, the courts have held that, because HIV infection carries grave consequences, even a theoretical risk of transmission can be sufficient to justify discrimination.[50] The courts have had little difficulty finding that HIV-infected HCWs pose a significant risk,[51] often resolving the issue through summary judgment without medical facts or expert testimony.[52] These courts have relied on the severity of harm *should the risk materialize*. One court allowed a hospital to reassign a surgical assistant to the procurement department despite the "small" risk, claiming: "The duration of infection is perpetual. And the virus inevitably leads to the fatal disease AIDS."[53]

This kind of reasoning perverts the significant risk standard because it means that individuals can be discriminated against in the absence of an appreciable public health threat. For example, a federal court of appeals upheld the segregation of HIV-infected inmates, arguing that they posed a threat to the prison population.[54] However, significant risk should be a product of four criteria (nature, probability, severity, and duration), and if any criterion demonstrates a very low chance of serious harm, then the risk should be "insignificant."[55] Notably, courts rely on the CDC guidelines to support their position.[56] The court in *Estate of Mauro v. Borgess Medical Center* found that a surgical technician posed a "direct threat to the health and safety of others" even though the technician had never placed his hands near the patient's wound and his duties consisted primarily of handing over the surgeon's instruments. The court concluded, "We must defer to the medical judgement in the report of the Centers for Disease Control."[57]

Even if HIV-infected HCWs pose a significant risk, hospitals have a duty to provide reasonable accommodations such as infection control, training, and a leave of absence for treatment.[58] If HIV-infected HCWs were to receive this kind of support, the great majority would be able to function effectively and safely.

Despite the potential of the ADA to safeguard the rights of HCWs, the courts and administrative agencies, with few exceptions, have upheld discrimination against HIV-infected HCWs.[59] The judiciary has permitted decisions to exclude HCWs from medical,[60] nursing,[61] and dental hygiene[62] practice. In response to concern about the Florida dental case, one court upheld the exclusion of an HIV-infected student from a dental school.[63] Despite the legal standard that the employer bears the burden of proving that the practice poses a significant risk of harm, in reality the courts have shifted the burden to HCWs to show that they pose virtually no risk.[64] The courts have approved discriminatory action not only for exposure-prone procedures, but also for less invasive procedures.[65] Notably, some courts have upheld restrictions despite expert review panel advice that the HCW should continue to practice.[66] These are cases where public health authorities have complied with the ADA's mandate for individualized determinations and the judiciary has nonetheless declined to protect HCWs' rights.

Privacy

The CDC requirement to disclose HCWs' HIV status to patients before they perform exposure-prone procedures has become common practice. Patient notification is supported by cultural, ethical, and legal reasoning.[67] American cultural thought strongly supports a patient's "right to know." Patients want to be informed and to decide for themselves whether to incur risks. A CDC survey in 2002, for example, found that 89 percent of patients would want to know if their doctor or dentist is infected with HIV.[68] Similarly, infected physicians may feel that they have an ethical duty to patients and the wider public to disclose their serologic status. Physicians may choose to "put patients first" by disclosing their serologic status, even if the risk of transmission is very low. Finally, the legal doctrine of informed consent appears to support disclosure. In many states, the law requires physicians to disclose risks that "reasonable" patients would want to know, and many patients do want to know if their physician is infected with HIV.[69]

Despite these significant arguments, the law should not *require* HCWs to disclose their HIV status to patients. A legal obligation to notify patients is an invasion of the HCWs' privacy. It is important to remember that the HCW is also a patient who is being treated for a stigmatizing disease. Forced disclosure of this sensitive information may be socially embarrassing and harm a HCW's livelihood and professional reputation.[70] Moreover, the invasion of privacy is extensive because patients have no duty of confidentiality and may spread the information to other patients and the media.[71] It is perhaps for this reason that Canada, which issued guidelines after the CDC guidelines were published, does not recommend notification to patients.[72]

The doctrine of informed consent also should not require HIV-infected HCWs to disclose their HIV status to patients. First, informed consent requires disclosure of "material" risks, not remote risks. The risk of HIV transmission from HCW to patient is too low to meet the legal standard for disclosure. If the risk were significant, the logical remedy would be to restrict the HCW's right to practice, not to notify the patient. Public health authorities would not permit a clinician to practice knowing that she poses a meaningful risk regardless of whether patients are notified. Second, informed consent usually requires disclosure of risks entailed in the medical procedure, not those posed by the HCW herself. Ordinarily, HCWs are not required to inform patients about their personal health status or disability (whether temporary or permanent). For instance, HCWs who have depression, have had insufficient sleep, or have had alcohol at a social occasion in the hours preceding a patient encounter are ordinarily not required to disclose these facts to patients. In each of these cases, the HCW may pose a risk that is the same as, or greater than, the risk of HIV transmission. Yet, provided the HCW is considered competent and reasonably safe, she is entitled to practice without a duty to disclose.

State courts have affirmed hospital decisions to disclose the HCW's HIV status to patients. Relying on CDC guidelines, these courts have required compulsory disclosure as part of the informed consent process.[73] Some courts even permit disclosure for the purposes of retrospective investigations.[74] In *Faya v. Almaraz*, an HIV-infected oncological surgeon performed partial mastectomies on two patients. When the patients read that the physician had died of AIDS, they brought a lawsuit alleging emotional distress. The court allowed damages for the period between the time that the patients learned of the physician's HIV status and their conclusively testing negative for HIV.[75] Similar results have occurred in other court decisions.[76] In these kinds of cases, hospitals and HCWs face liability even though patients suffer no tangible harm or infection.[77] This litigation, moreover, is not restricted to HIV but could apply equally to other infectious diseases such as HBV, HBC, or tuberculosis.

Fortunately, most state courts require plaintiffs to show actual exposure to HIV in order to recover emotional distress damages.[78] But even if litigation is unsuccessful, it can influence hospitals to restrict an HCW's rights more than they think may be justified in the public interest. Hospitals, fearing potential liability, may assume that it is less costly to mandate patient notification or to restrict an HCW's practice than to face litigation. Malpractice liability concerns exacerbate this problem if insurers urge screening out infected HCWs rather than incurring liability risks.

Compulsory Testing

The CDC does not recommend HIV testing in the absence of behavioral risk factors. Nor does it recommend mandatory testing. Nevertheless, hospitals occasionally require HCWs to be tested against their will, and courts have approved such policies. A federal court of appeals upheld a hospital's decision to fire a licensed practical nurse who was suspected of being HIV-infected but refused to be tested. The court reasoned that the hospital was prevented from "deciding what, if any, measures were necessary to protect the health of patients."[79] Courts also have held that HIV testing can be "job related and consistent with business necessity."[80] In one case, a training school obtained a medical assistant's blood purportedly to test for rubella but instead performed an HIV test.[81] The court found that this constituted an invasion of privacy. This case shows the lengths to which some facilities will go to identify HIV-infected HCWs. If the standard of care remains that HCWs must notify patients and possibly discontinue their practice, then health care organizations and the courts may believe that compulsory testing is an appropriate response.

HCWs' Rights and the Public's Health

HCWs living with HIV/AIDS face the loss of their livelihood, professional status, and self-image. They have been terminated, forced to resign, reassigned, denied rotations, or not permitted to continue their education.[82] To avoid discrimination, many HCWs do not seek diagnosis and treatment because they have greater legal protection if they can honestly say that they did not know their serologic status. Some pay for treatment out of their own pockets to avoid filing claims with their health insurance carriers. Others travel outside their geographic areas to protect their anonymity.[83]

Current policy and practice not only adversely affect the professional and personal interests of HCWs, but also may not be in the public interest. By denying talented health care professionals the opportunity to treat patients, the current policy may limit patients' ability to obtain care.[84] Punitive policies may serve as disincentives for HCWs to determine their HIV status or to disclose it to their employers or personal physicians. Consequently, the CDC's restrictive policy may reduce HCWs' opportunities for therapy, thereby increasing risks to patients.

Proposed Reform of National Policy

Current national policy offers no discernible risk reduction for patients—few, if any, new blood-borne infections are prevented by excluding HIV-infected HCWs. At the same time, the policy imposes human rights burdens, undermines efforts to retain experienced professionals, and poses liability risks. New national policy should focus on structural changes to make the health care workplace safer for both patients and HCWs rather than on identification and management of infected HCWs.[85] Certainly, patient safety remains the most important part of any national policy, but it ought to be possible to ensure patient safety while not undermining HCWs' interests in autonomy, privacy, and livelihood. The following five recommendations would ensure that patients receive care in a safe environment, while treating HCWs with respect and dignity:

1. *Establish programs to prevent blood-borne pathogen transmission.* Health care organizations should be responsible for planning, implementing, enforcing, and evaluating effective strategies for the prevention of blood-borne pathogen transmission. Prevention programs should include policies and procedures for (1) standard (universal) precautions (e.g., barrier equipment such as gloves, gowns, and face protection),[86] (2) reprocessing patient care equipment (e.g., cleaning, disinfecting, and sterilizing) and cleaning environmental surfaces, (3) infection control training (in professional schools and in the health care setting), (4) prevention and management of infectious conditions (e.g., HBV vaccination), (5) injury and exposure prevention during surgical, obstetric, and dental procedures—such as less invasive alternatives to conventional interventions (e.g., laparoscopy), practice changes (e.g., "no touch" techniques and double-gloving), and safer instruments (e.g., blunted suture needles and use of staples instead of sutures), and (6) surveillance for transmission of blood-borne pathogens (e.g., reporting and evaluating parenteral injuries).

2. *Define responsibilities of infected HCWs.* HCWs, as professionals, have ethical responsibilities to promote their own health and well-being and to ensure patient safety. HCWs should learn their serologic status through testing with informed consent. Infected HCWs should seek medical care and treatment, including ongoing monitoring of viral load, as well as evaluations of physical and mental health status. HCWs should notify patients and hospitals in all instances of significant exposure to the HCW's blood.

3. *Discontinue expert review panels and special restrictions for exposure-prone procedures.* Identifying infected physicians, requiring expert review panels, and adopt-

ing special restrictions for exposure-prone procedures have served to stigmatize HCWs. The term "exposure-prone procedure" has not been clearly defined, so the courts have erred on the side of restricting HCW practice. Expert review panels, moreover, are constituted differently in each state, so there are multiple standards of care; even when panels permit practice, health care organizations sometimes disregard their advice. Review panels, therefore, should be replaced by expert consultants who would provide advice on HCW health and patient safety but would not be empowered to restrict HCW practice.

4. *Discontinue mandatory disclosure of HCWs' infection status.* HCWs may feel morally obliged to voluntarily notify patients of their infection status, but the law should not require disclosure of very low-level risks. HIV is a highly personal, and sometimes stigmatic, health condition that usually has little relevance to patient safety. Because notification represents an invasion of privacy and may result in loss of livelihood, it should not be legally mandated.

5. *Impose practice restrictions to avert significant risks to patients.* Public health authorities have a public duty to ensure patient safety. Consequently, health care organizations and/or public health authorities should issue practice restrictions if an HCW (1) suffers from a physical or mental impairment that affects his professional judgment or practice, (2) has exudative lesions or weeping dermatitis, (3) has a history of poor infection control technique and practice, or (4) has had an incident of transmission of a bloodborne pathogen. In these cases, the HCW cannot practice competently and safely, and should be restricted from practice.

Conclusion

The health care system must be made as safe as possible for both patients and their care providers. The HIV epidemic has driven the public to demand a near zero risk. However, a standard of zero risk is impossible. In its effort to assuage the public, the government has imposed human rights burdens, driven qualified HCWs from the profession, and posed unfair liability risks. A new national policy, focused on management of the workplace environment and injury prevention, would achieve a high level of patient safety without discrimination or invasion of privacy.

Disease screening is one of the most basic tools of modern public health and preventive medicine. Screening programs have a long and distinguished history in efforts to control epidemics of infectious diseases and targeting treatment for chronic diseases. . . . In practice when screening is conducted in contexts of gender inequality, racial discrimination, sexual taboos, and poverty, these conditions shape the attitudes and beliefs of health system and public health decision-makers as well as patients, including those who have lost confidence that the health care system will treat them fairly. Thus, if screening programs are poorly conceived, organized, or implemented, they may lead to interventions of questionable merit and enhance the vulnerability of groups and individuals.
— Institute of Medicine, National Academy of Sciences (1999)

Chapter 13

Perinatal Transmission of HIV

Controversies in Screening and Policy

In 1994 AIDS law and policy were transformed with the scientific discovery that perinatal (mother-to-infant) HIV transmission could be dramatically reduced with treatment. AIDS Clinical Trials Group (ACTG) Study 076 determined that a regimen of antiretroviral therapy administered to women during pregnancy, labor, and delivery,[1] and to infants postnatally, could reduce the risk of perinatal transmission by two-thirds—from approximately 25 percent to 8 percent.[2] Since then, modern treatment regimens of combination antiretroviral medications have confirmed the results of ACTG 076[3] and reduced the risk even further.[4] Studies have shown that when viral loads are undetectable during pregnancy, mother-to-child HIV transmission rates are less than 2 percent.[5] For women with detectable viral loads, studies demonstrate the efficacy of elective cesarean section.[6] Without such interventions, a 25 percent mother-to-infant transmission rate would result in the birth of an estimated 1,750 HIV-infected

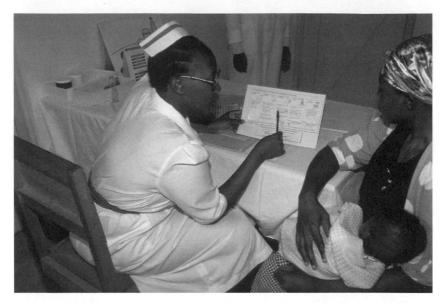

A nurse in Kenya teaches a mother how to breast-feed her newborn in 1996. Since the beginning of the epidemic, HIV transmission from mother to child during pregnancy, labor, and delivery or by breast-feeding has accounted for 91 percent of all AIDS cases reported among U.S. children.

infants annually in the United States and would yield lifetime medical costs of $282 million.[7] Globally, in the absence of effective maternal treatment, 800,000 HIV-infected infants would be born each year.[8]

The scientific knowledge that transmission from mother to infant could be substantially decreased set into motion fierce debates about HIV screening and treatment policy in the United States. (For a discussion of women and infants living with HIV/AIDS in resource-poor countries, see Chapter 16). Some politicians insisted that public health and health care professionals take active steps to identify infected mothers and babies. The moral belief that everything possible must be done to protect "innocent" children meant that these politicians were prepared to consider compulsory measures if necessary to accomplish that goal.

This chapter examines the legal, ethical, and policy debates surrounding perinatal HIV testing and screening in the United States. First, it explains the current status of HIV testing and counseling. Second, it canvasses existing law and policy, including recommendations by the Institute of Medicine (IOM) and the Centers for Disease Control and Prevention (CDC). The IOM and CDC recommendations raise critical issues concerning the appropriate population for screening and the perplexing problems of coercion and consent. Third, the chapter considers the lawfulness of routine HIV screening, particularly whether the IOM proposal could be implemented lawfully in the states. Finally, it provides proposals for reform of prenatal screening policy in the United States.

The analysis will reveal deep fault lines in politics and ethics relating to perinatal transmission of HIV. Because pregnant women and infants are highly vulnerable, their protection is often politically charged. To some, society's primary obligation is to respect the autonomy and privacy of pregnant women. They believe that women have interests that are separate from the fetus and that these interests deserve rigorous protection. Others argue that the fetus is the highest priority and that a pregnant woman does not have the freedom to act in ways that may endanger her fetus. These sharp differences of opinion have resulted in political struggles about what is the most appropriate policy for pregnant women at risk of HIV.

Current Status of HIV Testing and Counseling among Women

The prevention of vertical transmission of HIV from mother to infant is crucial because the spread of HIV among women is growing rapidly. Women represent about 20 percent of AIDS cases in the United States.[9] African American women and Latinas account for 25 percent of all U.S. women, but they represent 80 percent of AIDS cases among women.[10] Although women of all ages are affected by HIV/AIDS, the disease is most prevalent among women in their childbearing years. An estimated 120,000–160,000 HIV-infected women reside in the United States, 80 percent of whom are of childbearing age.[11] The CDC estimates that over a hundred perinatal transmissions continue to occur each year.[12] This is a dramatic decrease from 1991, when 1,760 newborns were born with HIV infection.[13] The potentially large number of pregnant women who are at risk of transmitting infection to their newborns gives urgency to the implementation of effective prevention policies.

The percentage of women of childbearing age and pregnant women that are screened and counseled for HIV infection is not fully known.[14] Although most parturient women are offered a prenatal HIV test and are tested, testing numbers have not reached national goals and differ significantly by location and health insurance status. Researchers have determined that the greatest barrier is failure of clinicians to recommend testing.[15] Moreover, studies indicate that universal testing would be accepted by most women.[16]

Routine Screening and Treatment of Pregnant Women

The U.S Public Health Service (USPHS) responded to ACTG 076 by issuing guidelines for the treatment of pregnant women in 1994,[17] for counseling and screening in 1995,[18] and for antiretroviral drug treatment in 2002.[19] In 1996 Congress required the secretary of health and human services to determine by 1998 whether HIV screening of infants was "routine practice." If so, funding under Title II of the Ryan White CARE Act (CARE) Amendments of 1996 would become contingent on the states demonstrating that perinatal transmission had declined by half, that 95 percent of women were being screened during prenatal care visits, or that a program of mandatory newborn screening had been instituted.[20] In January 2000 the secretary of health and human services determined that it "has not become routine practice to require testing of newborn infants for HIV infection in the United States."[21] Hence the secretary's finding nullified the contingent requirements of CARE Title II funding.

As stated in the secretary's determination notice, only New York and Connecticut "require mandatory HIV testing of all newborns whose mothers did not undergo prenatal HIV testing and only New York has fully implemented this requirement."[22] Additionally, six other states require providers to *offer* HIV testing (California, Florida, Indiana, Iowa, Rhode Island, and Texas).[23]

In 1996 New York enacted the "Baby AIDS" Bill, which gave women the option of "unblinding" the results of their infants' HIV screening tests; in 1997 New York required mandatory notification to the mother if the test was positive; and in 1999 the state mandated either voluntary testing of women in labor whose HIV status was undocumented or mandatory testing of their newborns.[24] The sponsor of the New York mandatory screening statute, Assemblywoman Nettie Mayersohn, reasoned that it was "criminal" to allow the suffering of "innocent and helpless victims."[25]

Despite political protestations to the contrary, policies that screen newborns do not prevent HIV infection. By the time infants are tested, they will already have been exposed to their mothers' infection. The only way to reduce perinatal transmission is to screen pregnant women and treat those who are HIV-infected. Although screening of pregnant women is imperative, policymakers have grappled with two perplexing questions: (1) Should all pregnant women be screened or just those who are at heightened risk of HIV? (2) Should screening be entirely voluntary, with informed consent, or should it be coercive in any way?

The Institute of Medicine recognized that pregnant women who do not know that they are HIV-infected cannot take advantage of antiretroviral therapy. The IOM panel concluded that existing requirements for pretest counseling and specific informed consent posed a barrier to prenatal HIV screening. Many health care professionals were deterred from offering the test because of the economic costs and legal obstacles involved in counseling women and documenting informed consent. Consequently, the IOM made a bold proposal for a national policy of universal screening. Every pregnant woman in the United States would be offered testing for HIV infection as a routine component of prenatal care—that is, as one of the battery of tests routinely conducted during pregnancy. The IOM's proposal departed substantially from previous HIV policies by making testing universal and eliminating requirements for pretest counseling and specific (often written) informed consent.

The IOM report has spurred changes in prenatal HIV testing policies. The motivation for change is strong because the path of perinatal transmission is clear, beneficial interventions exist, and the intended beneficiaries of the intervention—babies—cannot protect themselves. HIV screening and treatment programs for pregnant women are also cost-effective,[26] despite the small potential for harm to both mother and infant (i.e., drug toxicity and development of drug-resistant strains of the virus).[27] Accordingly, the American College of Obstetrics and Gynecology and the American Academy of Pediatrics have endorsed the IOM's recommendations.[28] The USPHS has similarly recommended universal antiretroviral treatment for pregnant women infected with HIV,[29] and, in the wake of the report, some states have adopted new prenatal HIV screening policies.[30]

On November 9, 2001, the USPHS issued revised recommendations for HIV screening of pregnant women that updated the CDC's 1995 guidelines.[31] The revised guidelines followed the IOM structure by recommending (1) HIV testing as a routine part of prenatal care, (2) simplification of the testing process so that pretest counseling would not be a barrier to testing, (3) increased flexibility of the consent process to allow for various types of informed consent (e.g., written or verbal), (4) provider exploration and redress of reasons for refusal of testing, and (5) HIV testing and treatment at the time of labor and delivery for women who did not receive prenatal testing and chemoprophylaxis.

The revised CDC guidelines departed from the IOM's proposal in important respects. The CDC explicitly recommended HIV prevention counseling with a minimum standard of information (e.g., a discussion of perinatal transmission, ways to reduce this risk, and the implications of HIV testing). More importantly, the CDC proposed informed consent before testing so that women could not be tested without their knowledge: "HIV testing should be voluntary and free of coercion. Informed consent before HIV testing is essential. Information regarding consent can be presented orally or in writing and should use language the client understands. Accepting or refusing testing must not have detrimental consequences to the quality of prenatal care. Documentation of informed consent should be in writing, preferably with the client's signature. State or local laws and regulations governing HIV testing should be followed."[32]

In 2003 the CDC announced a new initiative that brought it into closer conformance with the IOM. CDC appeared to change its recommendation for pretest counseling: "Because prevention counseling . . . should not be a barrier to testing, CDC will promote adoption of simplified HIV testing procedures in medical settings that do not require counseling before testing." CDC reemphasized its recommendation for "routine" HIV testing of all pregnant women, and, "as a safety net, for routine screening of any infant whose mother was not screened."[33]

The IOM and CDC proposals raise two important scientific and ethical dilemmas: (1) the problem of targeting—what is the appropriate population to screen? and (2) the problem of compulsion and consent—how much information should women receive before testing?

The Problem of Targeting

HIV screening is often fraught with political controversy. Legislatures may wish to appear to be "doing something" about the AIDS epidemic, especially where vulnerable children are at risk.[34] Screening, however, infringes on privacy since it reveals the serologic status of both mother and infant. Even if the mother is not tested, her status is revealed by testing her baby. (All infants with HIV-infected mothers initially test positive for HIV antibodies, even if they are not actually HIV-infected). An HIV antibody positive serologic status may subject the mother and infant to potential stigma and discrimination. Policymakers must also consider the cost-effectiveness of HIV screening. Because screening can be expensive and impose burdens, they must evaluate whether HIV screening programs are well matched to those at risk of infection. That is, will the screening program correctly identify persons with HIV infection at a reasonable cost?

HIV screening may not be cost-effective in a low-prevalence population, even though it is highly accurate. The use of an accurate test in a low-prevalence population is likely to identify few cases because relatively few people are infected with HIV. Moreover, the screening program will produce some false positive cases, particularly if there is insufficient confirmatory testing. False positive results for serious conditions such as HIV can have profound psychological effects, including suicidal behavior.[35]

From a scientific and public health perspective, therefore, screening in higher-prevalence populations is preferable (see Chapter 7). High-prevalence screening finds more cases, at less cost per case, and generates fewer false positive results. Given its clear advantages, one would expect that policymakers would almost always target populations at high risk of infection. But some have rejected this approach because of the human rights implications. If the risk group is vulnerable, narrowly targeted screening may expose the population to social risk. Consider the disproportionate social burden of HIV/AIDS on African American women and Latinas (80 percent of AIDS cases reported in U.S. women in 2000 were among these groups) if they are singled out for screening.

Policymakers face a dilemma. Targeting a narrow, high-risk population will reinforce existing bigotries and thereby create harm to individuals and to the group itself. If African American women and Latinas are targeted for HIV screening, the public may closely associate them with stigmatized behaviors such as drug use. Alternatively, public health authorities may choose to screen a much broader population that includes, but is not limited to, risk groups. This broad population–based approach, however, will unnecessarily test many individuals who are unlikely to be infected. There is no sure resolution to this dilemma because it involves a selection of competing values: the most efficient screening program versus the program that is least burdensome to vulnerable communities. In the end, policymakers must make a difficult choice and weigh the goals of public health against those of social justice.

The CDC and IOM faced just this sort of dilemma when drafting guidelines about how to target prenatal screening—to pregnant women living in neighborhoods with a high prevalence of HIV infection or to all pregnant women regardless of risk. From a public health perspective, the screening of pregnant women at greatest risk would result in the highest yield, the best predictive value, and the least cost. Narrowly targeted screening, however, would starkly acknowledge differences of class and race as well as the obvious gender discrimination inherent in all prenatal screening. It would effectively separate women by skin color and socioeconomic status, fashionable suburbs from inner cities, and rural from urban America. The symbolic value of broad, rather than narrow, screening therefore was obvious. Screening the entire population would convey the message that AIDS concerns all people. Public health measures, by design, would apply universally. Although the epidemiologic evidence had long demonstrated that HIV was a disease prevalent among racial minorities, the CDC and IOM preferred population-based screening.

Given the difficult tradeoff between cost efficiency and justice, public health organizations chose fairness. The choice was reasonable given the political and social realities of the HIV epidemic. Since the public associates AIDS with marginalized populations and the poor, policymakers would have perpetuated and exacerbated these harmful stereotypes by targeting low-income communities. Although some argued that targeted screening would lead to treatment, there was no guarantee that low-income women would have full access to culturally appropriate and scientifically modern HIV therapies. Moreover, to the extent that screening posed a burden (in terms of loss of autonomy or privacy), that burden should be fairly distributed. Screening mostly indigent, minority women while exempting those in middle- and upper-class communities would have appeared inequitable.

The Problem of Compulsion and Consent

Any effort by states to mandate specific courses of behavior for pregnant women, particularly for the benefit of their fetuses, raises grave concerns for the remaining degree of reproductive autonomy left for women by increasingly less sympathetic courts. Like fetal abuse cases that have opened a dangerous door for the erosion of reproductive autonomy, mandated medical treatment for pregnant women based on their HIV status does not bode well for the future of any reproductive rights, including and not limited to, a woman's right to choose to terminate her pregnancy.—Theresa McGovern, founder of the HIV Law Project (1997)

The politics of screening are especially volatile because policymakers are often attracted to the notion that identifying contagious persons promotes public well-being. Some elected officials regard pregnant women as vessels for transmission of infection to their newborns. However, the AIDS community insists on maintaining its personal autonomy and privacy—a claim that civil libertarians strongly support.

Chapter 7 reviews the various forms of screening, ranging from voluntary and routine to compulsory. A summary of this discussion will be helpful in examining the IOM and CDC proposals for screening pregnant women. As we will see, the IOM proposal was neither completely voluntary nor compulsory, but rather a form of routine screening. The CDC proposal, on the other hand, was explicitly informed and voluntary.

Voluntary Screening

Voluntary screening consists of information about the nature of the test in advance, full understanding by a competent person, and the freedom to choose or decline to be tested. Many HIV-specific statutes require pretest counseling by health care professionals and informed consent, often in writing. As the IOM proposal did not require hospitals to inform pregnant women before they were tested, many women would not have had a meaningful opportunity to decline the test.

Compulsory Screening

Compulsory screening occurs when the state requires persons to submit to testing without their informed consent. Government can only compel testing by enacting legislation through the democratic process. The IOM did not propose that pregnant women be forced to be tested against their will. If women were aware that testing would take place, they could theoretically decline the procedure without legal consequence.

Routine Screening

As described in Chapter 7, there are at least two forms of routine screening: screening with advance notification ("opt-in") and screening without advance notification ("opt-out"). The civil liberties paradigm that had been set for a generation was informed consent, with pre- and post-test counseling. This rights-oriented paradigm, however, has genuine defects from a public health perspective. An elaborate pretest process compromises the practicality of screening all, or even most, pregnant women. Such a process incurs considerable costs in training health care professionals and counseling women, creates disincentives for hospitals, and risks the possibility that women might decline testing, or worse, avoid prenatal care. Medical record data collected by the CDC suggest that opt-in voluntary testing is associated with lower testing rates than either opt-out or mandatory testing procedures.[36]

The IOM recommended a national policy of universal HIV screening with patient notification as a routine component of prenatal care. This proposal had natural attractions because it would maximize women's participation while nominally recognizing their right to consent. At the same time, the proposal omitted essential details about the theory and practice of notification. How would women be notified—individually or by public notice, orally or in writing, or with (or without) the opportunity to ask questions? What safeguards would be instituted to ensure that women were competent, understood the information, and gave voluntary consent? The IOM proposal, by abandoning explicit written consent, appears to ignore a broad consensus about the importance of pretest counseling, patient autonomy, and privacy. Many women would be tested for HIV infection without their full understanding or agreement.

It is also possible that prenatal HIV screening would be administered unfairly. Middle- or upper-class women (because they have the ability to pay and often have access to more caring and nurturing health care environments) would often be informed and counseled about HIV testing. Poorer women (because they are in "Medicaid mills" or busy emergency rooms) would be more likely to be tested without their knowledge and consent. In other words, physicians and nurses often spend more time explaining the implications of testing and treatment to higher socioeconomic classes than lower classes. This policy could undermine the fairness that the IOM so earnestly sought in its screening policy. At the same time, the IOM's proposal may well violate HIV-specific testing statutes, as the following discussion demonstrates.

The Lawfulness of Routine HIV Screening for Pregnant Women

The IOM panel did not consider how its recommendations might conflict with existing state statutes. An analysis of HIV statutes in the fifty states demonstrates that the IOM proposal, if implemented, would be unlawful in many places (see Table 13-1).[37] Thus, universal prenatal screening could not be adopted without reform of state law. Virtually every state has a statute governing HIV testing generally or prenatal HIV testing specifically. These laws stand as an obstacle to implementing the IOM proposal.

Pretest Counseling

Eighteen states have laws addressing HIV counseling and/or testing of pregnant women, the majority of which require some form of pretest counseling.[38] Some states require pretest explanations of the nature of the test, risks and benefits (including psychosocial harm), prevention information, and confidentiality of test results.

Informed Consent

The majority of states require specific consent to HIV testing, often in writing. States frequently require specific information to be conveyed as part of the informed consent process. For example, health care professionals may have to explain the nature of the test, the confidentiality of test results, reporting requirements, the availability of anonymous testing, and the right of the person to decline or withdraw consent.

Disclosure of Information and Offer of Testing

Eighteen states have laws that specifically address prenatal HIV screening of pregnant women, but none permits testing without pretest counseling and/or consent. At least six of these states have routine opt-out procedures, whereby providers are required by law to test pregnant women unless the woman specifically objects (see Table 13-1).[39] These states take a variety of approaches to testing. Most require health care professionals to provide information to pregnant women and/or offer testing. Depending on the state, such information must be in written or oral form and may have to cover specific topics such as the modes of HIV transmission, the availability of treatment, and the health of the fetus. Some states require health care professionals to offer testing to all pregnant women or to only those women with specific risk factors. No state requires compulsory prenatal testing, but Connecticut and New York require newborn testing that indirectly reveals maternal HIV status. Florida and Indiana also permit perinatal testing of newborns for medically necessary cases (see Table 13-1).

Privacy Safeguards

Many states protect the privacy of HIV data and prohibit disclosure except under specified circumstances (see Chapter 5). Similarly, some states protect HIV data from compelled disclosure through the legal process. Maryland offers the strongest privacy protection for pregnant women, holding that personally identifiable HIV testing data are "confidential and not discoverable or admissible in evidence in any criminal, civil, or administrative action."[40] Other states permit disclosure of test results to the woman's spouse or her sex or needle-sharing partner.

Many of the foregoing state statutes would make it difficult or impossible to implement the IOM's proposal. Since routine, opt-out screening does not require counseling, the provision of specific information, or explicit consent, it would be inconsistent with statutory requirements in many states.

TABLE 13-1. Perinatal Testing — State Policies, Laws, and Regulations

State/Jurisdiction	Testing of Pregnant Women	Testing of Newborns
Alabama	Voluntary	
Alaska	Voluntary	
Arizona	Voluntary	
Arkansas	Providers required to test as early as possible, or at time of delivery, unless woman refuses	
California	Providers required to offer HIV testing	
Colorado	Voluntary	
Connecticut	Providers required to test when woman is admitted for delivery, unless she objects	Required as soon as possible after birth
Delaware	Voluntary by law	
District of Columbia	Voluntary	
Florida	Providers required to offer HIV testing as a standard of care	Providers may test if medically necessary and parents not available for · consent
Georgia	Voluntary	
Hawaii	Voluntary	
Idaho	Voluntary	
Illinois	Voluntary	
Indiana	Providers required to offer HIV testing	Providers may test if mother has not been tested and it is medically necessary
Iowa	Providers required to offer testing to any woman who asks, and to encourage women with risk factors to be tested	
Kansas	Voluntary	
Kentucky	Prenatal clinics (1/3 of women who give birth) required to offer testing as part of diagnostic workup	

Table 13.1 (continued)

State/Jurisdiction	Testing of Pregnant Women	Testing of Newborns
Louisiana	Voluntary by law	
Maine	Voluntary	
Maryland	Voluntary by law	
Massachusetts	Voluntary	
Michigan	Providers required to test, unless woman objects	
Minnesota	Voluntary	
Mississippi	Voluntary	
Missouri	Voluntary	
Montana	Voluntary	
Nebraska	Voluntary	
Nevada	Voluntary	
New Hampshire	Voluntary	
New Jersey	Providers required to offer HIV testing	
New Mexico	Voluntary	
New York	Providers required to test woman, unless she refuses, at delivery, if her HIV status is unknown	Testing required
North Carolina	Voluntary	
North Dakota	Voluntary	
Ohio	Voluntary	
Oklahoma	Voluntary	
Oregon	Voluntary	
Pennsylvania	Voluntary	
Puerto Rico	Voluntary	
Rhode Island	Providers required to offer HIV testing	
South Carolina	Voluntary	
South Dakota	Voluntary	

Table 13.1 (continued)

State/Jurisdiction	Testing of Pregnant Women	Testing of Newborns
Tennessee	Providers required to conduct HIV testing, unless woman refuses	
Texas	Providers required to conduct HIV testing, unless woman objects	
Utah	Voluntary	
Vermont	Voluntary	
Virginia	Practitioners required to request that pregnant women consent to be tested	
Washington	Voluntary by law	
West Virginia	Voluntary	
Wisconsin	Voluntary	
Wyoming	Voluntary	

Source: Amanda Watson, *Reducing Perinatal Transmission* (Washington, D.C.: Health Policy Tracking Service, 2000), <http://stateserv.hpts.org>.

Proposals for Reform of Prenatal Screening Policy in the United States

The policy goal should be to reduce vertical transmission of HIV infection to extremely low levels, ideally under 2 percent of births. There is a growing conviction that transmission levels can be lowered to near zero.[41] To ensure that every woman infected with HIV has a 98 percent chance of delivering an uninfected child, it is necessary to have high standards of prenatal screening and treatment.[42] However, pregnant women should not be regarded purely as reproductive vessels, but as rights-bearing individuals to be treated with dignity and respect.[43] Consequently, perinatal screening policy should be reformed by affording women the following rights:

1. *Universal prenatal screening.* All pregnant women should know their serologic status as early in gestation as possible. This requires routine screening as a universal component of prenatal care.

2. *Informed decisions.* To ensure that pregnant women can make an informed choice, they should be told in advance of their right to refuse an HIV test, the benefits of treatment, and that they will not be denied care if they decline to be tested.

3. *Privacy and nondiscrimination safeguards.* Because women who receive routine HIV testing face social risks, they should receive strong protections for privacy and nondiscrimination. In particular, HIV test results should not be disclosed without the woman's consent to the courts, immigration officials, or social workers. Nor should the information be disclosed without the woman's consent to her spouse or partner. Studies have shown that women are often subjected to domestic violence if their HIV status is disclosed to their partners.[44] This potential for abuse may affect the pregnant woman and her baby in fundamental ways—causing the woman severe physical and mental harm, impeding her ability to receive regular prenatal care and antiretroviral therapy, and risking the health and safety of the fetus.

4. *Post-test care.* Prenatal HIV testing is only the first step in ensuring the health and well-being of women and children. Pregnant women and their babies also deserve ongoing health care and psychosocial support. This includes the right to receive state-of-the-art highly active antiretroviral therapy, viral load monitoring, elective cesarean section, and referral for support services.

Conclusion

U.S. programs to screen women and infants for HIV infection demonstrate that screening is far from a neutral scientific pursuit.[45] Rather, HIV screening is political—elected officials perceive some groups as blameworthy and some as innocent. Screening is also rich in symbolism—the public health response helps to construct disease socially on dimensions of race, gender, and socioeconomic status. Finally, screening is fraught with complex choices and a weighing of values—efficiency, cost, autonomy, and justice. Perhaps the lesson is that tidy evaluative criteria are only part of a textured understanding of screening. Politics, symbolism, and values appear to be just as important as science in understanding the complexities of perinatal HIV screening.

This nation is fighting two deadly epidemics—AIDS and drug abuse. They are robbing us of far too many of our citizens and weakening our future. A meticulous scientific review has now proven that needle exchange programs can reduce the transmission of HIV and save lives without losing ground in the battle against illegal drugs. It offers communities that decide to pursue needle exchange programs yet another weapon in their fight against AIDS.
—**Donna E. Shalala,** secretary of health and human services in the Clinton administration (1998)

Junk is a cellular equation that teaches the user facts of general validity. I have learned a great deal from using junk: I have seen life measured out in eyedroppers of morphine solution. I experienced the agonizing deprivation of junk sickness, and the pleasure relief when junk thirsty cells drank from the needle. Perhaps all pleasure is relief. I have learned the cellular stoicism that junk teaches the user. I have seen a cell full of sick junkies silent and immobile in separate misery. They knew the pointlessness of complaining or moving. They knew that basically no one can help anyone else. There is no key, no secret someone else has that he can give you. I have learned the junk equation. Junk is not, like alcohol or weed, a means to increased enjoyment of life. Junk is not a kick. It is a way of life.
—**William S. Burroughs,** Junky (1977)

Chapter 14

The Interconnected Epidemics of
AIDS and Drug Dependency

If junk is a way of life, as William S. Burroughs vividly conveys, then the critical inquiry for law and policy is whether to punish or rehabilitate the junky. In the United States, criminal justice authorities cast drug dependency as an evil or a moral wrong to be penalized. Public health professionals regard drug dependency as a medical condition to be prevented, treated, and, if possible, cured. These competing approaches have long spawned conflict between the criminal justice and public health systems, but never have the differences been more divisive than in the debate over syringe availability;[1] that is, the prescription, sale, distribution, and exchange of drug-injection equipment.

A syringe is a powerful symbol—as an essential tool of the medical profession and as an emblem in the bitter controversy surrounding drug policy in the United States.[2] Criminal justice and public health ideologies profoundly differ

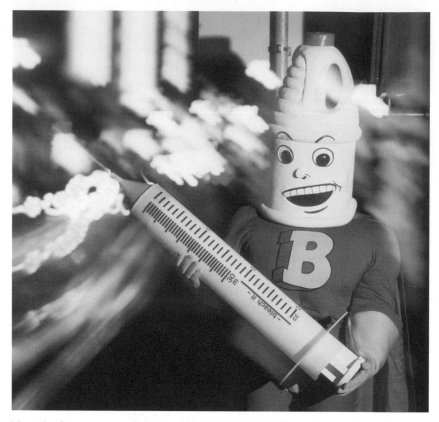

To make drug users aware that sterilizing needles with bleach can reduce the transmission of HIV, "Bleachman" became a spokesperson for the San Francisco AIDS Foundation in 1998. (© Roger Ressmeyer/CORBIS)

over the social and moral construction and meaning of syringes, as well as the desirable policy response to them.

The tenets of the criminal justice model hold that illicit drug use and its instrumentalities, including syringes, must be criminally proscribed. Syringes, essential for delivering injection drugs, are seen as an integral and pernicious part of the illegal drug trade and of the underground drug subculture. Syringes have become a metaphor for illicit drug use itself and associated criminal activity, family disintegration, child neglect, economic ruin, and social decay. To many people, legalizing, and especially promoting, the possession and use of sterile drug-injection equipment sends the wrong message by encouraging initiation into drug use and undermining moral and family values.[3] Historically, American drug policy has closely conformed to the criminal justice model. Legislation, regulations, and professional practice guidelines at the federal, state, and local levels comprise a complex, pervasive web of laws that severely restrict access to sterile injection equipment. Through this body of law, the United States has adopted a policy that consciously creates an artificial scarcity of syringes.

The public health approach, not unlike the criminal justice approach, recognizes the disutilities of drug use and supports interventions that prevent drug use or that facilitate treatment of drug users.[4] Unlike the criminal justice construct, however, the public health framework advocates harm reduction, a strategy that seeks to minimize health risks for injection drug users (IDUS).[5] Public health professionals reason that persons who persist in using drugs might nevertheless mitigate the considerable and demonstrable health risks of injection drug use. A key aspect of a harm reduction strategy for IDUS is to maximize the lawful distribution and use of sterile injection equipment. Accordingly, harm-reduction strategies embrace education, counseling, and the means for safer injection practices. These harm-reduction measures, designed to promote access to drug-injection equipment, encompass three interrelated policies: (1) permitting physicians to write prescriptions for syringes, (2) authorizing pharmacists to sell syringes over the counter, and (3) legalizing and funding syringe exchange programs (SEPS). From a public health perspective, physicians who prescribe syringes, pharmacists who dispense syringes, and IDUS who possess syringes should not face criminal penalties for complying with public health recommendations.

This chapter examines the legal environment for programs designed to prevent transmission of HIV/AIDS among IDUS. The discussion is also relevant for preventing the transmission of blood-borne diseases such as malaria, syphilis, hepatitis B and C, and endocarditis.[6] It demonstrates that public health efforts to facilitate access to sterile syringes may conflict with statutes and regulations at the federal, state, and local levels. Public health authorities, health care professionals, and community groups have sometimes creatively circumvented legal restrictions on the availability of drug-injection equipment. Even when these creative strategies have withstood legal challenges (and they have not always succeeded), criminal laws pose a chilling effect; the law makes it difficult for drug users to comply with public health advice to protect themselves and their partners from disease.

Public Health Dimensions

The conflict between law enforcement and public health becomes all the more acute in light of the profound health threat posed by blood-borne disease and the growing consensus that providing the means for safer injection is an effective prevention strategy. Injection drug use is the second most frequently reported risk for AIDS in the United States. The incidence rate among IDUS is approximately 10,000 new HIV cases per year.[7] As of December 31, 2001, of the 807,075 cumulative cases of AIDS reported to the Centers for Disease Control and Prevention (CDC), 284,176 were directly or indirectly associated with injection drug use.[8] This number represents 35 percent of all AIDS cases reported since the beginning of the epidemic. In contrast, in 1981 only 12 percent of all reported AIDS cases were associated with injection drug use.[9]

Prevalence of HIV infection among IDUS varies considerably by geographic location, with rates ranging from 0 to 65 percent.[10] Several large metropolitan areas in the United States, Europe, and Asia experienced rapid increases in seroprevalence among IDUS, demonstrating the possible explosive growth of disease in the absence of effective prevention.[11] Moreover, HIV/AIDS in the drug-dependent population disproportionately strikes the urban poor, including African Americans and Hispanics. African Americans account for 49 percent of the AIDS cases among IDUS; Hispanics, 23 percent; and whites, 26 percent.[12] African American IDUS are five times more likely to get AIDS than their white counterparts.[13] Ethnographic studies of IDUS living with HIV/AIDS describe them as "street drug abusers," the vast majority of whom are homeless, unemployed, or underemployed.[14] Many suffer from multiple physical dependencies on drugs and alcohol. These studies point to the vulnerability of the drug-dependent population and its frequent inability to meet its health care needs.

Blood-borne spread of HIV/AIDS has a cascading effect as infections are spread from IDUS to their sex and needle-sharing partners and to the children of HIV-infected mothers. Among women, 55 percent of the cumulative number of AIDS cases are IDUS or sex partners of IDUS.[15] The connection between pediatric AIDS and drug use is just as significant: 52 percent of the cumulative total of pediatric AIDS cases result from a mother who either was an IDU or had sexual relations with an IDU.[16] AIDS is the leading cause of death among Hispanic children under five in New York City; it is the second leading cause of death among African American children.[17] These data suggest that drug use— the use of crack among women, trading drugs for sex,[18] and needle sharing among heroin and cocaine users—is perhaps the most important catalyst for the spread of HIV throughout the population.[19] Approximately one-fourth of all the newly reported AIDS cases in 2001 were estimated to occur among IDUS.[20]

Provision of sterile injection equipment and community outreach are associated with lower incidences of HIV infection among IDUS.[21] Research suggests that SEPS helped to lower the rates of needle sharing in North America,[22] Europe,[23] and Australia;[24] provide a source of referrals for social services, health care, and drug treatment;[25] and offer a forum for testing, health education, and distribution of condoms.[26]

Reviews of the accumulated scientific data conclude that increased access to sterile drug-injection equipment is an effective component of a comprehensive strategy to prevent HIV and other blood-borne infectious diseases. Public health programs that offer sterile equipment, moreover, help bring difficult-to-reach populations into systems of care that offer drug dependency counseling, mental health treatment, medical advice, and support services.[27] More importantly, no credible evidence has been found that access to sterile syringes increases drug use.[28]

Legal Restrictions on Access to Sterile Drug-Injection Equipment

Everybody carried their works on them, until the head of the narcotics squad in Philadelphia finally got what he wanted, and they could lock you up for a mark. See, you could have a pin mark on you from where you stuck yourself from fixin' a button on your shirt, and, if they took you down and the doctor said that was a needle mark, you were a positive drug addict and you got time in Philadelphia. And don't get caught with no paraphernalia on you, or you're going to jail anyhow, whether you have a mark or not. All of this happened in the early forties. That's when addicts started leaving their works, or hiding their works somewhere. — Dusty, Addicts Who Survived (1989)

In light of the serious health impact of needle-borne disease and the scientific conclusions that legal availability of sterile injection equipment can reduce the spread of infection without increasing the use of drugs, it is important to understand the precise effects of current laws. Government has a responsibility to ensure that law enforcement does not undermine safe and effective prevention programs for the control of infectious diseases; it has a similar responsibility to ensure that public health measures do not unwittingly contribute to the use of illicit drugs.

The sharing of drug-injection equipment is a highly complicated behavior. It involves the direct sharing of needles and syringes between members of friendship or sex groups, anonymous sharing of pooled injection equipment in shooting galleries, and indirect sharing where drug paraphernalia, such as the cooker, cotton, and rinse water, are commonly used by the group to prepare drugs for injection. The reasons for sharing are equally complex. Sharing be-

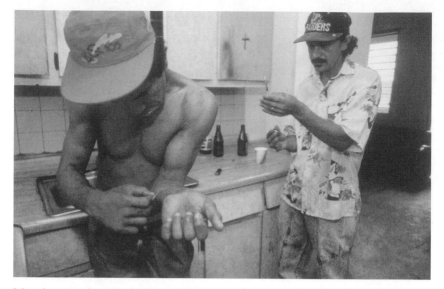

Men shoot up drugs in their home in Puerto Rico, 1993. Since the epidemic began, injection drug use has directly and indirectly accounted for more than one-third (35 percent) of AIDS cases in the United States. Of the 42,983 new cases of AIDS reported in 2001, 10,461 (24 percent) were IDU-associated. (CDC, September 2002; © *National Geographic*)

havior was originally reported as part of the subculture and routines of the drug world; it represented an initiation into drug use and a social bonding mechanism.[29] However, sharing is not merely part of the unfathomable world of drug subcultures but is principally caused by an artificially induced scarcity of injection equipment. Drug users commonly report that they share because of a limited supply of sterile needles and syringes.[30] This scarcity can deny IDUS a realistic opportunity to engage in safer behavior.

The limited supply of sterile injection equipment is the result of a conscious policy choice by government as part of its drug control strategy. Several inter-related legislative and regulatory provisions have the effect of systematically restricting the availability of syringes: state and municipal drug paraphernalia laws, the federal Mail Order Drug Paraphernalia Control Act, state syringe prescription laws, and regulations governing pharmacies.

Drug possession laws, although they do not explicitly regulate drug-injection equipment, are also relevant. Almost all states make it an offense to possess any measurable amount of an illegal drug.[31] Thus, IDUS could be prosecuted for the minute amount of drug residue that remains in a syringe that has been used for drug injection—for example, the traces of narcotic left in the barrel of a syringe. Under these laws, used syringes may help legally justify a search for drugs and possible arrest. The fear of prosecution may deter IDUs from possessing syringes.

In *Doe v. Bridgeport Police Department*, the clients of SEPs and legal pharmacy purchasers in Connecticut challenged prosecution based on drug residue found in a used syringe. The plaintiffs argued that such prosecutions were illegal under the state laws that had liberalized syringe access. The federal court held that the syringe access law not only eliminated criminal penalties for possessing fewer than thirty-one needles, but also necessarily decriminalized possession of any trace amounts of drug in the used syringe.[32]

A federal court in New York also upheld the "right to legally possess used hypodermic needles or syringes . . . containing a drug residue in the course of participating in a state-authorized needle exchange program."[33] In resolving the conflict between New York's penal law and public health law, the judge recognized that, to prevent the spread of HIV, needle exchange programs demanded that participants return used needles to the program and thus forced participants to carry syringes contaminated with drugs.[34]

Criminalizing the possession of trace amounts of narcotics within decriminalized, previously used hypodermic syringes and needles would thwart the public health purpose behind syringe exchange legislation. Such a policy discourages would-be SEP participants from transporting previously used injection equipment to the exchange and encourages all IDUs to hastily and likely improperly abandon now-easily-obtainable injection equipment after one use to avoid arrest.

Legal rules, of course, are not unequivocal and self-executing. The language of statutes and regulations is complemented by decisions by police in making arrests, prosecutors in charging IDUs, judges in sentencing and interpreting the law, and politicians in supporting or opposing public health activities.[35]

Drug Paraphernalia Laws

Drug paraphernalia laws followed the precipitous growth of the drug paraphernalia industry.[36] The industry began in "the late 1960's with the sale of cigarette rolling papers to drug-using college students and American GI's for 'rolling their own' marijuana."[37] As cocaine and other drug use increased, manufacturers developed accessories tailored to their use. By 1976 drug paraphernalia had become an estimated $3 billion industry. Nationwide, approximately 15,000–30,000 retail establishments known as "head shops" catered to persons seeking drug paraphernalia. As the industry expanded, numerous drug paraphernalia publications emerged; they ranged from pamphlets and books such as *The Co-*

caine Consumer's Handbook and *The Great Book of Hashish* to magazines like *Head, Rush, Stone Age, HiLife,* and *High Times.*

In an era where drug use was celebrated by the young and entrepreneurs openly flouted drug control efforts, drug paraphernalia laws appeared to be reasonable. Law enforcement and community leaders surmised that limiting the availability of drug paraphernalia would deny drug sellers and users the tools of their trade. Notably, the drug paraphernalia industry was the only interest group that opposed government restrictions, arguing that paraphernalia did not cause drug abuse. Inexplicably absent from the debate—both legislative and judicial—was a public health perspective on the effect that this legislation might have on the blood-borne transmission of disease.

Throughout the 1960s and 1970s, against the backdrop of concern about illegal drugs, states and municipalities enacted drug paraphernalia laws. Many legislatures drafted broadly worded statutes that would comprehensively cover various drug paraphernalia. Some of these statutes prohibited the mere possession of the "instruments of a crime."[38] Retailers and manufacturers responded by challenging the constitutionality of these early drug paraphernalia laws. The courts found that imprecisely worded laws encompassing an array of paraphernalia were unconstitutionally vague and overly broad.[39] To cure the constitutional flaws, in 1979, at the request of President Jimmy Carter, the Justice Department's Drug Enforcement Administration promulgated the Model Drug Paraphernalia Act (MDPA). Moreover, the Supreme Court advanced the trend toward comprehensive drug paraphernalia laws by upholding the constitutionality of broadly worded local laws that were not based on the MDPA.[40]

Drug paraphernalia statutes ban the manufacture, sale, distribution, possession, or advertising of a wide range of devices if knowledge exists that they may be used to introduce illicit substances into the body. The statutes typically define drug paraphernalia to include all equipment, products, and materials of any kind that are used to "manufacture, inject, ingest, inhale, or otherwise introduce into the human body a controlled substance."[41] They also provide an exemplary list of items such as "hypodermic syringes, needles, and other objects used, intended for use, and designed for use in parenterally injecting controlled substances into the human body."[42] Under this definition, the status of any item as paraphernalia depends not just on the characteristics of the item itself but also on the intention or acts of the defendant. To commit a crime, the seller must not only transfer possession of the syringe, but must do so knowing of the intended drug-related use.[43] The statute is not violated if the drug-injection equipment is sold without knowledge that it will be used to inject illegal drugs. Thus, a pharmacist who sells hypodermic syringes and needles over

Exempts Some or All Syringes (9)	Exempts Some Types of Sellers (9)	Omits Reference to Syringes or Injections (5)	Other Significant Exemption (6)
CT	CA (MDs & pharmacists)	CO	IA (syringes sold for "lawful purpose")
IN (items customarily used to inject lawful substances)	GA (pharmacists)	MI	LA (items for medical use)
ME	HI (MDs, pharmacists, and health care institutions)	NV	
MN		SC	MA (does not criminalize paraphernalia possession)
NH	MT (MDs and pharmacists)	WY	
NY (syringes legally obtained from pharmacy or SEP)	NM (pharmacists)		MI (does not criminalize paraphernalia possession)
OR	OH (MDs and pharmacists)		SC (does not cover items used with heroin)
RI	TN (MDs and pharmacists)		
WI	WA (pharmacists)		VA (does not criminalize paraphernalia possession)
	WV (licensees such as pharmacists)		

Source: Scott Burris, Steffanie A. Strathdee, and Jon S. Vernick, Syringe Access Law in the United States: A State of the Art Assessment of Law and Policy (Washington, D.C., and Baltimore: Center for Law and the Public's Health at Georgetown University Law Center and Johns Hopkins University, 2002).

the counter, believing that the purchaser is an insulin-dependent diabetic, commits no offense under drug paraphernalia laws.

Forty-nine states and the District of Columbia have enacted drug paraphernalia laws; only Alaska has no statewide statute. The broad wording of such laws led early commentators to conclude that they uniformly forbade syringe sale to, and possession by, IDUs. Scott Burris, Steffanie Strathdee, and Jon Vernick, however, have shown that there are small but important differences among state statutes.[44] Some states have fully or partially deregulated syringes as a public health measure or have provisions that, at least on paper, make it legal for an IDU to purchase a syringe (see Table 14-1).

Nine state paraphernalia laws explicitly or implicitly exclude syringes in at least some quantity. Indiana, for example, exempts items "historically and customarily used in connection with the . . . injecting . . . of . . . lawful substance[s]."[45] In nine states, pharmacists and in some instances other health care professionals are exempt from the law. Five state statutes do not mention injection or syringes explicitly, thus departing from the language of the MDPA. Although the broad definition of paraphernalia could be reasonably deemed to include syringes, a judge could read the statute more narrowly.

Drug paraphernalia laws have detrimental effects on the population's health. Public health officials, community-based organizations, and health care professionals may feel deterred by the potential sweep of these laws. The variability in the statutory language may slightly open the door to greater freedom in distributing injection equipment, but the prospect of legal penalties remains a serious public health problem.

The Federal Mail Order Drug Paraphernalia Control Act

The Mail Order Drug Paraphernalia Control Act (Mail Order Act), proposed by Representative Mel Levine of California in 1985, made it a federal felony to sell "drug paraphernalia in interstate and foreign commerce, through use of the Postal Service or other interstate conveyance or in importation or exportation of drug paraphernalia."[46] At the time, the MDPA was being hailed as a great success. But efforts to control drug paraphernalia on the state level led to a federal problem: as local head shops were being closed, federal mail-order businesses opened. The paraphernalia formerly sold through head shops were now available via mail-order catalogs or through classified advertising in certain publications.

The Mail Order Act was passed at the peak of the HIV epidemic in 1986.[47] Remarkably, despite the potential health effects of legislation restricting access to sterile injection equipment during the HIV epidemic, not a single public health voice was heard during congressional hearings.[48] Moreover, federal courts that subsequently reviewed the act expressed no reservations about the health consequences.[49]

The federal Mail Order Drug Paraphernalia Control Act, passed as part of the Anti-Drug Abuse Act of 1986, was expanded in 1990.[50] It prohibits the sale and transportation of drug paraphernalia, including syringes, in interstate commerce. The act also authorizes seizure and forfeiture of drug paraphernalia. The U.S. Supreme Court in *Posters 'N' Things, Ltd. v. United States* upheld the constitutionality of the Mail Order Act against a challenge that it was unduly vague.[51]

The terms of the Mail Order Act make it uncertain whether it regulates physician prescription or pharmacist dispensing of syringes to IDUs[52] The statute does not consider syringes provided by "legitimate suppliers" with "legitimate uses . . . in the community" to be drug paraphernalia.[53] It also relies on scientific evidence to determine whether an object is drug paraphernalia.

Nevertheless, the importance of the Mail Order Act is its introduction of federal jurisdiction in an area traditionally reserved for the states.[54] State legislatures and law enforcers, in deference to public health, may permit greater access to drug-injection equipment. This would not, however, preclude a decision by federal authorities to vigorously enforce the Mail Order Act. Since virtually all syringes pass through interstate commerce, it is possible that federal enforcement authorities would have the power to prosecute many activities relating to the exchange and possession of drug paraphernalia, irrespective of state enforcement decisions. Consequently, the public health approach to blood-borne disease requires federal as well as state cooperation.

Syringe Prescription Laws

The hypodermic syringe shares with the stethoscope the distinction of being almost a symbol of the practicing physician. There must be few people with access to medical care who have not received a hypodermic injection to protect them from disease or to give rapid relief from pain. . . . The main advantages of this method of administering drugs, which takes its name from the Greek words meaning under the skin, are that the active principles are quickly absorbed into the bloodstream from the subcutaneous tissue and that they are not altered or destroyed by the digestive juices.—Norman Howard-Jones, The Origins of Hypodermic Medication (1971)

In the United States, drug policy creating an artificial scarcity of sterile syringes can be traced to the mid-nineteenth through the early twentieth century. Hypodermic syringes, developed in the 1850s, were commonly used in medical practice by the 1870s. Their development and use coincided with a dramatic increase in the consumption of opiates, which were freely dispensed by physicians and pharmacists to treat a myriad of conditions (e.g., anxiety, cholera, food poisoning, and parasites).[55] A growing fear of the dangers of opiate addiction and other drug use eventually led to public demand that physicians be prohibited from freely dispensing narcotics.[56] The medical profession objected, reportedly reacting with "fear that the state would dominate the practice of medicine."[57]

Such was the environment in which New York State enacted a syringe prescription law as part of the Boylan-Town Act of 1914.[58] The act sought to reduce drug addiction by restricting access to narcotic drugs and the instruments necessary to administer them through five avenues of action: prevent pharmacists from dispensing narcotics or syringes to persons who did not hold a valid medical prescription; require physicians to issue prescriptions only after physically examining the patient; limit pharmacy and physician discretion in refilling narcotic prescriptions; mandate record-keeping of retail transactions for five years; and authorize revoking professional licenses for violations.[59] Other states followed suit, adopting prescription laws primarily to prevent drug abuse.[60] Many states that enacted syringe prescription laws—and those that have them still—have the most daunting problems with drug abuse.[61]

Syringe prescription laws proscribe the dispensing or possession of a syringe without a valid medical prescription. These laws differ from drug paraphernalia laws in that criminal intent is not required for a violation. Thus, in a state with a syringe prescription law, a pharmacist who dispenses a syringe without a prescription need not know that the buyer intends to use the syringe to inject illegal drugs; the very act of selling or dispensing the syringe without a prescription constitutes a violation. In this sense, prescription laws potentially encompass many more transactions than paraphernalia laws.

Twelve states have statutes prohibiting the dispensing of hypodermic needles and syringes without a valid medical prescription.[62] A thirteenth state, Michigan, does not have a syringe prescription law, but some of its cities and counties have ordinances that prohibit the sale of syringes without a prescription. (See Table 14-2.) In addition, Pennsylvania requires a medical prescription by regulation. Syringe prescription requirements pose a significant public health problem in only six of these states: California, Delaware, Illinois, Massachusetts, New Jersey, and Pennsylvania. In Florida and Virginia, a prescription is required only for minors; in Nevada, a favorable view of syringe sales from the pharmacy board has reportedly led to reasonably liberal syringe access in the state. The remaining four prescription law states—Connecticut, New Hampshire, Maine, and New York—have partially deregulated syringe sales and now allow nonprescription sale and possession of syringes in limited amounts (see Table 14-2 and Map 14-1). Courts have upheld the constitutionality of syringe prescription laws against public health challenges.[63] Other courts have held that the defendant bears the burden of proving by a preponderance of evidence that the hypodermic instrument was obtained legally.[64]

To limit physicians' and pharmacists' discretion in dispersing syringes, most syringe prescription laws require a "legitimate medical purpose." The "legitimate medical purpose" doctrine strengthens the regulatory effect of syringe prescription laws through dual mechanisms. First, the doctrine holds that a prescription is invalid unless it has been issued in good faith for a therapeutic

TABLE 14-2. State Syringe Prescription Statutes and Regulations, 2002

State	Sold at Pharmacy Only	Prescription Required	Information on Purpose Required	Record Keeping by Pharmacists Required	Syringe Purchasers Required to Show Identification	Display Limits
AL	S					
CA	S	S (except for use with insulin or adrenaline)		S (date and time of sale; type, size, and quantity of syringe; and signature of the pharmacist)	S (name, address, signature, and ID of purchaser required for nonprescription sales)	S
CT	S	S (for > 10 only)		S (prescriptions must be retained on file for not less than 3 years)		S
DE		S		S (date of sale, description of instrument sold, and prescription on file)	S (name, age, and address of purchaser)	S
FL		S (for sale to minors only)				
GA	R		R (no sale if seller has reasonable cause to believe syringe will be used for an "unlawful purpose")			R
IL	S	S		S (date of sale and desription of the instrument)	S (name and address of purchaser)	

Table 14.2 (continued)

State	Sold at Pharmacy Only	Prescription Required	Information on Purpose Required	Record Keeping by Pharmacists Required	Syringe Purchasers Required to Show Identification	Display Limits
IN	R			R (name and quantity of device, date of purchase, and name or initials of pharmacist who dispensed the device)	R (unknown purchasers must show ID)	
KY			S (pharmacists must determine purchaser's planned use of syringes)	S (purchaser name and address, quantity of syringes purchased, date, purpose)	S (ID)	S
LA	R		R (pharmacist must determine bona fide medical purpose)	R (date, item, quantity, and signature of pharmacist)	R (purchaser's name, address, and ID)	R
MA	S	S		S (date of sale and description of instrument and signature of pharmacist shall be recorded on face of prescription)	S (name and address of purchaser)	S
MD	R		R (sales shall be made in good faith by pharmacists to purchasers showing indication of need)	R (date of sale, item, quantity sold, and signature of pharmacist)	R (purchaser's name, address, and proper identification must be provided)	
ME	S	S (for > 10 only)			S (purchaser must be over 17 years old)	

Table 14.2 (continued)

State	Sold at Pharmacy Only	Prescription Required	Infomation on Purpose Required	Record Keeping by Pharmacists Required	Syringe Purchasers Required to Show Identification	Display Limits
MN	S					
NH	S	S (for > 10 only)		S (date of sale and number of instruments sold shall be recorded on prescription)		
NJ	S	S		S (date of sale recorded on prescription)		
NV	S	S (Except for asthma or diabetes)				
NY	S	S (for > 10 only)		S & R (date of sale recorded and signature of pharmacist)		
OH	S (and authorized dealers)		S (Seller must know or reasonably believe that purchaser is not an unauthorized user)			S
PA		R				
RI	S	S				S

Table 14.2 (continued)

State	Sold at Pharmacy Only	Prescription Required	Information on Purpose Required	Record Keeping by Pharmacists Required	Syringe Purchasers Required to Show Identification	Display Limits
SC			R (pharmacists must obtain written or oral affirmation that sale is for a legitimate medical use)	R (type and quantity of needles/syringes sold)	R (signature, address, sex, age, and ID)	R
TN	R		R (proof of medical need)			
VA	S	S (for minors over 16 only)	S (purchaser must furnish written legitimate purpose)	S (date of sale, name, quantity, and price of device)	S (name, address, and ID, including proof of age)	R
WA			S (pharmacist must be satisfied that device is for a "legal use")			
WV	R					
Total	20	13	9	14	11	11

R = requirement imposed by regulation

S = requirement imposed by statute

Source: Scott Burris, Steffanie A. Strathdee, and Jon S. Vernick, Syringe Access Law in the United States: A State of the Art Assessment of Law and Policy (Washington, D.C., and Baltimore: Center for Law and the Public's Health at Georgetown University Law Center and Johns Hopkins University, 2002).

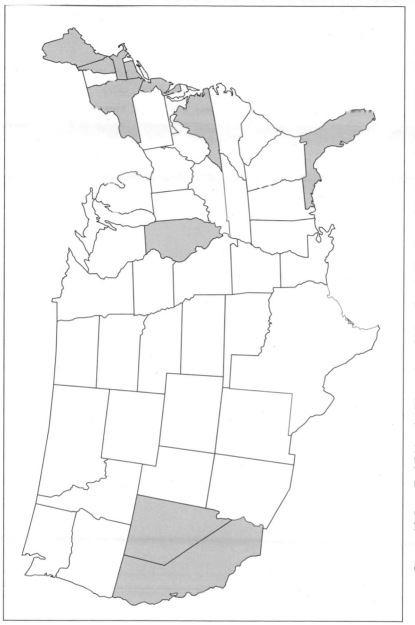

MAP 14-1. States with Laws Prohibiting the Dispensing of Hypodermic Needles and Syringes without a Valid Medical Prescription

purpose. Physicians have been convicted or have had their licenses revoked for improperly prescribing drugs or drug paraphernalia.[65] Second, the laws in some states require pharmacists to document syringe and needle sales, together with the intended medical purpose.[66]

Physicians and other health professionals who prescribe syringes, or directly assist IDUS in injection practices, face potentially dire legal consequences. Several courts have held that physicians who issue prescriptions for "nonmedical purposes" are not acting in the course of a professional duty, and at least one court has held that issuing a prescription to an addict "for the purpose of maintaining his or her habit" does not constitute a prescription within the meaning of public health law.[67] Syringe prescription statutes pose a conflict between law and medical ethics.[68] The law criminalizes the physician for writing a prescription even if the intention is to reduce the risk of blood-borne transmission of HIV. Medical ethics, however, requires physicians to do everything possible to safeguard the health and well-being of their patients.[69]

Pharmacy Regulations and Practice Guidelines

Pharmacy regulations are established under state law by pharmacy boards or other governmental agencies, such as the Department of Consumer Protection, the Department of Health, or the Department of Drug Control. Pharmacists are legally required to comply with the rules regulating the sale of syringes. In addition, state pharmacy boards typically establish practice guidelines. Although these guidelines lack the force of law, a pharmacist who fails to comply with them could be found civilly liable under state tort law or be subject to professional sanction.[70] Legal and public health scholars are beginning to recognize the significance of pharmacy regulations and practice guidelines in restricting access to sterile injection equipment. Over-the-counter sales of syringes were at one time thought to be regulated by syringe prescription laws in only a small minority of states, primarily in the Northeast and California. Now it is generally understood that legal restrictions on syringe access are far more extensive.

Pharmacy regulations or guidelines significantly affect the practices of pharmacists in dispensing syringes in a majority of states. First, these rules or guidelines may prevent pharmacists from dispensing syringes if they have knowledge that the syringes will be used to inject illegal drugs. For example, they often require the seller to determine, or the buyer to produce information about, the use to which the syringes will be put. Second, they often restrict the display of syringes in retail establishments, normally requiring that they be kept behind the counter. Third, and importantly, they frequently require that persons buying syringes present identification or record their name and address in a record book kept by the pharmacist. The effect of these regulations or guidelines, then, may be to discourage IDUS from buying syringes over the counter for fear that their names and addresses will be kept and perhaps sent to government health or criminal justice officials. Thus, even if drug paraphernalia or syringe prescription laws are not an issue in some states, pharmacy regulations and guidelines may create obstacles to the purchase and sale of sterile injection equipment.

This discussion reveals a pervasive network of laws, regulations, and practice guidelines that severely restrict the sale and possession of sterile drug-injection equipment. Forty-nine states and the District of Columbia have drug paraphernalia statutes or local ordinances; only Alaska has not enacted such provisions. Twelve states have statutes that require a prescription for the purchase of syringes; in five of them, the legal problem for IDUS is particularly acute. Numerous other states have regulations that restrict the sale and purchase of syringes in pharmacies.

The Chilling Effects of Legal Restrictions on Sterile Syringes and Needles

Because I obtain my morphine supplies from bottles of kaolin purchased in sundry chemists (if the bottles sit for long enough most of the morphine rises to the top), the stuff still contains an appreciable amount of chalk. Months of injecting have given my body an odd aspect. With every shot, more chalk has been deposited along the walls of my veins, much in the manner of earth being piled up to form an embankment or a cutting around a roadway, mapping out the history of my addiction....

I have been driven to using huge five millilitre barrels, each one fitted with the long, blue-collared needles necessary for hitting the arteries. Should I miss, the consequences for my circulatory system could be disastrous. I might lose a limb; there could be tailbacks. I wonder sometimes if I may be losing my incident room.—Will Self, *Scale* (1993)

Legal restrictions on access to sterile injection equipment present formidable obstacles to public health promotion and disease prevention. These restrictions make it much more difficult for pharmacists to sell syringes over the counter, pose a chilling effect on IDUS seeking to comply with public health advice, and place significant obstacles in the way of public health authorities and community activists in exchanging injection equipment.

Pharmacy Sales of Syringes

Pharmacy syringe sales, capable of reducing risky injecting behavior, have been found to be more cost-effective than syringe exchange programs and can reach IDUs in areas that cannot sustain an SEP.[71] A study in Baltimore found that if legal restrictions were lifted, pharmacies would be a viable source of syringes, particularly for women.[72] Under New York's Expanded Syringe Access Demonstration Program, pharmacies have in fact become an important source of sterile injection equipment.[73]

Yet prescription statutes prohibit pharmacists from selling syringes to customers who are unable to produce a medical prescription. Drug paraphernalia statutes prohibit pharmacists from selling syringes with knowledge that they will be used for the injection of illicit drugs. Finally, pharmacy regulations require pharmacists to obtain proof of medical need, to ask the customer personal questions, or to maintain a registry of buyers. The law, therefore, may prevent pharmacists from playing an active role in the prevention of blood-borne disease.[74]

Pharmacists retain considerable discretion in deciding whether they will sell injection equipment and to whom they will sell it, leading to wide variations in syringe availability.[75] Biases against, for example, racial minorities, young people, or the homeless potentially can limit the opportunities for IDUs to purchase syringes at pharmacies.[76] Professional training of pharmacists in providing sterile syringes and condoms, and in referring people for education and counseling, is an important part of a comprehensive prevention strategy.[77]

Drug User Compliance with Public Health Advice

Even the simple act of counseling IDUs to possess new syringes or to sterilize their equipment can result in legal problems. The IDU who complies with public health advice can be prosecuted for possessing drug-injection equipment. An IDU is unlikely to be able to demonstrate a valid medical reason for possessing a syringe and so is likely to be found in violation of both needle prescription and drug paraphernalia laws. Sometimes IDUs are arrested for carrying syringes or even bottles of bleach.[78]

It may appear peculiar that IDUs would be dissuaded from carrying sterile injection equipment when they are engaged in far more serious criminal behavior. From the IDU's perspective, however, laws penalizing the possession of syringes are a serious concern. Drug users arrested on a drug paraphernalia charge are identified by police and subject to fines and possible incarceration. Moreover, this may invite more intense police surveillance and make it more difficult to avoid arrest and prosecution for future offenses. Police are more apt to search for illicit drugs once they find that a person is in possession of drug paraphernalia. Indeed, possession of a syringe and needle, or even bleach, may provide probable cause under the Fourth Amendment for a wider search of drug users and their personal property.

Drug users are well aware of the consequences of paraphernalia laws. Ethnographic studies have vividly shown that IDUs fear detection while in possession of drug-injection equipment and often fail to carry syringes because of local enforcement of these laws.[79] Paraphernalia laws, therefore, create a marked disincentive for IDUs to have sterile injection equipment on their person when they go to places where they buy or inject drugs. It is precisely at this time that users need sterile syringes and needles. To arrest and prosecute an IDU for following the safer injection practices encouraged and aided by the health department undermines the public's health.

The Lawfulness of Syringe Exchange Programs

SEPs provide sterile syringes in exchange for used syringes to reduce the transmission of blood-borne infections. Just as important, they serve as community-based prevention and health promotion centers for IDUs. SEPs offer male and female condoms, education and counseling, vaccinations, STD screening, and referral to health care programs, including substance abuse treatment.[80]

The lawfulness of SEPs is uncertain because of the lack of legal clarity in many jurisdictions; several legal surveys have been undertaken but are likely outdated.[81] The most recent study from the Center for Law and the Public's Health divides SEPs into four categories: specifically authorized by state law, specifically authorized by local law, no applicable law making SEPs unlawful, and SEPs operating without a specific claim of legal authority (see Table 14-3).[82]

The District of Columbia and nine states explicitly recognize SEPs (Connecticut, Hawaii, Maine, Maryland, New Mexico, Rhode Island, and Vermont) or authorize local governments to do so (California and Massachusetts). In New York, SEPs are authorized by the commissioner of health exercising power granted in the paraphernalia law.[83] In Washington State, local health officials secured a declaratory judgment from the state supreme court,[84] a ruling that was later codified by the legislature (see Table 14-3).

SEPs in three cities (Philadelphia, Cleveland, and Chicago) are authorized by local government without explicit permission from the state.[85] In five states

TABLE 14-3. Legal Status of Syringe Exchange Programs, 2002

SEP Authorized by State Law (13)	SEP Authorized by Local Government Based on Its Interpretation of State Law (3)	Free Distribution of Syringes Not Restricted by State Law (5)	SEP (s) Operating Without Specific Claim to Legality, 1998 (19)
CA, CT, DC, HI, MA, MD, ME, NH, NM, NY, RI, VT, WA	IL, OH, PA	AK, LA, OR, RI, WI	AZ, CO, GA, IN, KS, MA, MI, MN, MT, NC, NJ, NY, OK, PA, PR, TN, TX, UT, WA

Source: Scott Burris, Steffanie A. Strathdee, and Jon S. Vernick, *Syringe Access Law in the United States: A State of the Art Assessment of Law and Policy* (Washington, D.C., and Baltimore: Center for Law and the Public's Health at Georgetown University Law Center and Johns Hopkins University, 2002).

(Alaska, Louisiana, Oregon, Rhode Island, and Wisconsin), there are no relevant laws prohibiting syringe distribution, so SEPs are probably lawful.

In nineteen states, SEPs operate without a specific claim of legal authority.[86] Where there is no explicit authorization, the lawfulness of SEPs depends on the provisions in syringe prescription, drug paraphernalia, and pharmacy practice laws.

Restrictions on the Use of Federal Funds for Syringe Exchange

Since 1988, Congress has enacted numerous statutes that contain provisions prohibiting or restricting the use of federal funds for SEPs and their activities. The ban applies regardless of the lawfulness of the SEP. For some time, annual federal appropriations statutes have contained restrictions for funding SEPs.[87] The U.S. General Accounting Office concluded that the Department of Health and Human Services (HHS) is authorized to conduct demonstration and research projects involving the provision of syringes but is prohibited from using certain funds to support SEPs directly; this may prevent HHS from funding ancillary support services provided by SEPs.[88] Accordingly, SEPs must rely on state, local, or philanthropic funds for their operations, which is problematic given their uncertain legal status.

Under current law, before the federal government can fund SEPs, the secretary of health and human services must find that the programs effectively prevent the spread of HIV and do not encourage the use of illegal drugs. The National Academy of Sciences recommended that the surgeon general make such a determination.[89] An NIH consensus panel concurred: "An impressive body of evidence suggests powerful effects from needle exchange programs. . . . Can the opposition to needle exchange programs in the United States be justified on scientific grounds? Our answer is simple and emphatic—no. Studies show reduction in risk behavior as high as 80 percent, with estimates of a 30 percent or greater reduction of HIV in IDUS. The cost of such programs is relatively low."[90] The secretary of HHS determined that SEPs probably reduce the risk of blood-borne infections and do not encourage illicit drug use. Nevertheless, the secretary declined to authorize federal funding for SEPs, despite specific authority to do so.[91]

Judicial Declaration of Lawfulness

Public health and law enforcement are frequently unable to agree on which set of statutes takes precedence. Rather than having two government agencies engage in efforts that undermine the goals and programs of the other, it may be desirable to have the courts decide which set of laws should be enforced. Courts have the power to declare the lawfulness of SEPs, but much depends on judges' views concerning drug control and AIDS prevention in a particular jurisdiction. In two cases in Washington State, the courts affirmed the power of health officials to establish SEPs. In the first case, the Tacoma County Board of Health in January 1989 voted to formally endorse and fund a syringe exchange that had been conducted by a community activist. In July of that year, the state attorney general issued an opinion that the program violated the state's drug paraphernalia law. A court issued a declaratory judgment that the SEP did not violate the law, as that statute provided an exemption from liability for government officials who were engaged in the lawful performance of their duties.[92] The court also noted that Washington's AIDS statute authorized local programs to prevent needle-borne HIV.[93]

In the second case, the Spokane County Health District Board of Health in July 1990 adopted a resolution directing its health officer to set up an SEP. However, the state prosecuting attorney stated that he would authorize the prosecution of SEP clients. The state supreme court declared the SEP program to be lawful. Although the legislature had not explicitly authorized such programs, it had enacted an Omnibus AIDS Act that empowered the health department to prevent the spread of needle-borne HIV infection. The health department also possessed broad constitutional public health powers that included all reasonable activities to stop the spread of HIV/AIDS.[94] This case illustrates the inherent powers of health departments to take reasoned actions in defense of public health.

Programs that would otherwise be criminal may be upheld if they are ordered in accordance with public health laws.[95] It is by no means clear, however, that all state courts would support the supremacy of public health powers over prosecutory powers under drug paraphernalia laws. Even if the courts were to uphold the power of public health officials to establish SEPs in reliance on health and AIDS statutes, they could continue to permit enforcement of drug paraphernalia laws against the clients of such programs. It is, therefore, imperative to secure the cooperation of public health and law enforcement in the development of HIV prevention programs.

Toward a Synergistic Relationship between Public Health and Law Enforcement: Proposals for Law Reform

Public health and law enforcement authorities exist for similar reasons: to ensure the community's health and safety. It is desirable and possible for society and government to embrace both health and safety in ways that respect the moral force of each and do not undercut their efforts or enforcement. The regulation of drug paraphernalia can assist law enforcement in its attempt to prevent and punish the sale and use of illicit drugs, but it should not interfere with public health measures to prevent needle-borne disease. The regulation of drugs must be directed toward the criminal enterprise of importation, sale, and use of illegal drugs, not toward empirically valid public health activities (e.g., pharmacy sales and exchanges of sterile syringes and needles). To this end, syringe prescription statutes should be repealed or significantly modified, and drug paraphernalia statutes should focus on drug dealers and street sellers of syringes and needles rather than on public health officials, health care professionals, and SEP participants.

Public health,[96] medical,[97] and legal[98] organizations have all supported the deregulation of drug-injection equipment. Most laws, regulations, and practice guidelines that restrict the sale, possession, or distribution of syringes were promulgated before blood-borne diseases among IDUs were recognized as a pressing public health problem and without careful contemplation of the health implications. Since the laws were enacted, the dual epidemics of drug use and HIV/AIDS have produced illness and death, particularly among poor, urban, minority communities. Research indicates that many drug users will alter their behavior if given the opportunity and the means.[99] States that have deregulated access to drug-injection equipment have substantially reduced multiperson use of contaminated syringes, the primary factor in the blood-borne spread of infection.[100] Despite careful study, researchers have found no correlation between greater availability of syringes and increased drug use.[101] Moreover, since legal access to syringes, particularly through SEPs, affords greater opportunities for referral to drug treatment and counseling about the harms of drug use, SEPs and deregulation of syringes may facilitate, rather than hinder, drug control efforts. To harmonize the interests of law enforcement and public health, I propose the following legal reforms:

1. *Clarify the legitimate medical purposes of sterile syringes.* Unlike other forms of drug paraphernalia, sterile syringes serve a legitimate medical purpose beyond the administration of drugs: use of sterile syringes helps to protect the public health. Data suggest that possession and use of new syringes by IDUs promotes the valid medical purpose of preventing blood-borne diseases. Drawing a legal distinction between syringes and other drug paraphernalia would facilitate this medical objective in several ways. First, a legal distinction sanctioning the procurement and possession of sterile syringes would allow IDUs to access sterile equipment at the point at which they inject, the time at which they are most vulnerable for using contaminated equipment. Second, legal recognition of the unique medical advantages of sterile syringes would legitimize the practice of physicians and pharmacists who dispense sterile syringes in a good-faith exercise of their professional duties but fear criminal or professional repercussions. It would also clarify the law on which criminal justice and public health authorities rely, and align the law as written with its enforcement in practice. Finally, a legal distinction would eliminate the need for legal machinations to justify SEPs.

2. *Modify drug paraphernalia laws.* Drug paraphernalia laws should exempt authorized sellers, distributors, or possessors of syringes (e.g., pharmacists, physicians, public health officials, registered SEPs, and their patients/clients). Permitting IDUs to obtain syringes from reliable sources would enable them to comply with public health directives to use a new sterile syringe for each injection. Legislators, law enforcement officials, and community leaders should acknowledge that the criminal law is an inappropriate tool to wield against health professionals who are attempting to reduce the incidence of blood-borne disease by dispensing sterile injection equipment.

With this reform, the law could justifiably continue to criminalize the unauthorized sale of drug paraphernalia by drug dealers, shooting galleries, head shops, and mail-order firms. From an economic perspective, unauthorized sellers ought not to profit from the sale of drug paraphernalia. From a public health perspective, unauthorized sellers remain dubious sources of sterile injection equipment where, in an environment of limited supply and continuing demand for needles and syringes, they reportedly repackage contaminated syringes and sell them as new.

3. *Repeal syringe prescription laws.* Repealing syringe prescription laws would legalize over-the-counter sales of syringes in pharmacies and would promote several public health benefits. This legislative reform would enable IDUs and the public to secure sterile equipment for safer injections, free physicians and pharmacists from risking criminal liability or professional sanctions simply for prescribing or dispensing syringes for a legitimate medical purpose, and allow pharmacists to participate in public health efforts by educating and counseling customers about safer sex and drug-injection practices.

Rigidly regulating physician and pharmacist prescription and retail sales is counterproductive. If permitted to perform within the scope of their professional practices, physicians and pharmacists could assist drug users in adopting safer injection techniques and could serve as a link to drug treatment and education.

Medical and pharmacy boards would retain the authority to sanction unprofessional behavior (e.g., physicians or pharmacists who improperly encourage or assist the illicit sale or use of drugs). Moreover, legalizing over-the-counter sale of syringes constitutes one of the most cost-effective means of increasing syringe availability.[102] Pharmacies are well-suited distribution points for injection equipment. Their extensive network, diverse locations, hours of operation, and professional resources would help ensure wide access to supplies and expertise. Furthermore, over-the-counter syringe sales would remain within the private sector, so the state itself would neither be involved in distributing nor incur the cost of drug-injection equipment.

4. *Repeal restrictive pharmacy regulations and practice guidelines.* The repeal of restrictive pharmacy regulations and practice guidelines would enable IDUs and the general public to obtain sterile syringes more readily. States should repeal onerous regulations and guidelines that require purchasers to present prescriptions or other proof of legitimate medical need, to proffer identification, or to sign a register prior to buying sterile injection equipment. Arguably reasonable on their face, these regulations and guidelines

impede both pharmacists and their clients in transactions involving sterile equipment. Reasonable practice guidelines should be retained to maintain high professional standards and to ensure appropriate and exclusive
display of injection instruments in retail pharmacies.

5. *Promote and fund professional training.* Professional training for pharmacists,
other health professionals, and criminal justice personnel would advance
public health goals. Successful implementation of this proposal rests on
the active participation of professionals in each of these disciplines. For
instance, educating pharmacists about the transmission of blood-borne
infections would equip them to make well-informed decisions about the
sale of syringes. In addition, the pharmacist's role need not be limited to
distribution of sterile syringes. Ideally, pharmacies could offer or refer
customers for education and counseling on safer drug-injection and sexual practices, and assist in safely disposing of used syringes. Informing
criminal justice personnel about public health prevention strategies would
prepare them to direct IDUs to appropriate programs. Instructing health
care professionals about blood-borne infections would enable them to
offer the best preventive education to IDUs.

6. *Permit local discretion in establishing SEPs.* Allowing public health officials to establish SEPs would augment the public health arsenal to prevent blood-
borne diseases. Many communities have found SEPs to be an essential element in a comprehensive HIV prevention program. Local health officials
are best situated to assess the community's response to, and the potential
effectiveness of, such a program. Moreover, ample data have been collected to satisfy the statutory requirements for permitting federal funding
of SEPs (e.g., reduction in the incidence of HIV and absence of evidence
of increased drug use). Federal funds for SEPs would inject needed resources into state and local HIV prevention programs, help SEPs secure
matching funds from philanthropic sources, and assure SEP operators and
clients of the legality and long-term stability of the programs.

7. *Design programs for safe syringe disposal.* Programs that ensure the safe disposal of used drug-injection equipment would decrease dissemination of
contaminated syringes—either shared or discarded—and reduce health
risks to the public. Although many syringe prescription laws dictate safe
disposal, rarely do these laws specify the parties responsible for initiating
or implementing such schemes. Public health officials, health care professionals, and pharmacists are well situated to collaborate in designing and
directing effective programs for safe syringe disposal.

Conclusion: Harmonizing Perspectives on Drug Use and HIV/AIDS

Too often the public health perspective discounts the legitimate concerns of the community and law enforcement about the moral and social aspects of drug use. Some communities are understandably threatened by proposals to improve IDUS' access to drug-injection equipment (e.g., through deregulation of SEPS or syringe sales). Law enforcement officials and church, school, and community leaders may believe that allowing access to sterile injection equipment conveys the wrong message, promotes initiation into drug use, and accelerates the disintegration of families. Residents and business owners may fear increased street crime, lower property values, and heightened health risks from discarded syringes. A considerable amount of careful research, however, does not support these conclusions.

To the contrary, the data indicate that the restriction of access to sterile injection equipment has produced unnecessary illness and death. The prevailing policy inflicts significant harms without concomitant benefits. On the other hand, empirical evidence suggests that an alternate approach of enabling access to sterile syringes, executed through legal reform, would likely reduce bloodborne disease without expending scarce resources. Certainly, legal measures alone are not likely to be universally embraced or fully effective; deregulation of syringe sales must constitute but one component of a comprehensive, well-financed program to impede the interconnected epidemics of drug use and HIV/AIDS.

An earnest national effort would devote ample resources to education and counseling regarding the harms of illicit drugs, effective community ventures to discourage drug sellers, crime prevention measures in schools and housing projects, drug treatment on demand, rehabilitation for offenders, and community activities and support for families and young people. Ultimately, both law enforcement and public health draw their moral authority from their charge to protect the health and welfare of the community. Instead of undertaking singular and countervailing approaches, these two disciplines must devise a coherent policy to reduce morbidity and mortality from the dual epidemics of HIV and drug dependency, a policy grounded in science and realized through law.

The final part of this book expands the examination of AIDS policy from the United States to the global effects of the pandemic. Chapter 15 explores the issue of international travelers and immigrants, arguing that screening and exclusion does not serve a legitimate public health purpose and violates the human rights of persons living with HIV/AIDS. Chapter 16 focuses on three fundamental issues: the absence of political will to confront the HIV/AIDS pandemic in a serious way; drugs, patents, and international trade law; and research ethics in international collaborative AIDS research. Finally, Chapter 17 reviews the effect of the AIDS pandemic on policy, politics, and the law.

Part 5 AIDS in the World

The last few years have not been good for immigrants seeking refuge in the United States. ... HIV-positive immigrants seeking entry to the United States are worse off than when we began the litigation in 1991. While they can still obtain [HIV] waivers for entry, the exclusion has now been legislated by Congress, and only Congress can lift the ban.—**Michael Ratner,** Center for Constitutional Rights (1998)

Chapter 15

Screening and Exclusion of
Travelers and Immigrants

Global strategies to control infectious disease historically have included the erection of barriers to international travel and immigration.[1] All too often immigrants have been stigmatized and blamed for a wide variety of biological and social ills. Anti-immigrant rhetoric and policy have been framed in public health language and justifications.[2] Keeping people with infectious diseases outside national borders reemerged as public health policy in the HIV pandemic. Sixty-one countries have introduced border restrictions on foreigners infected with HIV, usually those planning an extended stay in the country, such as students, workers, or seamen.[3]

In the early period of the HIV pandemic, travel restrictions were established primarily by countries in the western Pacific and Mediterranean regions, where HIV seroprevalence was relatively low.[4] Today, travel restrictions sweep more broadly throughout the world. One of the most comprehensive systems of

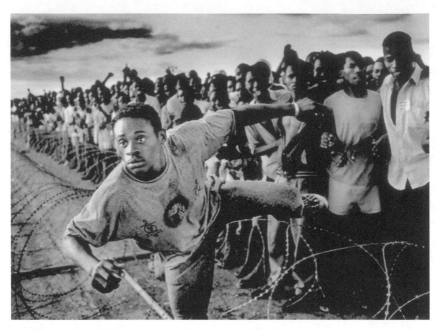

In 1992 the United States prohibited HIV-infected Haitians from entering the country and quarantined many refugees in this camp at Guantánamo Bay, Cuba. In 1993 a Brooklyn U.S. District Court judge ruled that the United States could no longer detain 158 Haitian HIV-infected refugees at the Guantánamo Bay Military Camp.

HIV testing and restricting persons seeking immigration is in the United States. In fact, similar restrictions were rejected in Canada in 2001. The Canadian Health Department proposed HIV testing for all prospective immigrants and planned to exclude those who tested positive.[5] After vigorous dissent within Canada and internationally, the minister of health proposed a revised plan, conceding that if HIV-infected immigrants received information and counseling, they did not pose a public health threat. Other countries, such as Costa Rica, France, and the United Kingdom, have lifted immigration bans based on HIV infection.[6] These policies may still be the subject of debate. In January 2003 Lord Thurnberg, former chair of Britain's Public Health Laboratory Service, called for medical testing of immigrants. In the United Kingdom, 92 percent of the people diagnosed with HIV in 2002 were immigrants.[7]

National[8] and international[9] organizations have sharply criticized U.S. immigration policy for its inconsistency with public health goals and human rights principles. In protest of the U.S. policy, for example, the Eighth International Conference on AIDS, scheduled to be held at Harvard University in July 1992, was moved to Amsterdam. To this day, many AIDS and human rights organizations boycott international meetings held in the United States. These conferences are vital for the study of prevention, education, and treatment of HIV infection. The United States has not hosted an official international AIDS conference since it imposed immigration restrictions on persons with HIV.

This chapter examines the fairness and effectiveness of immigration policy in the United States as it relates to people living with HIV/AIDS. It describes the current law, including testing and restrictions on temporary visitors and permanent residents; the public health consequences of U.S. policy, including the scope of restrictions and the accuracy of tests; and the harms of this policy, notably the infringement of human rights. The chapter concludes by recommending repeal of screening and restrictions on travel and immigration. The government should adopt policies that promote global health and freedom of travel.

Current Law

The U.S. Immigration and Nationality Act decrees that any applicant who has a communicable disease of public health significance is ineligible for admission or a visa to the United States.[10] By the mid-1980s there were seven designated diseases—five of them sexually transmitted (chancroid, gonorrhea, granuloma inguinal, lymphogranuloma venereum, and infectious syphilis) and two non-venereal (infectious leprosy and active tuberculosis [TB]). Louis Sullivan, secretary of health and human services in the first Bush administration, publicly stated that only TB should be a designated disease. Ignoring the secretary's advice, Senator Jesse Helms (R-N.C.), a well-known antagonist of gay rights and AIDS prevention, introduced a bill in 1987 mandating the inclusion of HIV/AIDS on the list of infections that would restrict entry into the country. On June 9, 1987, in response to congressional direction in the Helms Amendment,[11] the U.S. Public Health Service (USPHS) added HIV infection to the list of communicable diseases of public health significance;[12] HIV infection remains on the list as of this writing. The Immigration and Nationality Act, however, provides for waivers of inadmissibility for both nonimmigrant (travelers) and immigrant applicants, as explained below. But even with these waivers, public health advocates have condemned the policy. June Osborn, chair of the National Commission on AIDS, said in 1989 that the policies "fly in the face of strong opinion and practice and lead to unconscionable infringement of human rights and dignity, and they reenforce a false impression that AIDS and HIV infection are a general threat when in fact they are sharply restricted in their mode of transmission."[13]

Temporary Visitors

Persons who seek entry into the United States for a temporary stay are not routinely tested for HIV, although they must declare their serologic status when applying for a visa. An immigration officer may require a test if there is suspicion that the person is infected. "Suspicion" has been triggered in the past by the possession of antiretroviral medication, a medical alert card or bracelet for hemophilia, or the intention to attend an AIDS conference.[14]

Two waiver policies apply to applicants for admission as nonimmigrants: routine waivers and "designated event" waivers. A routine waiver of exclusion can be granted by the attorney general at the time of the visa application or by an immigration judge if the risk of spread of HIV is considered minimal and there is no cost incurred at any level by a government agency. The individual can then enter the United States for up to thirty days to attend conferences, receive medical treatment, or conduct business. If a waiver is granted, the alien's passport has a removable document stamped with a code indicating that the exclusion of a person with a communicable disease of public health significance has been waived. Persons infected with HIV must obtain an approved waiver in advance each time they wish to travel to the United States.

The "designated event" policy allows a blanket waiver for HIV-infected persons to enter the United States to attend events considered to be in the public interest, including academic and educational conferences and international sports events. To obtain this waiver, the Department of Health and Human Services writes a letter to the Department of State (DOS) regarding the event. The DOS must recommend the event to the attorney general, who then authorizes a blanket waiver. The waiver allows HIV-infected applicants who are seeking admission to the United States specifically to participate in the event to be admitted for the duration of the event without being questioned about their HIV status. This policy was first implemented in June 1990, when the Immigration and Naturalization Service (INS) automatically granted waivers to all persons attending the Sixth International Conference on AIDS in San Francisco.[15]

Permanent Residents

All persons applying for permanent residence (a "green card") must undergo a medical examination that includes chest radiography for TB and serological tests for venereal diseases and HIV infection.[16] Those who test HIV positive must be denied permanent residence unless they can meet the stringent requirements for an exclusion waiver.

Persons can apply for permanent residence under three categories: visa applicants, applicants for legalization, and applicants for refugee status or asylum. All visa applicants must be tested for HIV and are automatically refused permanent residence if the results are positive. To obtain an exclusion waiver, applicants are required to establish the existence of a family relationship with a U.S. citizen or lawful permanent resident. The applicant must be the spouse, unmarried son or daughter, or lawfully adopted minor, of a U.S. citizen or permanent resident or have a son or daughter who is a U.S. citizen or permanent resident. The Department of Homeland Security's Bureau of Citizenship and Immigration Services (BCIS) (formerly the INS)[17] has three additional criteria that an immigration applicant has the burden of demonstrating to obtain a waiver: (1) the danger to the public health created by the alien's admission is minimal, (2) the possibility of the spread of the infection created by the alien's admission is minimal, and (3) no expense will be incurred by any government agency without that agency's prior consent.[18] The message is clear: immigrants with financial resources are welcome, but impoverished and potentially ill immigrants would likely become a public charge.

HIV testing is also required of all applicants under the legalization ("amnesty") program. Applicants who test positive for HIV can be excluded from the United States, but they are eligible for waivers on the grounds of family unity, public interest, or humanitarian concerns.

Refugees (who apply from abroad) and people seeking asylum (who are already in the country) are permitted to enter or remain in the United States after proving that they have a well-founded fear of persecution in their own countries. In 1996 the INS recognized persecution based on HIV infection as a basis for granting asylum in the United States.[19] To qualify for asylum on this basis, the applicant must demonstrate that his home government causes "extreme harm" to HIV-infected individuals. However, the INS specifically noted that inadequate medical treatment and social ostracism are not by themselves sufficient to establish persecution.[20] An HIV test is required of applicants for refugee status but not asylum. If the asylee wants to apply for permanent residence after one year, a test is required.

Public Health Consequences

The BCIS is conducting one of the largest HIV screening programs in the world, yet the program has never been carefully evaluated for its appropriateness or effectiveness. From a global perspective, the testing and exclusion of international travelers is a specious public health policy.[21] Restricting travel is unlikely to reduce the reservoir of infection in the world. More importantly, the absence of provisions for education and counseling suggests that the program is not intended to reduce the global burden of HIV/AIDS. Furthermore, there is no attempt to identify and educate HIV-infected citizens who leave the United States to travel abroad. The only potential global effect of restrictions on international travel, then, might be to shift the geographic distribution of infection marginally.

Efficacy in public health is often viewed from the insular perspective of individual countries rather than that of the international community as a whole.[22] The most persuasive case for HIV screening and exclusion could be made for countries with very low HIV prevalence. However, even in countries with low prevalence, such a policy is unlikely to be effective. No policy can eliminate the introduction of infection because countries cannot lawfully exclude returning nationals,[23] nor can they practically screen all visitors and exclude those who test positive. Persons recently infected with HIV, moreover, might not be excluded because they would not have produced antibodies to HIV. More importantly, if citizens were given the false sense that all foreign visitors were free of infection, they might be less likely to avoid high-risk behavior with those visitors. The United States, a country with a reservoir of approximately 800,000 to 900,000 infected people,[24] has even more difficulty in demonstrating the public health benefits of screening.

The Scope of the U.S. Restrictions

Every year, many people move from countries all over the world to the United States. Most come to live permanently, but many also seek temporary asylum. In fiscal year 2003 (October 1, 2001, through September 30, 2002), the INS received 6,324,496 applications for immigration benefits. Of these, 5,691,715 were approved.[25] The INS received 66,577 applications for asylum and approved 19,611.[26] The latter individuals were allowed to enter the United States as asylees and remain without being tested for HIV unless they apply for permanent residence, which is possible after one year. However, all of those who obtained permanent legal status as immigrants had to first test negative for HIV. Unfortunately, the BCIS does not compile statistics on the number of people rejected because of positive-HIV test results or for other medical reasons.

In addition, many people from other countries are temporary visitors to the United States every year. In fiscal year 2001, there were 32.8 million nonimmigrant admissions. Though few of these travelers were tested for HIV, some were subjected to questioning based on their possible HIV status. In the same year over 16.4 million visitors were admitted to the United States without visas under the Visa Waiver Pilot Program.[27] These individuals did not need visas to enter the country and, therefore, did not have to undergo HIV testing.

In sum, many millions of immigration applicants are required to undergo HIV testing annually. Although the great majority of nonimmigrants do not have to be tested for HIV, they still may be asked intrusive questions and are subject to screening at the discretion of BCIS officials.

Accuracy of Tests

HIV antibody tests are very accurate, but, like any complicated series of biological tests, a certain number of the results are incorrect.[28] In addition, an unknown proportion of those who are infected with HIV do not yet have antibodies or no longer have them.[29] Although carefully developed and monitored programs can substantially reduce the number of testing errors,[30] such ideal conditions are rarely obtained. The BCIS, for example, provides applicants for immigration with a list of "civil surgeons" who are authorized to conduct tests for a variety of conditions, including HIV infection. These physicians are in private practice, clinics, and hospitals and need only four years of professional service. Civil surgeons are not required to have any experience in interpreting the results of HIV laboratory tests. Furthermore, because of the diverse circumstances in which testing is performed, numerous laboratories in various parts of the United States and in other countries are used. There is no comprehensive program to monitor the quality of the tests. Thus, there is a possibility for substantial violations of recommended technical protocols, misreading of test results, and transmission of inappropriate or inaccurate information to applicants and immigration authorities.

An optimistic assumption is that the sensitivity and specificity of a series of HIV antibody tests are 99.99 percent. Even if one assumes this level of accuracy, however, it is still likely that there will be a number of inaccurate test results in a low-risk population. If we assume that the prevalence of HIV infection is 1.5 per 1,000, then for a series of tests with a sensitivity and specificity of 99.99 percent, there might be as many as 100 false-positive tests for every million people tested. Even a slight decrease in overall test performance would result in a markedly larger number of errors. For example, if the sensitivity and specificity were 99.90 percent, there would be 0.7 false-positive results for every true positive (998 vs. 1,499). This situation results in the unfair denial of entry to uninfected applicants without any mechanism to rectify the error.

Harms of the Screening Program

Even if the immigrant screening program was able to achieve a sensitivity and specificity of 99.99 percent, it would not provide an effective response to the information provided by the test.[31] Certainly, no systematic effort is currently made to provide travelers and immigrants with the type of information needed to help them avoid behaviors that put them at high risk of further spreading HIV. Indeed, rather than promoting testing and changes in behavior, the nature of the program actually causes people to avoid testing or to falsify their test results. Persons who have engaged in risky behaviors are advised by immigration lawyers to stay underground rather than apply for permanent residence.[32] Such people may therefore avoid using health care facilities where they could be identified and reported to public health or immigration authorities. If individuals living with HIV/AIDS do not receive effective treatment, they pose a risk to their own health and to their sex and needle-sharing partners. Persons who are not treated effectively have significantly higher levels of circulating virus, thus rendering them more infectious.[33]

Travelers to the United States are also discouraged from being tested because they have to declare their serologic status openly when applying for entry.[34] Travelers who declare a positive test result may be required to undergo an arduous process, including an administrative hearing, before being granted a waiver. If a waiver is granted, a document is inserted in the traveler's passport marked with a code denoting the communicable disease. The restrictions on travelers, moreover, are easily flouted by people who are asymptomatic; because of the reliance on an open declaration to immigration authorities, an infected person could easily go through passport control without being identified and turned back.

In the xenophobic context of testing "outsiders," it is all too easy to forget that (except when used to protect the blood supply) an HIV test is primarily a clinical test designed to promote the health and well-being of the patient. The U.S. policy provides no constructive response to the test results except to restrict travel. A positive HIV test does not trigger any of the services recommended by the USPHS, including appropriate immunization against specific infections (such as influenza), prospective monitoring of CD4 cell counts, early intervention with antiviral drugs, and prophylactic use of medications for pneumocystis.[35] Indeed, immigration regulations specify that persons must not be a financial burden on U.S. services and programs.[36] Immigrants who are infected with HIV and who are therefore ineligible for permanent residence are disqualified from Medicaid and other public benefits.[37] Moreover, visa applicants may harm their cases by taking visible precautions to protect their health, such as carrying medications for treating HIV-related diseases. Persons infected with HIV may therefore decide not to come to the United States for necessary treatment, or may stop taking medication during their stay, to the detriment of their health. Identifying cases with the express intention of excluding, rather than including, people from benefits and services is contrary to the traditions of medicine.

Infringements on Human Rights

The exclusion of persons living with HIV/AIDS reiterates a recurrent theme in America—"undesirable" groups are labeled "high risk," often based on fears and stereotypes. HIV/AIDS was perniciously conflated with sexual deviancy and racial discrimination. From 1990 to 1993, for example, the INS quarantined HIV-infected Haitian immigrants at the U.S. Marine Base at Guantánamo Bay, Cuba. They were confined in such abysmal conditions that a federal district court judge, Sterling Johnson, ruled that they were denied adequate health care and legal counsel.[38] Thereafter, Congress refused to revoke the policy that restricted persons living with HIV/AIDS from immigrating to the United States. In 1993 Senator Don Nickles (R-Okla.) sounded a hateful warning: "If we change this policy, it will almost be like an invitation for many people who carry this dreadful, deadly disease, to come into the country because we do have quality health care in this country" and will "jeopardize the lives of countless Americans and will cost U.S. taxpayers millions of dollars."[39]

A public health program should adhere to basic principles of justice. The BCIS program excludes people on the basis of their serologic status, not their risk to others. Restrictions based on infection rather than risky behavior are discriminatory and overly inclusive. The law penalizes those who behave responsibly and safely, as well as those who do not. The screening program is arbitrary because it does not include lawful visitors without visas and returning nationals who may be as (or more) likely to spread infection through sexual relations or intravenous drug use. The net effect of mandatory screening, health declarations, and deportation is that many people visiting or living in the United States may forgo the testing, counseling, and education that are so important in encouraging safer behavior concerning drugs and sex. Worse still, travelers and immigrants may avoid treatment, harming their own health and rendering them more infectious.

U.S. policy restricting travel and immigration violates international law and global health guidelines. The International Health Regulations provide that the only document that can be required in international traffic is a valid certificate of vaccination against yellow fever.[40] The World Health Organization has stated that "no country bound by the Regulations may refuse entry into its territory to a person who fails to provide a medical certificate stating that he or she is not carrying the AIDS virus."[41]

Restrictions on the freedom to move between countries because of serologic status interfere with a wide range of human endeavors, including business enterprise, cultural and scientific exchange, access to specialized medical care, and family unity. Moreover, as governments erect such restrictions, it becomes more likely that other governments will impose retaliatory restrictions, escalating the social cost to the global community.

Except under the legalization program, moreover, U.S. policy does not guarantee confidentiality.[42] The possibility that highly sensitive information may be disclosed to third parties, even to other government agencies, only broadens the concern for human dignity. If an application for immigration is denied, the BCIS can use the information to locate, arrest, and deport the applicant. Persons infected with HIV outside the United States may be permanently barred from entry.

Conclusion

A just and effective travel and immigration policy would not exclude people because of their serologic status unless they posed a danger to the community through casual transmission. U.S. regulations should list only active TB as a contagious infectious disease.[43] An appropriate program would protect the health of travelers infected with HIV through immunization and prophylactic treatment and would reduce behaviors that may transmit infection.

Undoubtedly, treating patients infected with HIV who immigrate to the United States will incur costs for the public sector. It is inequitable, however, to use cost as a reason for exclusion, for there are no similar exclusionary policies for those with other costly chronic maladies, such as heart disease or cancer. Rather than arbitrarily restrict the movement of a subgroup of infected people, we must dedicate ourselves to the principles of justice, scientific cooperation, and a global response to the HIV pandemic.

Screening and exclusion of travelers and immigrants are symptoms of the irrational fears and prejudices that have characterized the HIV/AIDS pandemic. The next chapter discusses deeper and more intractable problems: the lack of political will, the global trade system, and international collaborative research.

A constant theme in all our messages has been that, in this inter dependent and globalized world, we have indeed again become the keepers of our brother and sister. That cannot be more graphically the case than in the common fight against HIV/AIDS. —**Nelson Mandela,** former president of South Africa (2001)

Chapter 16

The Global Reach of HIV/AIDS

Science, Politics, Economics, and Research

HIV/AIDS affects people throughout the world—their health, communities, and economic structures. It is truly a global epidemic, imposing a burden on all countries and regions and leaving none immune from its devastating impact.[1] Forty-two million people are infected with HIV,[2] with one-third of the cases between the ages of 15 and 24.[3] The highest infection rates are concentrated in countries that can least afford the sickness, death, and loss of productivity associated with the epidemic; the vast majority (95 percent) of people living with HIV/AIDS reside in developing countries (see Map 16-1).[4]

If the current trend continues, 100 million people will be infected by 2006, thereby making HIV/AIDS the worst pandemic since the bubonic plague swept through Europe in the fourteenth century, killing one in four people. More than 20 million people have already died from AIDS since it was first identified in the early 1980s.[5] In 2002 alone, 3 million people died from AIDS (see Map 16-2).[6]

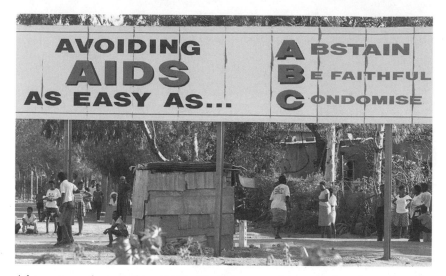

A banner near the township of Naledi in Gaborone advises people on how to avoid AIDS. Botswana now has the world's highest incidence of infection.

The continent of Africa has experienced the greatest burden of disease. Botswana has the highest prevalence of HIV, with almost 40 percent of its adult population infected. For the first time since 1950, the average life expectancy in Botswana is now below forty years of age.[7] The HIV/AIDS epidemic is the reason that the average life expectancy in southern Africa is expected to drop to under thirty by 2010 (see Figure 16-1).[8]

The fastest-growing rate of HIV infection is in the former Soviet Union, with Russia experiencing a fifteenfold increase during 1998-2001; the second fastest rate of growth is in the Caribbean, and the third fastest is in India.[9] At the beginning of the twenty-first century, the Chinese government acknowledged that 600,000 to 1 million of its people were living with HIV/AIDS.[10] Yet only 4 percent of the adults in the world's most populous country knew how HIV is contracted and spread (see Table 16-1).[11]

The epic tragedy of HIV/AIDS in Africa and the tragedy unfolding in other regions is, in the words of Kofi Annan, a product of "simultaneous catastrophes": famine and armed conflict.[12] More than 30 million people are at risk of starvation in southern Africa and the Horn of Africa. Agricultural production has declined because of AIDS, and nutritional requirements for whole communities have increased because people are sick and need more food.[13] The AIDS epidemic has sapped the strength and eroded the skills of land workers, retarded agricultural development, and reduced rural livelihoods.[14] War and civil strife also contribute to the tragedy of AIDS. The population lives in stressful

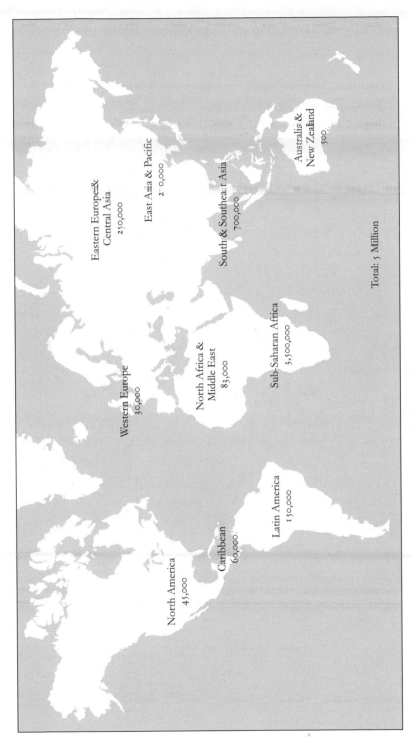

Eastern Europe &
Central Asia
250,000

East Asia & Pacific
2 0,000

South & Southeast Asia
700,000

Australia &
New Zealand
500

Western Europe
30,000

North Africa &
Middle East
83,000

Sub-Saharan Africa
3,500,000

North America
45,000

Caribbean
60,000

Latin America
150,000

Total: 5 Million

MAP 16-1. Estimated Number of Adults and Children Newly Infected with HIV during 2002

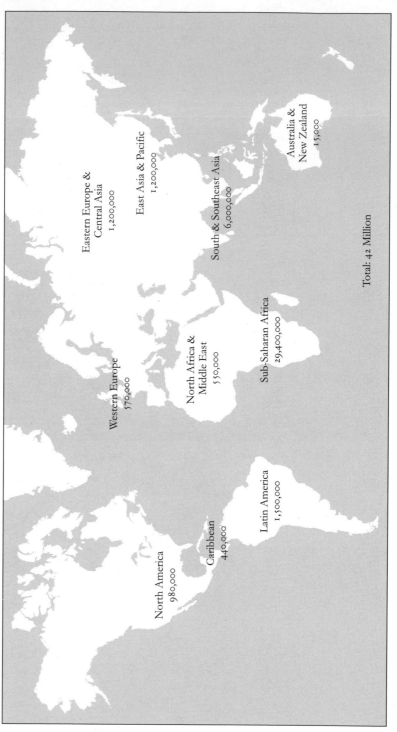

Eastern Europe &
Central Asia
1,200,000

East Asia & Pacific
1,200,000

South & Southeast Asia
6,000,000

Australia &
New Zealand
15,000

Western Europe
570,000

North Africa &
Middle East
550,000

Sub-Saharan Africa
29,400,000

North America
980,000

Caribbean
440,000

Latin America
1,500,000

Total: 42 Million

MAP 16-2. Adults and Children Estimated to Be Living with HIV/AIDS as of the End of 2002

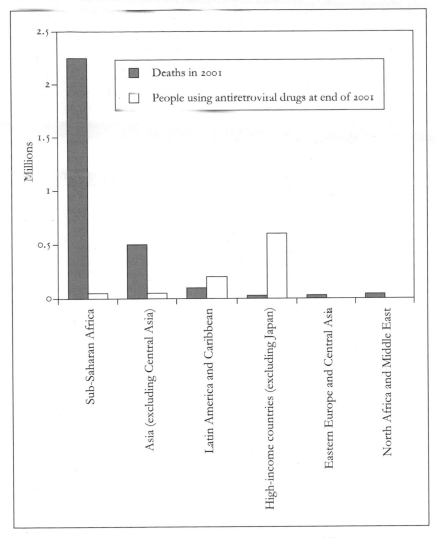

FIGURE 16-1. Deaths from AIDS and People Using Antiretroviral Drugs

and dangerous conditions; is subjected to human rights abuses, including sexual violence; and is left in conditions of poverty that might lead to commercial sex to survive. The massive displacements of people are associated with disruption of social cohesion and relationships, fostering promiscuity and commercial sex. Large population movements, moreover, facilitate the geographic spread of HIV infection.[15]

Societies are altered fundamentally as a result of HIV/AIDS penetrating through various populations: among young adults, HIV/AIDS weakens the labor force

TABLE 16-1. Regional HIV/AIDS Statistics and Features, 2002

Region	Epidemic Started	Adults & Children Living with HIV/AIDS	Adults & Children Newly Infected with HIV/AIDS	Adult Prevalence Rate (%)	HIV-positive Adults Who Are Women (%)	Main Modes of Transmission for Those Who Are Living with HIV/AIDS
Sub-Saharan Africa	late 1970s/ early 1980s	29.4 million	3.5 million	8.8	58	Hetero
North Africa & Middle East	late 1980s	550,000	83,000	0.3	55	Hetero, IDU
South & Southeast Asia	late 1980s	6.0 million	700,000	0.6	36	Hetero, IDU
East Asia & Pacific	late 1980s	1.2 million	270,000	0.1	24	IDU, Hetero, MSM
Latin America	late 1970s/ early 1980s	1.5 million	150,000	0.6	30	MSM, IDU, Hetero
Caribbean	late 1970s/ early 1980s	440,000	60,000	2.4	50	Hetero, MSM
Eastern Europe & Central Asia	early 1990s	1.2 million	250,000	0.6	27	IDU
Western Europe	late 1970s/ early 1980s	570,000	30,000	0.3	25	MSM, IDU
North America	late 1970s/ early 1980s	980,000	45,000	0.6	20	MSM, IDU, Hetero
Australia & New Zealand	late 1970s/ early 1980s	15,000	500	0.1	7	MSM
Total		42 million	5 million	1.2	50	

Source: UNAIDS, AIDS Epidemic Update (Geneva: UNAIDS and WHO, December 2002), 6.
Hetero = heterosexual transmission; IDU = transmission through injection drug use; MSM = sexual transmission among men who have sex with men.

and destabilizes the economy;[16] among mothers and fathers, it creates parent less children and dislocated families;[17] among infants and youth, it diminishes hope and possibilities for the future.[18] In short, the pandemic destroys families and social networks, diminishes economic growth, and creates pessimism about the future.[19]

Prevention of HIV/AIDS would benefit all regions and countries, irrespective of the prevalence or incidence of HIV/AIDS in the population. All countries should be concerned about the pandemic, as all social and economic life in the early twenty-first century is interconnected. HIV/AIDS in one part of the world is bound to affect the health, economy, and security of countries everywhere. The health of all people is affected by modern travel and migration patterns. HIV/AIDS, and the interconnected epidemics of tuberculosis (TB), sexually transmitted diseases (STDs), and drug dependency, can spread across countries and regions.[20]

The economy of all countries is affected because of the complex economic and trade relationships that exist in the modern world. Countries and regions with a heavy burden of HIV/AIDS often have weaker economies, impeding their ability to import and export essential products and services. This has a cascading effect on the economies of other countries.

The security of countries and regions is affected because HIV/AIDS can have a destabilizing effect on society. HIV/AIDS creates poverty, a sense of vulnerability and hopelessness that feeds conditions leading to feuds, violence, and dislocation. In turn, wars and armed conflict exacerbate conditions of poverty, powerlessness, and social instability, all of which facilitate HIV transmission.[21] A healthier, more prosperous, and stable Third World would experience fewer conflicts and disasters.[22]

In recognition of these substantial harms, the United States has declared HIV/AIDS a threat to national security.[23] The strength of American sentiment was clear in the words of Secretary of State Colin Powell: "From this moment on, our response to AIDS must be no less comprehensive, no less relentless and no less swift than the pandemic itself. I was a soldier and I know of no enemy in war more insidious or vicious than AIDS, an enemy that poses a clear and present danger to the world."[24]

Given the undeniable global effects of HIV/AIDS, one might expect the international community to unite in an effort to reach the common goal of preventing and treating HIV/AIDS. In June 2001 the United Nations General Assembly adopted by consensus the Declaration of Commitment on HIV/AIDS: "Global Crisis—Global Action." In the declaration, 189 governments pledged to reduce HIV prevalence among young people by 25 percent in the worst-affected countries by 2005 and globally by 2010. International organizations, such as the Joint United Nations Programme on AIDS (UNAIDS),[25] the World Health Organization (WHO),[26] and the World Bank,[27] have also issued warnings and calls for action (see Figure 16-2). Yet the responses by governments have been fragmented. There is often an absence of political will, an unwillingness to share strategies and resources, and wide philosophical and pragmatic differences principally among countries in the North/West and those in the South/East.[28] This unwillingness to cooperate is caused, in part, by insular attitudes toward world health, economics, and politics. A certain narrow self-interest seems to prevent many countries from engaging in truly global cooperative approaches. The unwillingness to cooperate may also be due to the fact that resource-rich and resource-poor countries have markedly different priorities tailored to the different dynamics of the epidemic in their regions.[29]

This chapter examines the major social, political, economic, and ethical issues involved in the global HIV pandemic. First, it considers the steps needed to prevent and treat HIV effectively and explores why many leaders have not responded more forcefully. This section discusses the intangible, but crucial, aspect of political will.[30] Second, the chapter looks at the divisive issue of drugs, patents, and international trade law. Highly developed countries usually want to uphold the patent system to protect the proprietary interests of drug companies. This keeps the price of HIV/AIDS drugs high, placing them out of the reach of resource-poor countries. In conclusion, the chapter focuses on the vexing issue of research ethics. The research community has struggled with one overriding question in international collaborative investigations: Should the ethical standards applicable in developed countries be used when engaging in research in less developed countries? Stakeholders are at odds and struggle to find the balance between ensuring strong ethical standards and expediting access to cost-effective treatments in poor countries.

Science, Politics, and Money: Understanding the Problem and Working toward a Solution

Individually, we must demonstrate the qualities of courage, integrity and respect for others. Collectively, our governments must recognize that leadership means abandoning rhetoric and taking action. They must energize our people and mobilize the necessary resources to conduct the campaign against HIV/AIDS.—Graça Machel, African Development Forum (2000)

National governments have unique responsibilities for preventing and treating HIV/AIDS and mitigating its public health and economic effects. Only govern-

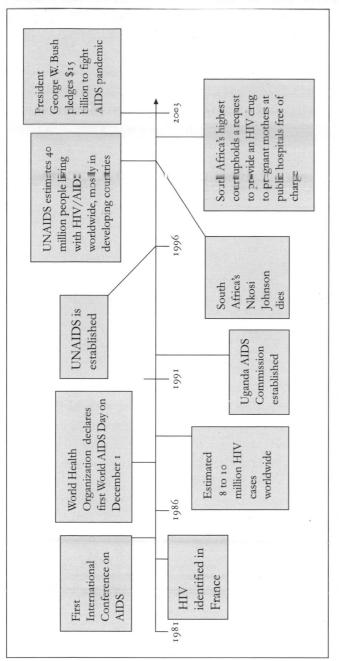

FIGURE 16-2. The HIV/AIDS Pandemic: International Timeline

1981

First International Conference on AIDS

HIV identified in France

1986

World Health Organization declares first World AIDS Day on December 1

Estimated 8 to 10 million HIV cases worldwide

1991

UNAIDS is established

Uganda AIDS Commission established

1996

UNAIDS estimates 40 million people living with HIV/AIDS worldwide, mostly in developing countries

South Africa's Nkosi Johnson dies

2003

President George W. Bush pledges $15 billion to fight AIDS pandemic

South Africa's highest court upholds a request to provide an HIV drug to pregnant mothers at public hospitals free of charge

TABLE 16-2. Ten-Step Strategy for HIV Prevention among Youth

1. End the silence, stigma, and shame

2. Provide young people with knowledge and information

3. Equip young people with life skills to put knowledge into practice

4. Provide youth-friendly health services

5. Promote voluntary and confidential HIV counseling and testing

6. Work with young people; promote their participation

7. Engage young people who are living with HIV/AIDS

8. Create safe and supportive environments

9. Reach out to young people most at risk

10. Strengthen partnerships, monitor progress

Source: United Nations Children's Fund, UNAIDS, World Health Organization, Young People and HIV/AIDS: Opportunity in Crisis (Paris: UNICEF, UNAIDS, WHO, 2002).

ments have the means and mandate to provide for "public" goods—services that benefit society but that the market will not provide due to insufficient incentives.[31] The role of government is to advance the well-being of its citizens and promote a fair distribution of social benefits. Governments, acting for the people, should adopt the most effective strategies and marshal the resources needed to reduce the burden of the epidemic. The public health community has long agreed on the appropriate response to HIV/AIDS (see, e.g., the ten-step strategy proposed by UNICEF, UNAIDS, and WHO for HIV prevention among youth in Table 16-2).

While strategies vary according to local conditions and cultures, the need for surveillance, prevention, treatment, and protection of human rights is the same everywhere. Most importantly, governments should act as soon as possible. Nearly half the world's population lives in areas where HIV is rare. For instance, at the end of 2002 the adult infection prevalence in North Africa and the Middle East was 0.3 percent; in East Asia and the Pacific, the proportion of infected adults was a mere 0.1 percent.[32] Investments in prevention and education at the earliest stages of an epidemic are the least expensive and most effective actions available to a government.[33] Decisive action could have saved countless lives in populous countries like India[34] and South Africa.[35] It could still save lives in China, the former Soviet Union, and other regions where poverty and lack of

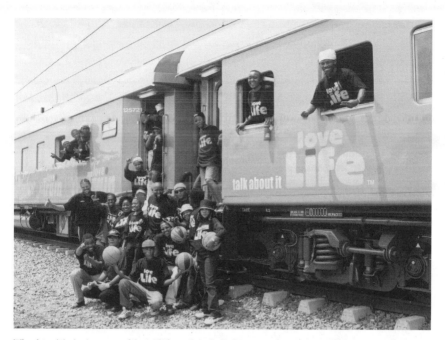

The loveTrain is part of loveLife—South Africa's national HIV prevention program for youth. This program began in 1999 and is supported by the Henry J. Kaiser Family Foundation and the Bill and Melinda Gates Foundation.

education lead to drug use and the spread of disease.[36] As Peter Piot, UNAIDS executive director, told an audience at the Fourteenth International Conference on AIDS: "It is now clear that the AIDS epidemic is still in its early stages. And let us be equally clear: our fight back is at an even earlier stage."[37]

Public health authorities cannot develop appropriate policies for prevention and treatment without accurate data about the prevalence and incidence of HIV/AIDS in the general population and within specific communities. Through comprehensive screening, reporting, and active surveillance, policymakers can ascertain the scope and direction of the epidemic in their country. Surveillance provides clear information about the growing burden of HIV/AIDS on women, youth, and ethnic minorities, and within groups at heightened risk in the society, such as gays, injection drug users, and sex workers. The information gathered can then be used to assist groups most affected by the disease.

Understanding the risks and realities of HIV/AIDS is a necessary precursor to behavioral change. Accordingly, information to the public about health risks is vital. This should include education, counseling, and other methods of targeted health promotion. It is crucial that individuals understand the methods of contracting and transmitting HIV. Educational messages should target the specific needs of individuals and groups. AIDS education should be culturally and linguistically appropriate but sufficiently explicit to convey the information clearly.

Politicians can thwart AIDS education by imposing societal prohibitions. For example, educational materials targeting gay men should not avoid specific, often graphic discussion of risk behaviors as a concession to the morality of the wider population. There may also be a pervasive culture of silence that excludes discussion of HIV/AIDS. A brave action to break this silence took place at the Thirteenth International Conference on AIDS in Durban, South Africa. Nkosi Johnson, a boy living with HIV/AIDS, criticized his president for neglecting the epidemic in South Africa.[38] Advocates and role models like Johnson are instrumental in raising awareness about HIV/AIDS and highlighting government denial of the true facts of the epidemic.

Although the risks of certain behaviors may be understood, avoiding risky activities is not always possible or realistic. Experience demonstrates that prohibition messages—"just say no"—are not effective.[39] Since individuals will continue to engage in risk behaviors, it is necessary to provide them with the means to protect themselves, such as condoms or sterile drug-injection equipment. These "harm reduction" strategies have been shown to be effective in reducing risk behaviors.[40]

Prevention of HIV infection is not always possible. Therefore, government policies should address both prevention and postinfection health care. As President Clinton observed, "Historians will look back on our time and see that our civilization spends many millions of dollars educating people about the scourge of HIV . . . but what they will find not so civilized is our failure to treat 95 percent of people with the disease."[41] In September 2002 the Office of the United Nations High Commissioner for Human Rights (OHCHR) and UNAIDS published updated guidelines on HIV/AIDS and human rights declaring that access to HIV/AIDS treatment is fundamental to realizing the right to health and that access to medication is one element of a comprehensive program of treatment, care, and support.[42]

Individuals can lead healthier, longer lives if they receive treatment for HIV. However, the levels of health care offered by states vary widely. Resource-poor countries generally focus their efforts on education and basic medical treatment. More developed countries commonly offer sophisticated treatments, including antiretroviral therapy and treatment of symptoms. Antiretroviral therapy can reduce viral load, boost the immune system, and reduce contagiousness.[43] Health care can alleviate symptoms and reduce the likelihood of opportunistic infections. Despite the different emphasis, access to health care is a primary objective in all countries. Persons living with HIV/AIDS should not be neglected or forgotten.

The public health strategies discussed above are insufficient to reduce the burden of HIV/AIDS. People also need to be empowered to protect their health. One of the primary strategies in the fight against HIV/AIDS is to safeguard the human rights of those who are infected or are at risk of infection (see Chapter 4). This is especially true of girls and women who are highly vulnerable. They may understand the risks and have access to condoms, but they may not be able to control safer sexual practices. Women's relationships may be controlled by violence, cultural expectations, or economic dependence. When their husbands leave or die, women may be deprived of credit, distribution networks, or land rights.[44] Improving the status of women and strengthening their social, political, and economic rights would allow them to protect themselves against HIV and other health threats.[45]

Governments are using these well-established public health and human rights strategies to mitigate the impact of HIV/AIDS in countries as varied as Senegal, Thailand, Uganda, Brazil, Zambia, and Cambodia. For example, Uganda, with limited access to high-technology medicine, has reduced the national average prevalence of HIV among adults from 18.5 percent in 1995 to 8.3 percent in 2000.[46] The government's response to the epidemic dates back to 1986, when an AIDS Control Programme was created in the Ministry of Health. The Uganda AIDS Commission (UAC) was constituted in 1992 and placed under the Office of the President.[47] The UAC created an atmosphere of openness and effective political commitment to HIV/AIDS control that has created high levels of public awareness about the dangers of the epidemic and means of prevention.[48]

A similar picture of success can be found in Senegal, where the government acted rapidly to develop a national program to prevent HIV, beginning with the screening of blood in 1987. The government in Dakar was the driving force behind a declaration on AIDS made by heads of member states of the Organization of African Unity in June 1992. In the mid-1990s Senegal invested significant resources to increase AIDS awareness so that by the late 1990s, over 95 percent of secondary school pupils and 99 percent of sex workers knew about HIV and methods of prevention.[49]

The Absence of Political Will

Above all, the challenge of AIDS is a test of leadership. — Kofi A. Annan, secretary general, United Nations (2001)

The strategies for prevention and treatment of HIV/AIDS are well accepted and have been proven in practice. However, they are only rarely implemented due to an absence of committed political leadership and inadequate funding. One might expect political leaders to concentrate on prevention and treatment of HIV/AIDS, given the epidemic's potential impact on the health and economy of a country. Yet, despite compelling reasons for careful attention, many national leaders demonstrate a benign neglect of the epidemic. The reasons are complex. HIV/AIDS is perceived to interfere with other priorities such as national image, tourism, and trade. Because HIV/AIDS is associated with unlawful or stigmatized behaviors such as drug use, homosexuality, and promiscuous heterosexuality, some political leaders seek to deemphasize its importance in society. This absence of political leadership occurs regardless of culture or region. Political inaction was as evident in the United States in the 1980s and in Kenya and Zimbabwe in the 1990s, as it is in India and China today.[50]

The inaction of some leaders is exemplified by South Africa's President Thabo Mbeki. He has expressed concerns about the link between race and HIV/AIDS and, in one speech, argued that AIDS advocates viewed black people as "germ carriers and human beings of a lower order."[51] Mbeki has questioned whether HIV actually causes disease, stating that "you cannot attribute immune deficiency solely and exclusively to a virus."[52] Such skepticism of science by a respected political leader seriously undermines AIDS education and prevention. President Mbeki has also openly doubted the accuracy of his own Department of Health estimates of the national HIV prevalence among pregnant women. The data, based on annual unlinked, anonymous HIV surveys among women attending antenatal clinics, demonstrate a thirtyfold increase in HIV prevalence —from 0.7 percent in 1990 to 22.4 percent in 1999.[53]

For several years, Mbeki resisted full implementation of UNAIDS guidelines for short-course antiretroviral therapy for pregnant women,[54] even though its cost-effectiveness had been demonstrated in South Africa.[55] Fortunately, there have been competing voices about the dangers of political inaction from the African National Congress. Former South African president Nelson Mandela observed: "Nothing threatens us more today than HIV/AIDS. AIDS is a scourge threatening to undo all the gains we made in our generations of struggle."[56] More radically, the premier of KwaZulu Natal, the South African province most affected by HIV/AIDS, declared that he would distribute drugs to pregnant women in direct violation of central government policy.[57] The government policy was altered by a 2002 court case, *Minister of Health and Others v. Treatment Action Campaign [TAC] and Others*, whereby the Constitutional Court of South

Africa upheld a request by TAC to provide nevirapine, an antiretroviral drug, to pregnant mothers at public hospitals free of charge.[58]

The politics of AIDS, of course, are complex and dependent on culture, experience, perception, and resources. Political leaders must have discretion to allocate resources according to the most pressing needs in their country, and HIV/AIDS is not always the single greatest need. Poor countries have urgent requirements for education, transportation, sanitation, security, and other necessities. Major threats are posed to the population from violence, dislocation, and infectious diseases such as malaria and TB. Spending substantial sums of money on high-technology HIV medications, for example, may not save the most lives given scarce resources. But political leaders should recognize the current or potential devastation of HIV/AIDS. There is never an excuse to ignore or underestimate the scope and impact of the pandemic. Basic AIDS education, prevention, and treatment can help produce the conditions in which people can lead healthy lives.

Even with the political will, the least developed countries still need economic assistance for HIV prevention and treatment.[59] In the world's sixty poorest nations, the average annual per capita health spending is $13. WHO recommends that, at a minimum, this should rise to $34.[60] (In the United States, the figure is $4,500.) Consequently, the United Nations established a Global Fund to Fight AIDS, Tuberculosis, and Malaria (these three diseases account for 24 percent of deaths worldwide). This global collaboration addresses joint concerns on penetrating the obstacles to HIV prevention and AIDS treatment. United Nations Secretary General Kofi Annan announced that this fund needed $7–$10 billion a year for AIDS alone,[61] but donors pledged only $1.4 billion in 2001,[62] and funding diminished further in the aftermath of the events on September 11, 2001.[63] By the time of the Fourteenth International Conference on AIDS in Barcelona in the summer of 2002, the fund had reached only about $2.8 billion.[64] As of February 2003, about $3.2 billion had been pledged, including the U.S. renewal pledge of $1 billion announced by President Bush in his 2003 State of the Union address.[65]

The need for donor funding is even more acute if all health problems (beyond HIV/AIDS) in resource-poor countries are considered. WHO's Commission on Macroeconomics and Health estimated that, to substantially improve global health, donor funding to all low-income countries would have to increase from current levels of approximately $6 billion to $27 billion by 2007.[66]

Strategies to reduce the impact of HIV/AIDS have not been universally implemented due to ignorance, fear, and uninspired leadership. Public health strategies also require resources, and many countries in the South and East cannot afford the cost. Countries in the North and West have not made the political and economic commitment to international aid that is necessary to reduce the global burden of the disease.[67] There are compelling reasons to provide this kind of international assistance. The most fundamental reason is humanitarianism—the understanding that preventing suffering and promoting human welfare is a reward in itself. Countries may also be motivated by their own self-interest, because HIV/AIDS in the developing world deeply affects the health, economy, and security of people globally.

Pharmaceuticals, Intellectual Property, and International Trade

Basic forms of HIV education, prevention, and treatment do not require sophisticated technologies. Most countries have the capacity to implement these public health strategies with little economic and technical assistance. Whereas comprehensive prevention programs in Thailand, Uganda, and other countries have significantly reduced the incidence of HIV,[68] more advanced treatments for HIV, as well as future vaccines, are highly technical and prohibitively expensive for poorer countries. Few people living with HIV/AIDS in resource-poor settings are receiving drug therapy, such as highly active antiretroviral therapy (HAART); HAART reaches fewer than 5 percent of those whose lives it would save. Arguments against the use of HAART in resource-poor countries have been based on the high cost of medications and the lack of infrastructure necessary for using them properly.[69] Should the most modern HIV treatments be available to people irrespective of the country in which they live?

An ethical argument could be made that a child or adult in a poorer country should have an entitlement to life-prolonging medications. If a highly effective treatment such as antiretroviral therapy is available and commonly used in developed countries, shouldn't it also be accessible in less developed countries? The benefits of treatment are no less clear and the lives of people in Africa or Asia are no less important than those in North America and Europe. Antiretroviral therapies not only enhance the lives of individuals, but they also promote the public's health. Individuals who are in treatment, with low viral loads, are less likely to transmit the infection to sex or needle-sharing partners or to newborns through childbirth or breast-feeding. Treatment, therefore, is clinically beneficial to individuals and a valuable component of a comprehensive HIV prevention program.

The problem, of course, is that resource-poor countries cannot afford adequate health care. The difficulties are deeply rooted in a combination of household poverty, inadequate publicly supported health care, and the high price of essential medicines. Consider the fact that combination HIV therapy in the United States costs $12,000 per patient per year,[70] while the average per capita health expenditure in the least developed countries is $13.

Tragically, high infection rates are found in countries least able to cope with the financial burden of providing health care. In 2000 Zimbabwe had an adult infection prevalence of 25.06 percent and a GNP per capita of $720;[71] Mozambique's adult infection rate was 13.22 percent with a GNP per capita of $140.[72] Compare this with Germany, which had an adult infection rate of 0.10 percent for the equivalent period and an economy generating a per capita GNP of $28,280.[73] Obvious consequences flow from these figures about a country's ability to provide expensive treatments for its citizens. Further, if modern therapies are not provided by government, they are even more unattainable for many individuals residing in poor countries. Personal wealth is very low and health insurance of any kind is scarce. At the end of 2001, for example, an estimated 4 million South Africans were infected with HIV, but only about 10,000 had the personal resources to pay for treatments.[74]

International agencies,[75] nongovernmental organizations,[76] and AIDS activists[77] have drawn attention to the urgent need for the dramatically increased availability of medications in developing countries. They have concentrated, moreover, on the high price of therapy, which is perceived as the major barrier to access. The United Nations conducts a program of "Accelerated Access" in collaboration with five pharmaceutical companies. The program assists countries with implementing comprehensive packages of care, treatment, and support for their citizens living with HIV/AIDS, including advocacy for significantly reduced drug prices.[78]

Patent Protection and the Artificially High Price of AIDS Medications

Pharmaceutical companies, supported by advanced industrialized countries, often seek to maintain a high price for HIV medications. These largely northern-based transnational firms claim that a market price is necessary to recoup the substantial costs of research and development. The pharmaceutical sector argues that intellectual property protection stimulates investment and innovation. Failure to safeguard commercial interests, they suggest, would chill entrepreneurs and provide disincentives for inventors.

The international trade system is specifically designed to safeguard the proprietary interests of corporations.[79] There are basically three levels of international trade agreements: bilateral relationships (e.g., Canada–United States Free Trade Agreement), regional agreements (e.g., North America Free Trade Agreement—NAFTA), and multilateral arrangements (e.g., World Trade Organization/General Agreement on Tariffs and Trade—WTO/GATT). The defense of intellectual property is embedded in each level, making it difficult for developing countries to violate patents without the imposition of trade sanctions.

The WTO's Agreement on Trade-Related Aspects of Intellectual Property Rights (TRIPS) establishes minimum standards for intellectual property protection, including the right to exclusively market a patented product for a minimum of twenty years. Northern governments use bilateral and regional trade agreements to negotiate even more stringent protection for patents under so-called TRIPS plus agreements. By restricting the right of governments to allow the production, marketing, and import of low-cost copies of patented medicines (generic drugs), international trade rules restrict competition, increase prices, and further reduce the already limited access of poor people to vital medicines. Patented medicines typically cost between three and fifteen times as much as their generic equivalents.[80] Although there are relatively few patents for HIV medicines currently in force in Africa,[81] international trade rules may militate against the availability and affordability of AIDS treatments in the future.

The United States and other developed countries argue for the "harmonization" of intellectual property rules with the goal of conforming the patent laws of least developed countries to their own.[82] According to proponents, harmonization of strong patent laws facilitates rapid economic development of poor countries through increased trade and foreign investment. Indeed, Article 7 of TRIPS states: "The protection and enforcement of intellectual property rights should contribute to the promotion of technological innovation and to the transfer of technology, to the mutual advantage of producers and users of technological knowledge and in a manner conducive to social and economic welfare, and to a balance of rights and obligations."[83]

In contrast, least developed countries typically resist harmonization and perceive the process as harmful to their interests. As these countries often lack a scientific infrastructure, they are predominantly consumers of foreign technology. For them, enforcing foreign patents dramatically increases the cost of imported drugs and inhibits local industry. Moreover, lacking patents of their own, least developed countries receive few reciprocal benefits by supporting strong international patent protection.[84]

The tension between developed and developing world perspectives is reflected in the Universal Declaration of Human Rights (UDHR) (see Chapter 4).

On the one hand, the UDHR guarantees the right to property (Article 17) and the protection of material interests resulting from scientific discovery (Article 27[2]). On the other hand, it guarantees the right to health (Article 25) and education (Article 26), and to share in scientific advancement and its benefits (Article 27[1]).[85] Developed countries seek the right to protect their proprietary interests resulting from scientific discovery, while least developed countries seek the right to share in scientific discoveries and to promote the right to health of the population.

WTO rules do provide limited methods of circumventing intellectual property law where necessary to protect the public's health. Article 31 of TRIPS provides for compulsory licensing—a government may transfer patent rights to itself or a third party without the patent holder's consent under specified circumstances. One of the designated circumstances is when the public interest necessitates abrogation of patent rights—for example, in a national health emergency.[86]

Although compulsory licenses are enshrined in TRIPS, pharmaceutical companies, supported by northern governments, have strongly resisted claims of a national health emergency, preferring to maintain their patents. For example, Thailand, under intense U.S. pressure, amended its law in order to provide patent protection for drugs and to limit compulsory licensing and importation of patented drugs.[87] This occurred against a backdrop of an epidemic in which one million people were infected with HIV and where AIDS was the leading cause of death.[88]

Many of the least developed countries have a powerful argument that the AIDS pandemic has caused a national health emergency. For example, in Kenya, 15 percent of the adult population is infected with HIV,[89] but fewer than one in one thousand of those infected receives antiretroviral treatment.[90] The U.S. Census Bureau estimates that the HIV/AIDS epidemic has reduced life expectancy in South Africa by fifteen years and in Zimbabwe by thirty-two years (see Figure 16-1).[91] Compare these justifications for compulsory licenses with those made by political leaders in the United States in response to the intentional release of anthrax in 2001. U.S. politicians suggested that the country exercise its compulsory licensing privilege under the TRIPS agreement to permit cheap production of the antibiotic Cipro, without the consent of Bayer Pharmaceuticals, even though there were only a half-dozen deaths from anthrax.

There are creative ways to relax rigid trade rules to allow less developed countries to obtain essential medicines at a more affordable cost. Through the innovative thinking of political leaders in developed and less developed countries, the criteria for the issuance of compulsory licenses under Article 31 of TRIPS could be clarified. The international trade system should recognize the devastating public health effects of HIV/AIDS in resource-poor countries.

Poor Countries Making AIDS Treatments Available and Affordable

Several countries have already asserted the right to produce or purchase generic drugs at significantly reduced cost.[92] For example, low-cost drugs are manufactured by Brazil, Thailand, and India.[93] Generic medications can reduce the cost of a daily treatment of AZT, 3TC, and nevirapine from $3.20 to $1.55. Countries like Nigeria conducted research trials to determine the safety and efficacy of imported generic HIV/AIDS drugs[94] and decided to begin importing them.[95] The actions of these states are driven by the need and desire to provide for their citizens.[96]

These actions, however, have been contested. The United States has attempted to use the WTO to force conformity with international patent law. It began proceedings—later dropped—against Brazil for production of HIV/AIDS generics.[97] In 2001 a conglomerate of thirty-nine major drug companies sued the South African government in its own courts to block the 1997 Medicines Act on the grounds that it was a breach of international patent protection. Following intense international pressure, culminating in a petition to "Drop the Case" signed by 260,000 people and 140 organizations in 130 countries, the companies withdrew the lawsuit.[98]

Surprisingly, despite the consistently negative response of the United States and multinational companies, international law experts have supported the right of least developed countries to circumvent patent rights to safeguard the public's health.[99] The decision to drop the litigation in South Africa was also greeted by positive responses from bodies as diverse as Oxfam,[100] UNAIDS,[101] and the WTO itself, whose director general, Mike Moore, felt the settlement proved that "WTO Agreements, such as TRIPS, contain the necessary flexibility to meet the needs of developing countries."[102]

The HIV/AIDS pandemic has turned the patent question into an explosive issue, and the WTO has been forced to resolve the problem. In November 2001, in Doha, Qatar, the Fourth WTO Ministerial Conference declared that TRIPS should be interpreted to support public health and allow for patents to be overridden if required to respond to emergencies such as the AIDS epidemic. But this ignored one significant problem. Countries with little or no manufacturing capability must import drugs. The Doha rules allowed them to break patents to import but did not authorize countries to override patents for the purpose of export to countries in need. In December 2002 in Geneva, 143 of the WTO's 144 members agreed on a solution. The lone holdout—the United States—obstructed the agreement. American negotiators lobbied to limit covered medicines to those for HIV/AIDS, malaria, TB, and a few diseases that affect primarily Africa. Other countries wanted a more flexible approach on access to medicines that would allow nations to protect public health as they saw fit.[103] In late August 2003, the United States finally relented and a deal was struck at the WTO that should allow resource-poor countries to import generic versions of some patented drugs.

Nonprice Barriers to Treatment Access: Infrastructure and National Priorities

Much of the discourse on barriers to access to HIV treatments has concentrated on the issue of price. But price is not the only barrier, and it is probably not even the most difficult one to overcome. The problems of fair and efficient methods of dissemination to people in need remain. Allocation and distribution of drugs within crowded cities, among homeless people, and in remote villages require organized transportation and communication systems. The health care system may not be capable of accurately diagnosing HIV, monitoring viral load, and checking for adverse reactions. Patients must also be educated correctly about the strict regimen of taking medication.

Taken together, these problems mean that, even if distribution can be achieved, the drug may not be prescribed or taken appropriately. Incorrect or intermittent use of antiretroviral medications would create serious health risks for individual patients and pose a wider risk to the population; public health agencies are concerned that the virus could become resistant to existing medicines, rendering them less effective. The problems of resistance to antiretroviral medication already exist.[104] They would be exacerbated by large-scale distribution to patients who do not have the health care and support systems needed to ensure appropriate use. These concerns are legitimate and often on the minds of northern states and aid donors. However, care must be taken as they touch on sensitive issues, as is seen in the reaction of Zimbabwe health minister Timothy Stamps to a comment by USAID director Andrew Natsios that Africans could not handle antiretroviral drugs because they had no concept of time: "Though we do not have clocks and roads in Africa we do know the time and time is ticking away inexorably for some of our states."[105] In response to legitimate demands, researchers are developing cheap, simple, and effective alternative treatments and monitoring technologies to improve the medical management of patients on antiretroviral therapy.[106] In Haiti, for instance, researchers successfully used a directly observed therapy program to monitor HAART (DOT-HAART) administered to HIV patients.[107] The public health community must reexamine the issue of HIV/AIDS medications in poor countries in the setting of rising mortality, falling drug prices, and innovative methods of drug delivery.

Making expensive HIV medications widely available would also raise questions of equity and cost-effectiveness. No one doubts that the appropriate use of these drugs would provide substantial benefits to patients and their communities. But some may ask why persons living with HIV/AIDS should receive special consideration. Many endemic diseases in developing countries could be prevented or treated with vaccines or pharmaceuticals that are not accessible to the population, including simple interventions such as penicillin and oral rehydration. For example, isoniazid and co-trimoxazloe prophylaxis against TB[108] and pneumonia respectively are highly effective but rarely available to poor people in less developed countries.[109] Similarly, almost 18 million people, mostly in Africa and Central and South America, are infected with river blindness (onchocerciasis), which is curable by administering a single oral dose of Ivermectin (trade name—Mectizan) per year.[110] Interventions for these and many other diseases may be more cost-effective and entail less risk than for the most expensive HIV therapies. Similarly, if the extensive resources needed to buy, distribute, and monitor HIV drugs were used for other pressing needs such as food, sanitation, and primary health care, lives might be saved at a lower cost. For example, in Sub-Saharan countries up to 40 percent of children are malnourished,[111] 30 percent of inhabitants do not have access to safe water,[112] and the lifetime risk of maternal death due to inadequate family planning and health care can be as high as one in nine.[113]

These difficult problems of resource allocation are endemic in the developing world and in the response to HIV/AIDS specifically. They have been a recurring theme of this chapter and raise several important questions. What are the best uses of scarce public health and health care resources? Should significant funding be devoted for, say, high-cost antiretroviral treatment or for more basic health services, including antenatal care, primary health care, and TB and STD treatments? Should intellectual property be protected to spur investment and innovation, or should patents be relaxed to ensure access to lifesaving medications in the least developed countries?

There are no easy answers to these and other dilemmas, but one thing is clear. The most developed countries of the North and West have failed utterly to see the critical need for sharing resources with the South and East. These highly industrialized countries may have articulated the humanitarian argu-ments that lie at the heart of international aid, but they have provided only a small fraction of the resources necessary to implement them. This is not only a tragedy for resource-poor countries, but it also will affect the health, econ-omy, and security of people everywhere.

Reduction of Perinatal Transmission in Resource-Poor Countries: The Ethics of Human Subject Research

Global success in combating HIV/AIDS must be measured by its impact on our children and young people. Are they getting the information they need to protect themselves from HIV? Are girls being empowered to take charge of their sexuality? Are infants safe from the dis-ease, and are children orphaned by AIDS being raised in loving, supportive environments? These are the hard questions we need to be asking. These are the yardsticks for measuring our leaders. We cannot let another generation be devastated by AIDS.—Carol Bellamy, executive director, UNICEF (2002)

UNAIDS and WHO estimate that of the over two million HIV-infected women giving birth each year, approximately 600,000 transmit the infection to their children.[114] Over 90 percent of the world's HIV-infected children live in Sub-Saharan Africa. The rate of HIV infection among women attending antenatal clinics in this region ranges from 10 to 50 percent,[115] with an average rate in some countries around 30 percent or more.[116] Vertical transmission of HIV oc-curs in utero, intrapartum during labor and delivery, and postpartum during breast-feeding (see Chapter 13).[117] Studies suggest that in Africa, approximately 65–70 percent of HIV transmission occurs intrapartum, 19–23 percent intra-uterine, and 11–12 percent postpartum. In the absence of intervention, peri-natal transmission is estimated to be 14–25 percent in developed countries and 21–43 percent in less developed countries;[118] the difference in rates of trans-mission are due mostly to breast-feeding in less developed countries.

Interventions that reduce vertical transmission include administration of antiretroviral agents to mother and child around the time of birth, substitution of formula feeding for breast-feeding, and cesarean section. Numerous inter-national observational studies have reported significant reductions in perinatal transmission with treatment.[119] In 1994 the AIDS Clinical Trials Group (ACTG) Study 076 showed a two-thirds reduction in transmission from HIV-infected women who received a complex regimen of zidovudine (AZT) for themselves and their infants (see Chapter 13).[120] Impressive decreases in perinatal HIV transmission have been achieved in North America and Europe based on these clinical trials.[121] Formula feeding can reduce the risk of HIV transmission but creates other risks.[122] Breast-feeding has nutritional, immunological, and birth-spacing benefits that deserve preservation if possible. In addition, formula feeding requires access to nutritionally sound formulas and potable water, which may be scarce in some regions. Cesarean section also reduces vertical transmission, although its cost-effectiveness has not been established and it is infeasible in areas with few resources.[123]

The success in reducing transmission in industrialized countries through antiretroviral therapy stands in stark contrast to the continuing perinatal HIV epidemic in less developed countries.[124] In low-resource settings, where infants of infected mothers are continuously exposed to HIV, the cost of the ACTG 076 regime is too expensive and too complex. The estimated cost of the regimen is $200 (with discounts in pricing to less developed countries), which makes the treatment unavailable to most people in Sub-Saharan Africa, where the annual health expenditure per person is between $2 and $40.[125] Additional barriers include the difficulty in compliance with a regimen entailing administration of a drug four or five times daily for weeks, limited infrastructure for distributing drugs and monitoring compliance, and inadequate maternal-child health care services.

Research in Sub-Saharan Africa and Southeast Asia has demonstrated that less expensive short-course antiretroviral regimens diminish perinatal transmission by one-third to one-half.[126] A trial in Uganda of a single oral dose of nevirapine given to the mother and newborn had similar benefits.[127] These results applied to women who did,[128] and did not,[129] breast-feed, although the formula-fed groups had greater reductions in transmission. Economic analyses have suggested that short-course therapies can achieve significant health and financial benefits considering the cost of the therapy.[130] As a result, WHO and UNAIDS recommend short-course perinatal antiretroviral therapy and advice to HIV-infected women not to breast-feed their infants where this can be accomplished safely.[131]

Despite clinical research, economic analysis, and public health guidance, few developing countries (with the exception, for example, of Botswana, Thailand, and Brazil) have national policies for the integration of preventive antiretroviral therapy in antenatal clinics.[132] As discussed below, those resisting these kinds of interventions object on grounds of economics[133] and ethics.[134] Neither the economic nor the ethical arguments are convincing. In fact, citizens and advocacy groups have powerfully influenced governmental policy, as exemplified by the successful suit by the Treatment Action Campaign in South Africa.[135]

Economic objections understandably rest on the still relatively high cost of short-course therapies, when compared to meager health budgets, and on the need to have a reasonably well-functioning health care system. There are also arguments based on distributive justice—for example, why HIV should hold a special status. But prevention of perinatal transmission, which can be achieved sometimes with a single dose, will save countless lives of young people with productive futures. The economic benefits of preventing perinatal transmission cannot be compared with therapy once the disease has taken hold, which requires far more expensive, complex, and arduous treatment regimes over the course of a lifetime.

The ethical objections to short-course therapy rest primarily on the need for voluntary counseling and testing before administration of antiretrovirals. Some believe that poor, uneducated women cannot give fully informed and voluntary consent to testing and treatment. Yet informing women in ways that are culturally and linguistically appropriate can ensure voluntary and informed consent.[136] Another alternative is to routinely offer a single dose of nevirapine orally to the mother and once to the infant without the need for an HIV test. Given the devastation of the perinatal HIV epidemic and the availability of uncomplicated, inexpensive interventions, it ought to be possible to relieve the suffering and loss of life in developing countries.

Women and children, wherever they live, deserve a comprehensive package of care in pregnancy, during delivery, and after birth. UNAIDS, UNICEF, and WHO recommend early access to antenatal care, voluntary and confidential counseling and HIV testing for women and their partners, antiretroviral preventive therapy, care during labor and delivery, and counseling on alternative methods of infant feeding including support for those who choose breast-feeding replacements.[137] Additionally, women deserve access to methods of family planning, children deserve postnatal care, and families deserve nutritional and social support.[138]

The Controversy over Research Ethics in International Collaborative Research

It is clear that short-course antiretroviral therapy can have enormous benefits for less developed countries. But this utilitarian argument has been challenged as an insufficient justification for conducting research trials in Africa, Asia, and the Caribbean to determine the efficacy of a low-dose regimen of AZT in pregnant women. In the middle-to-late 1990s fifteen placebo-controlled trials (PCTS) were conducted in the Ivory Coast, Uganda, Tanzania, Malawi, Ethiopia, Burkina Faso, Zimbabwe, Kenya, Dominican Republic, and South Africa.[139] A sixteenth trial conducted in Thailand was an equivalency trial in which a regimen that had already been proven effective (ACTG 076 regime) was compared with a second regimen (low-dose antiretrovirals) to determine if it was as effective but less toxic or expensive. Most of the studies were funded by the National Institutes of Health (NIH) and the Centers for Disease Control and Prevention (CDC); the others were funded by European countries, South Africa, and UNAIDS.[140]

There is no doubt that if these PCTs had been conducted in the United States, they would have been regarded as unethical. No trial would be ethically approved in a developed country if it denied access to an intervention thought to hold promise of being at least as effective as, if not more effective than, the prevailing standard of care. The question posed is whether it is ethical to withhold a treatment in a poor country when the treatment is used as the standard of care in developed countries but is not attainable in the country in which the research is taking place.[141] The issue is not whether it is ethical for First World researchers to investigate a therapy that would be out-of-reach or unimportant in the country in which the research takes place (e.g., testing high-technology interventions for cancer in the least developed countries). International collaborative research that is of little benefit to the host country arguably is unethical, but the short-course protocols were designed to find affordable treatments in developing countries.[142]

The short-course studies provoked a storm of controversy.[143] Critics argued that placebo controls are never justified when an effective treatment exists; subjects in the control group must receive the "best known treatment," meaning the highest standard that would be available in developed countries.[144] Critics argued that high levels of care for research subjects were mandated by the Helsinki Declaration as revised in 2000: "A new method should be tested against . . . the best current prophylactic, diagnostic, and therapeutic methods. This does not exclude the use of placebo, or no treatment, in studies where no proven prophylactic, diagnostic or therapeutic method exists."[145] Critics also cited the Council of International Organisations of Medical Societies (CIOMS) Guidelines on Biomedical Research, which state that ethical and scientific review should be conducted according to the standards of the sponsoring agency and should be "no less exacting" than if conducted in the sponsoring country.[146] In draft revisions to the guidelines, CIOMS asserts that the Helsinki standard should be adopted unless there are sound reasons to use a control, such as when withholding the best current treatment would result in no serious adverse effect and a comparative study of two treatments would yield no reliable scientific results.[147] Other scholars have elaborated on the ethical conditions that would justify use of PCTs in cases where there is a proven treatment.[148]

Marcia Angell, then editor of the *New England Journal of Medicine*, harshly compared the short-course trials to the infamous study in Tuskegee, Alabama, where African American men with syphilis were simply observed and left untreated: "Women in the Third World would not receive antiretroviral treatment anyway, so the investigators are simply observing what would happen to the subjects' infants if there were no study. And a placebo-controlled study is the fastest, most efficient way to obtain unambiguous information that will be of greatest value in the Third World."[149] Angell criticized this logic: "All the rationalizations boil down to asserting that the end justifies the means—which it no more does in Africa than it did in Alabama."[150]

Harold Varmus and David Satcher, then heads of NIH and CDC respectively, responded vigorously: "[Critics] allude inappropriately to the infamous Tuskegee study, which did not test an intervention. The Tuskegee study ultimately deprived people of a known, effective, affordable intervention. To claim that countries seeking help in stemming the tide of maternal-infant HIV transmission by seeking usable interventions have followed that path trivializes the suffering of the men in the Tuskegee study and shows a serious lack of understanding of today's trials."[151]

Varmus and Satcher, supported by a broad array of AIDS researchers in developed[152] and less developed[153] countries, strongly defended the trials on the grounds that PCTs were scientifically necessary; an equivalency study between two interventions of unknown benefit would not make clear whether either intervention was more effective than no intervention. There were also confounding factors such as the relative toxicity of the interventions. Further, they argued, an ACTG 076 regimen group would be of little use since the regimen was unaffordable and unavailable in the host country.

As Ronald Bayer suggests, this was not a clash over first principles, but a dispute over the application of agreed-upon principles in different social conditions.[154] The established ethical principle is that human research subjects should not be denied the standard of care, but which standard—the prevalent standard achievable in the most advanced industrialized economy or the standard in the host country? In this context, policymakers had to make treatment decisions under conditions of poverty, scarcity, and urgent need. Everyone felt conflicted making these critical choices and would have liked to have had a uniform standard everywhere. The research subjects were informed, consented, and not exposed to risk; the study was designed to benefit host countries, which desired the research and ethically approved the protocol; and the results may vastly improve the lives of the world's poorest and most disadvantaged mothers and children. Given the social and economic context, it may have been unethical not to conduct the most rigorous and efficient international studies to prevent perinatal transmission in the least developed countries.[155] Ethical questions surrounding HIV/AIDS research in resource-poor countries will continue to arise as the world struggles with the disease.[156]

Conclusion

Secretary General Kofi Annan's asked for seven billion dollars a year for a global fund to fight infectious diseases. I tell you, I've done a lot of work in this area. We can turn this epidemic around in three years. Brazil cut the death rate in half in three years with medicine and prevention. Uganda, with no medicine, cut the death rate in half in five years. We do not have to have 100 million AIDS cases in five years. We do not have to let countries be consumed by this. I promise you, fledgling democracies will be destroyed by this. They will not be able to sustain an AIDS caseload of 100 million. And we don't have to have it happen. We ought to fund this program. It's not very much money.—William Jefferson Clinton, former president of the United States (2001)

The world is in the midst of one of the great pandemics in human history with untold suffering, illness, and death. The devastating social and economic effects are just as sobering as the health effects. One would expect the international community to mobilize against a threat of this magnitude, but somehow there is complacency, even indifference, when there should be resolve and unity. As the toll of the pandemic rises, particularly in the poorest regions, there remains fierce debate about humanitarian assistance, property rights, and ethics.

Given the level of need, there ought to be little disagreement that the more prosperous countries of North America and Europe should be devoting significant resources for education, prevention, and treatment in the poorer countries of Africa and Southeast Asia. Yet political leaders in developed countries have not viewed it in their self-interest to provide the kind of resources needed. Nor have many leaders in less developed countries given HIV/AIDS the kind of priority necessary to reduce the burden of disease. For complex and not-well-understood reasons, there has been an absence of political will to confront the HIV/AIDS pandemic.

There is some hope that political will in developed countries could be changing. In his State of the Union address in January 2003, President Bush asked

Congress to commit $15 billion over the next five years "to turn the tide against AIDS in the most afflicted nations of Africa and the Caribbean."[157] The funding will go to initiatives to prevent new infections, treat, and care for those in countries where the disease has taken its greatest toll, including Botswana, Côte d'Ivoire, Ethiopia, Guyana, Haiti, Kenya, Mozambique, Namibia, Nigeria, Rwanda, South Africa, Tanzania, Uganda, and Zambia.

In May 2003 President Bush signed the U.S. Leadership against HIV/AIDS, Tuberculosis, and Malaria Act of 2003, the first step in turning his promise into law. While the world is enthusiastic about the act, some skepticism remains. Critics are concerned that the full amount will not be appropriated by Congress, and that the funding will be phased in too slowly.[158] Up to $1 billion per year could go to the Global Fund to Fight AIDS, Malaria, and Tuberculosis, which was designed to be an efficient method of dispersing AIDS funds. This is an improvement from the president's suggested $200 million, but still only one-third of the total funding.[159] The plan has also met with resistance because some countries greatly affected by the pandemic are left out. For example, Zimbabwe, where one in three adults is HIV-infected, borders three countries named in the plan but will not receive any funding. Finally, the bill requires that one-third of the amount designated for prevention must be set aside for programs that promote abstinence and not other proven preventions such as condom use.[160] The forces of moralism in the Bush administration and in Congress conflict with the humanitarian needs of countries devastated by HIV/AIDS. It remains to be seen whether the new funding will encourage other nations to provide funding and have an impact on the crisis or end up another lost opportunity to make a real difference.[161]

The private sector has also been unwilling to make the sacrifices necessary to make drugs and potential vaccines available in resource-poor markets. Transnational corporations, often supported by industrialized countries, have used international trade rules to safeguard their proprietary interests in AIDS medicines. This has resulted in higher prices and less access to these essential drugs in developing countries. Certainly, international public health agencies and some pharmaceutical companies have been working to reduce prices and increase access. Yet most modern medications are still out-of-reach for the poor.

There has even been sharp disagreement among ethicists. Some would require research subjects in the least developed countries to receive the standard of care available in the most developed countries. Although this might benefit persons directly participating in research trials, it might not be the best way to study the safety and efficacy of drug regimens that would be affordable in poor countries. This disagreement has distracted attention from the vital issue of preventing perinatal transmission in less developed countries by ensuring that women and their infants have access to a range of care and services.

The strategies needed to significantly reduce the burden of HIV/AIDS are well known and demonstrated to be effective. What is still needed are the economic resources and political will necessary to implement comprehensive programs for AIDS prevention and treatment in every region.

Chapter 17

AIDS Policy, Politics, and Law

Reflections on the Pandemic

This book has explored the HIV/AIDS pandemic in five areas: (1) AIDS litigation (the story of people and communities seen through the lens of the courtroom), (2) the rights and dignity of persons living with HIV/AIDS in domestic law and international human rights law (notably, the fundamental rights to privacy and nondiscrimination), (3) HIV/AIDS policies in conflict (the tensions between public health and civil liberties relating to some of the most divisive issues —screening, reporting, partner notification, and compulsory state powers), (4) special populations that have been subject to neglect, exclusion, or punishment (survivors of sexual assault, health care workers, pregnant women, and injection drug users), and (5) HIV/AIDS in the world (the problems of political will, global trade, and international collaborative research).

HIV/AIDS has deeply affected people and social institutions throughout the

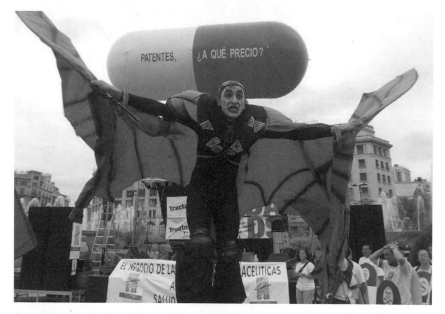

An AIDS protest takes place in Barcelona's Plaza de Catalunya, Saturday, July 6, 2002, under a giant balloon in the shape of a medicine capsule. The protest, coinciding with the Fourteenth International Conference on AIDS in Barcelona, highlighted the fact that only a tiny amount of medicine available for AIDS sufferers reaches the world's poor countries where the pandemic is the most deadly. Words on the balloon read "Patents: At What Price?" (© AP/Wide World Photos)

world. In concluding this examination of the pandemic, it will be helpful to briefly look back at the salient issues of policy, politics, and law.

The Legal Sphere

It is no exaggeration to say that HIV/AIDS has profoundly affected legal structures in the United States and internationally. No disease in modern history has provoked more domestic legislation and litigation. In the United States alone, the federal government and the fifty states have enacted HIV-specific legislation covering almost every conceivable aspect of AIDS policy.[1] Statutes and regulations govern the approval and oversight of vaccines and pharmaceuticals; set policy relating to casefinding and public health interventions; affect the organization of social institutions such as the health care system, the military, and prisons; and restrict the autonomy or liberty of persons engaging in risk behaviors. Similar patterns of HIV-specific legislation are found in most regions of the globe.[2]

The judiciary has been just as important as the legislature in setting policy and resolving disputes arising from the HIV/AIDS epidemic. Thousands of court cases have been decided affecting virtually all social groups and institutions (e.g., sex partners, families, hospitals, and blood suppliers). These cases have profoundly influenced the development of legal doctrine in areas as diverse as torts, family law, and constitutional law. AIDS policies have resulted in censorship, restraints, and discriminatory treatment. Courts have been called upon to resolve disputes involving bathhouses, adult cinemas, and AIDS advertising and education (see Chapters 2 and 3).

The HIV/AIDS pandemic also has affected international legal structures. Countries throughout the world have imposed travel and/or immigration restrictions on persons living with HIV/AIDS (see Chapter 15). Many countries have enacted HIV-specific criminal laws, and one country (Cuba) has even implemented universal screening and isolation.[3] International organizations, such as the World Health Organization (WHO) and the Joint United Nations Programme on AIDS (UNAIDS), have actively opposed these and other legal restrictions, often without complete success.[4]

In response to these and other repressive policies and practices, the AIDS community has embraced the promotion of human rights. Beginning with the pioneering work of the late Jonathan Mann, scholars and advocates have used human rights law to stress the importance of civil, political, social, and economic rights as tools of public health.[5] The HIV/AIDS pandemic has significantly influenced international law, which is exploring the interconnections between human rights and public health. Notably, the AIDS community has demanded that international agencies develop a more robust conception of the human right to health (see Chapter 4). In response, the Office of the High Commissioner for Human Rights (OHCHR) and UNAIDS updated human rights guidelines in 2002, proclaiming a right to HIV/AIDS treatment.[6] The United Nations issued a General Comment on the Right to Health in 2000,[7] and appointed a Special Rapporteur in 2002.[8] The human right to health has the potential for improving the lives of persons living with HIV/AIDS. This is illustrated by the ruling of South Africa's Constitutional Court in 2002 that the government must ensure greater access to antiretroviral medication for pregnant women.[9]

Human rights law, particularly the right to health, often conflicts with international trade law. Whereas proponents of human rights favor greater access to vaccines and drugs for all those in need, world trade law vigorously defends the proprietary interests of transnational pharmaceutical companies. Patents and trade are complex and evolving areas of international law. There are creative ways to ensure that protecting intellectual property does not mean reducing access to vaccines and drugs (see Chapter 16). Still, some of the most bitter disputes between highly developed and resource-poor countries involve access to affordable AIDS medications. These disputes are distinctively legal in nature, demonstrating the importance of the legal sphere in the AIDS pandemic.[10]

The Sociopolitical Sphere

The social and political dimensions of HIV/AIDS are profound and enduring. This observation should not be surprising given the fact that AIDS has deep associations with many of the social taboos of humanity—the fear of epidemics and death; the symbolism of blood as a protector or destroyer of life; the significance of sex in love, passion, and reproduction; and the euphoria, fear, and devastation of illicit drugs.[11]

These social dimensions are universal and explain many of the sociopolitical responses to HIV/AIDS around the world. Societies, irrespective of cultural tradition, have shunned, stigmatized, or excluded persons living with HIV/AIDS. The public has claimed a "right to know" who is infected and a right to discriminate based on serological status. Politicians have denied the full reality of AIDS, questioned scientific fact, and stubbornly refused to act. To some elected officials, the negative associations of HIV/AIDS have been more important in shaping their political agendas than the urgency of saving lives (see Chapter 16).

HIV/AIDS transforms life stories for those affected. The disease saps individuals of strength and vitality and creates gaping holes in the fabric of community life. Lovers lose their partners, children lose their parents, and communities lose their friends, families, and coworkers. As HIV/AIDS affects the health and longevity of more people (particularly the young) in a community, it is bound to deeply affect social life.[12]

The sociopolitical effects of the epidemic are not purely negative. The HIV/AIDS epidemic also has changed society and politics for the better. At the beginning of this book I asserted that as families and communities begin to see AIDS within their own members, they will become less fearful and exclusionary and more compassionate and welcoming. That certainly has been the experience in many societies once the human costs of the epidemic have become internalized. HIV/AIDS should not be seen as a disease of "the other"; if the burdens are shared among us all, they become more bearable.

At the same time, elected officials slowly have come to see the salience of HIV/AIDS in the political culture. In the early stages of the epidemic, elected officials often ignored the problem or, worse, focused on moralism rather than the public's health. Over the long term, however, they have been forced to act. Persons living with HIV/AIDS and their advocates have demanded that the political community engage in HIV prevention and treatment. For the most part, the wider public has concurred, especially as they see HIV/AIDS as part of the human condition.

The Economic Sphere

The economic sphere is closely related to the social and political spheres. The health effects of HIV/AIDS often render individuals unable to work and contribute to the nation's economy. This is the case in poorer countries experiencing higher levels of morbidity and mortality. In these countries, HIV/AIDS harms the economy in multiple ways. It lowers productivity as men and women with skills and energy are taken from the workforce, contributing to food emergencies and famine.[13] HIV/AIDS also vastly increases costs for health care and social support, especially given the high price of AIDS medications. Finally, the private sector is often discouraged from investing in countries with high burdens of HIV/AIDS. Cumulatively, these financial impediments can devastate the economic systems of poor nations.[14]

International economic systems are even more complex and important. Resource-poor countries have paltry sums to spend on health. Many urgent health needs compete with HIV/AIDS for resources.[15] It is in this context that poorer countries look to the more industrialized countries of North America and Europe for financial and technical assistance. Recognizing this, the United Nations established a Global Fund to Fight AIDS, Tuberculosis, and Malaria.[16] Yet donor countries have not found it in their self-interest to contribute generously to this fund or to global efforts to fight HIV/AIDS generally.[17] This failure to recognize the urgent health needs in poor countries is lamentable from a humanitarian perspective. But it is also shortsighted because, in a world of international travel and migration, HIV/AIDS and other infectious diseases (e.g., severe acute respiratory system) cannot be contained within country borders. President Bush's 2003 promise of $15 billion over five years to fight AIDS in Africa and the Caribbean may signal a new commitment to combat the epidemic. Time will tell if, in the third decade of the disease, leaders are willing to expend the resources necessary to turn the tide.

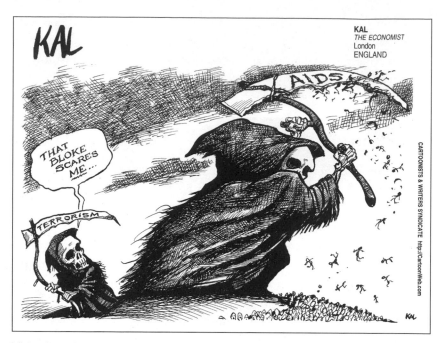

This editorial cartoon ran in the *Baltimore Sun* in July 2002 following reports from the Fourteenth International Conference on AIDS in Barcelona that over 3 million people died from HIV/AIDS in 2001 alone.

The Scientific Sphere

Science and public health have come a long way since the beginning of the HIV/AIDS epidemic.[18] For many years, the only vaccine for HIV was education and the only treatment was prophylaxis against opportunistic infections.[19] As a result, persons living with HIV/AIDS had a feeling of hopelessness and despair. It was thought that deteriorating health, and ultimately death, would occur in only a matter of time. This feeling of despair turned to near euphoria for the decade beginning in 1987. This was a time of rapid advances in the treatment of HIV/AIDS. The use of highly active antiretroviral therapy (HAART) seemed to create miracles, making viral loads of individuals virtually undetectable. Persons infected with HIV were living active, healthy lives. New therapies also offered the hope of significant declines in the transmission of HIV.[20] Notably, antiretroviral treatment administered to pregnant women and newborns significantly reduced the rate of mother-to-child HIV transmission.[21]

Looking back at the advances in treatment, we can now see that the promise of HAART was premature and exaggerated. Certainly, AIDS treatments remain highly effective, but they are not cures or panaceas. Many people experience serious side effects, their viral loads increase, and their health deteriorates.[22] Newly diagnosed drug-resistant strains of HIV more than tripled between 1995 and 2000, and the problem continues to escalate.[23] At the same time, science still has not yet developed a safe and effective vaccine.[24]

AIDS Today

Perhaps the most salient reality of HIV/AIDS in the world is the disproportionate burden it places on poor and powerless populations. When AIDS first appeared in North America, it affected primarily gay men and recipients of blood transfusions, particularly persons with hemophilia. The demographics of HIV/AIDS today are quite different. Worldwide, women now account for half of new HIV infections.[25] Like so many other diseases in the past, the burden of HIV/AIDS has fallen principally on the poor and on people of color. That is the demographic pattern in the United States as well as in other developed countries.[26]

Reducing the burden of HIV/AIDS is achievable. If countries raise awareness of risk behaviors, educate the public, and provide the means by which individuals can protect themselves (e.g., condoms and sterile drug-injection equipment), the spread of HIV can be markedly reduced.[27] We have the medications to dramatically decrease perinatal HIV transmission and improve the lives of persons living with HIV/AIDS. We also have to understand the powerful connections between health and human rights. By ensuring the dignity and rights of persons at risk for HIV and those already infected, we can enable people to better protect their health and prevent the spread of infection to others.

The policies for preventing and treating HIV infection are clear and effective. What is still lacking is the political will and the financial commitment necessary to safeguard the public's health in the United States and globally.

Notes

Abbreviations

AJPH	*American Journal of Public Health*
APPJ	*AIDS and Public Policy Journal*
ASTHO	Association of State and Territorial Health Officials
BWHO	*Bulletin of the World Health Organization*
CSIS	Center for Strategic and International Studies
H/ASR	*HIV/AIDS Surveillance Report*
JAIDS	*Journal of Acquired Immune Deficiency Syndromes*
JAMA	*Journal of the American Medical Association*
JAPA	*Journal of the American Pharmaceutical Association*
JHHR	*Journal of Health and Human Rights*
MMWR	*Morbidity and Mortality Weekly Report*
NEJM	*New England Journal of Medicine*
NYT	*New York Times*
UNICEF	United Nations Children's Fund

Preface

1. CDC, "*Pneumocystis* Pneumonia—Los Angeles," *MMWR* 30 (June 5, 1981): 250–52.

2. CDC, "Current Trends Update on Acquired Immune Deficiency Syndrome (AIDS) —United States," *MMWR* 31 (September 24, 1982): 507–14.

3. Luc Montagnier, "A History of HIV Discovery," *Science* 298 (November 29, 2002): 1727–28; Robert C. Gallo, "The First Human Retrovirus," *Scientific American* 255 (December 1986): 88–98; Stanley B. Prusiner, "Discovering the Cause of AIDS," *Science* 298 (November 29, 2002): 1726.

4. Michael T. Osterholm et al., "Screening Donated Blood and Plasma for HTLV-III Antibody: Facing More Than One Crisis," *NEJM* 312 (May 2, 1985): 1185–89.

5. CDC, *H/ASR* 13 (Atlanta: CDC, December 2001): 6.

6. CDC, "Advancing HIV Prevention: New Strategies for a Changing Epidemic— United States, 2003," *MMWR* 52 (April 18, 2003): 329–32.

7. Patricia Fleming et al., "HIV Prevalence in the United States, 2000" (paper presented at the Ninth Conference on Retroviruses and Opportunistic Infections, Seattle, Wash., 2002); Lawrence K. Altman, "Many in US with HIV Don't Know It or Seek Care," *NYT*, February 26, 2002.

8. Thomas American Health Consultants, "HIV Prevention Efforts Reach a Crossroad as Signs Point to Rising Infections," *AIDS Alert* 18 (June 2003): 70–73; Michael Gross, "The Second Wave Will Drown Us," *AJPH* 93 (June 2003): 872–81.

9. United Nations, *National Population Policies, 2001* (Geneva: United Nations Population Division of the Department of Economic and Social Affairs, 2001).

10. UNAIDS and WHO, *AIDS Epidemic Update* (Geneva: UNAIDS and WHO, December 2002), ⟨http://www.unaids.org/worldaidsday/2002/press/Epiupdate.html⟩.

11. Karen A. Stanecki, *The AIDS Pandemic in the 21st Century* (Washington, D.C.: U.S. Census Bureau, 2002).

12. Liz McGregor, "Botswana Battles against 'Extinction,'" *The Guardian*, July 8, 2002.

13. UNAIDS, *AIDS Epidemic Update* (Geneva: UNAIDS, December 2000).

14. UNAIDS and WHO, *AIDS Epidemic Update* (December 2002); Lawrence K. Altman, "Women with HIV Reach Half of Global Cases," *NYT*, November 27, 2002.

15. UNAIDS, UNICEF, and USAID, *Children on the Brink 2002: A Joint Report on Orphan Estimates and Program Strategies* (Washington, D.C.: UNAIDS, UNICEF, and USAID, July 2002).

16. Randy Shilts, *And the Band Played On: People, Politics, and the AIDS Epidemic* (New York: Penguin Books, 1988); David Altman, *AIDS in the Mind of America* (Garden City, N.Y.: Anchor Press/Doubleday, 1986).

17. Lawrence O. Gostin and David W. Webber, "The AIDS Litigation Project: HIV/AIDS in the Courts in the 1990s, Part 1," *APPJ* 13 (Spring 1998): 105–21; Gostin and Webber, "The AIDS Litigation Project: HIV/AIDS in the Courts in the 1990s, Part 2," *APPJ* 13 (Summer 1998): 3–19.

18. Barton Gellman, "AIDS Is Declared Threat to Security," *Washington Post*, April 30, 2000.

19. Editorial, "An Anti-Life Crusade," *NYT*, December 20, 2002.

20. Sheryl Gay Stolberg and Richard W. Stevenson, "The President's Proposals: AIDS Policy; Bush AIDS Effort Surprises Many, but Advisors Call It Long Planned," *NYT*, January 30, 2003.

21. Garance Franke-Ruta, "The Fakeout: Bush Promised Billions for AIDS—But Not until He's Left Office," *American Prospect*, April 2003.

22. Scientifically, it was also a period of intense research but little apparent success.

See Robert C. Gallo, "The Early Years of HIV/AIDS," *Science* 298 (November 29, 2002): 1728–30.

23. Charles J. Cooper, Assistant Attorney General, Office of Legal Counsel, U.S. Department of Justice, "Memorandum for Ronald E. Robertson, General Counsel, HHS, Re: Application of Section 504 of the Rehabilitation Act to Persons with AIDS, AIDS-Related Complex, or Infection with the AIDS Virus," Washington, D.C., June 20, 1986.

24. Douglas W. Kmiec, Acting Assistant Attorney General, Office of Legal Counsel, U.S. Department of Justice, "Memorandum for Arthur B. Culvahouse, Jr., Counsel to the President, Re: Application of Section 504 of the Rehabilitation Act to HIV-infected Individuals," Washington, D.C., September 27, 1988.

25. Supplemental Appropriations Act of 1987, P.L. 100–71, § 518, 101 Stat. 391, 475 (1987) (codified at 52 Fed. Reg. 32,540) (August 28, 1987).

26. Ryan White and Ann Marie Cunningham (contributor), *Ryan White: My Own Story* (New York: Penguin Books, 1992).

27. Charles Marwick, "FDA Seeks Swifter Approval of Drugs for Some Life-Threatening or Debilitating Diseases," *JAMA* 260 (November 25, 1988): 2976.

28. The FDA did not approve a rapid HIV diagnostic test kit until 2002. CDC, "Approval of a New Rapid Test for HIV Antibody," *MMWR* 46 (November 22, 2002): 1051–52.

29. Edward M. Connor et al., "Reduction of Maternal-Infant Transmission of Human Immunodeficiency Virus Type 1 with Zidovudine Treatment: Pediatric AIDS Clinical Trials Group Protocol 076 Study Group," *NEJM* 331 (November 3, 1994): 1173–80.

30. CDC, "Recommendations for Preventing Transmission of Infection with Human T-Lymphotropic Virus Type III/Lymphadenopathy-Associated Virus in the Workplace," *MMWR* 34 (November 15, 1985): 682–86, 691–95.

31. CDC, "Perspectives in Disease Prevention and Health Promotion Public Health Service Guidelines for Counseling and Antibody Testing to Prevent HIV Infection and AIDS," *MMWR* 36 (August 14, 1987): 509–15.

32. Presidential Commission on AIDS, *AIDS and Government: A Plan of Action?* (Washington, D.C.: GPO, 1988).

33. National Commission on AIDS, *First Interim Report to the President and the Congress: Failure of U.S. Health Care System to Deal with HIV Epidemic* (Washington, D.C.: National Commission on AIDS, December 1989).

34. Presidential Advisory Council on HIV/AIDS, *Progress Report: Implementation of Advisory Council Recommendations* (Washington, D.C.: Presidential Advisory Council on HIV/AIDS, July 8, 1996).

35. HOPE Act of 1988, P.L. 100–607, 102 Stat. 3048 (codified as amended in scattered sections of 42 U.S.C.).

36. CARE (1990), P.L. 101–381, 104 Stat. 576 (codified as amended in scattered sections of 42 U.S.C.).

37. ADA of 1990, P.L. 101–336, 104 Stat. 327 (codified as amended in scattered sections of 42 U.S.C.).

38. *Bragdon v. Abbott*, 524 U.S. 624 (1998).

39. HOPWA, 42 U.S.C. § 12912 (1991).

40. CDC, *H/ASR* 10 (Atlanta: CDC, June 1998): 36, ‹http://www.cdc.gov/hiv/stats/hasr1001/table28.htm›.

41. Ricky Ray Hemophilia Relief Fund Act, 42 U.S.C. § 300c–22 (1998).

42. Global AIDS and Tuberculosis Relief Act of 2000, P.L. 106–264, 114 Stat. 748 (codified as amended in scattered sections of 22 U.S.C.).

43. CDC, "Advancing HIV Prevention: New Strategies for a Changing Epidemic—United States, 2003," *MMWR* 52 (April 18, 2003): 329–32.

44. Linda A. Valleroy et al., "HIV Prevalence and Associated Risks in Young Men Who Have Sex with Men," *JAMA* 284 (July 12, 2000): 198–204; CDC, "HIV Incidence among Young Men Who Have Sex with Men—Seven U.S. Cities, 1994–2000," *MMWR* 50 (June 1, 2001): 440–44.

45. Charles F. Turner, Heather G. Miller, and Lincoln E. Moses, eds., *AIDS: Sexual Behavior and Intravenous Drug Use* (Washington, D.C.: National Academy Press, 1989).

46. Susan J. Little et al., "Antiretroviral-Drug Resistance among Patients Recently Infected with HIV," *NEJM* 347 (August 8, 2002): 385–94; Joan Stephenson, "'Sobering' Levels of Drug-Resistant HIV Found," *JAMA* 287 (February 13, 2002): 704–5.

47. The results for some ethnic subgroups were inconclusive, and more analysis is needed. AVAC, "Understanding the Results of the AIDSVAX Trial," March 11, 2003.

48. CDC, "Unrecognized HIV Infection, Risk Behaviors, and Perceptions of Risk among Young Black Men Who Have Sex with Men—Six U.S. Cities, 1994–1998," *MMWR* 51 (August 23, 2002): 733–36.

49. UNAIDS and WHO, *AIDS Epidemic Update* (December 2002).

50. Stanecki, *AIDS Pandemic*.

51. Robert Steinbrook, "Beyond Barcelona—The Global Response to HIV," *NEJM* 347 (August 22, 2002): 553–54.

52. Todd Summers, J. Stephen Morrison, et al., *The Global Fund to Fight AIDS, TB, and Malaria Progress Report* (Washington, D.C.: CSIS, February 2003).

53. Jim Lobe, "Health Activists Slam Bush AIDS Initiative," *Inter Press Service*, June 19, 2002.

54. Franke-Ruta, "The Fakeout."

55. Lawrence O. Gostin, William J. Curran, and Mary E. Clark, *Acquired Immunodeficiency Syndrome: Legal, Regulatory, and Policy Analysis* (Washington, D.C.: HHS, 1986; reprint, University Publishing Group, 1988).

56. Lawrence O. Gostin, William J. Curran, and Mary Clark, *Global Survey of AIDS Legislation* (Geneva: WHO, 1990).

57. Lawrence O. Gostin and Lane Porter, eds., *International Law and AIDS: International Responses, Current Issues, and Future Directions* (Washington, D.C.: ABA, 1992).

58. Jonathan Mann, Lawrence O. Gostin, Sofia Gruskin, et al., "Health and Human Rights," *JHHR* 1 (1994): 6–22; Gostin and Mann, "Towards the Development of a Human Rights Impact Assessment for the Formulation and Evaluation of Health Policies," *JHHR* 1 (1994): 58–81.

59. Lawrence O. Gostin and William J. Curran, eds., "The Harvard Model AIDS Legislation Project," *American Journal of Law and Medicine* 16 (1990): 1–278.

60. Lawrence O. Gostin, Lane Porter, and Hazel Sandomire, *U.S. AIDS Litigation*

Project I: A National Survey of Federal, State, and Local Cases before Courts and Human Rights Commissions, 2 vols. (Washington, D.C.: GPO, 1990).

61. Lawrence O. Gostin, Zita Lazzarini, Kathleen Flaherty, and Robert Scherer, *The AIDS Litigation Project III: A Look at HIV/AIDS in the Courts in the 1990s* (Menlo Park, Calif.: Henry J. Kaiser Family Foundation, 1996).

62. Lawrence O. Gostin and David W. Webber, "HIV Infection and AIDS in the Public Health and Health Care Systems: The Role of Law and Litigation," *JAMA* 279 (April 8, 1998): 1108–131; Gostin and Webber, "The AIDS Litigation Project: HIV/AIDS in the Courts in the 1990s, Part 1," *APPJ* 12 (Winter 1997): 105–21; Gostin and Webber, "The AIDS Litigation Project: HIV/AIDS in the Courts in the 1990s, Part 2," *APPJ* 13 (Spring 1998): 3–19.

63. Lawrence O. Gostin and Zita Lazzarini, *Public Health and Human Rights in the HIV Pandemic* (New York: Oxford University Press, 1997).

64. Lawrence O. Gostin, Zita Lazzarini, Verla S. Neslund, and Michael T. Osterholm, "The Public Health Information Infrastructure: A National Review of the Law on Health Information Privacy," *JAMA* 275 (June 26, 1996): 1921–27.

65. Lawrence O. Gostin and James G. Hodge Jr., "Piercing the Veil of Secrecy in HIV/AIDS and Other Sexually Transmitted Diseases: Theories of Privacy and Disclosure in Partner Notification," *Duke Journal of Gender Law and Policy* 5 (Spring 1998): 9–88.

66. Lawrence O. Gostin and Zita Lazzarini, "Prevention of HIV/AIDS among Injection Drug Users: The Theory and Science of Public Health and Criminal Justice Approaches to Disease Prevention," *Emory Law Journal* 46 (Spring 1997): 587–696; Gostin, Lazzarini, T. Stephen Jones, and Kathleen Flaherty, "Prevention of HIV/AIDS and Other Blood-borne Diseases among Injecting Drug Users: A National Survey on the Regulation of Syringes and Needles," *JAMA* 277 (January 1, 1997): 53–62; Gostin, "The Inter-connected Epidemics of Drug Dependency and AIDS," *Harvard Civil Rights–Civil Liberties Law Review* 26 (Winter 1991): 113–84.

67. Lane Porter and Lawrence O. Gostin, "The Application of United States Protection of Human Subjects Regulations and Ethical Provisions to United States Funded or Conducted HIV-Related Research in Foreign Countries: A Comprehensive Reference Guide for Researchers and the United States Public Health Service," September 1994.

Chapter 1

1. Thomas A. Delaney, "Actual Exposure or Reasonableness?: Policy Issues Drive the Ongoing Debate over What Standards Should Govern the Recovery of Emotional Distress Damages for Fear of Contracting Infectious Disease," *Health Lawyer* 13 (August 2001): 11–17.

2. *New York v. New St. Mark's Baths*, 497 N.Y.S.2d 979 (Sup. Ct. 1986).

3. *Ben Rich Trading v. City of Vineland*, 126 F.3d 155 (3d Cir. 1997).

4. CDC, "Acquired Immunodeficiency Syndrome—United States, 1992," *MMWR* 42 (July 23, 1993): 547–51, 557.

5. *Doe v. American Nat'l Red Cross*, 34 F.3d 231 (4th Cir. 1994).

6. Eric A. Feldman and Ronald Bayer, eds., *Blood Feuds: AIDS, Blood, and the Politics of Medical Disaster* (New York: Oxford University Press, 1999); Lauren B. Leveton, Harold C. Sox Jr., and Michael A. Stoto, eds., *HIV and the Blood Supply: An Analysis of Crisis Decision Making* (Washington, D.C.: National Academy Press, 1995).

7. *Paramo v. Matthew*, No. 92–3144, 1992 U.S. App. LEXIS 26256 (10th Cir. Oct. 9, 1992).

8. *Walker v. Peters*, 233 F.3d 494 (7th Cir. 2000).

9. *Herring v. Keenan*, 218 F.3d 1171 (10th Cir. 2000).

10. See, e.g., *Doe v. Coughlin*, 697 F. Supp. 1234 (N.D.N.Y. 1988) (holding that assignment of all inmates suspected of being HIV positive to a central facility for testing and evaluation amounted to an unconstitutional constructive disclosure of the inmate's medical status); *Woods v. White*, 689 F. Supp. 874 (W.D.W.I. 1988) (holding that medical staff violated the inmate's constitutional right to privacy by wrongfully communicating his medical status to nonmedical staff and other inmates).

11. *New York State Court Guidelines* (Albany, January 1988).

12. "Re: Jefferson County District Court Judges," *AIDS Litigation Reporter*, January 1989.

13. Charles Rosenberg, *The Cholera Years: The United States in 1832, 1849, and 1866* (Chicago: University of Chicago Press, 1987).

14. Allan M. Brandt, *No Magic Bullet: A Social History of Venereal Disease in the United States since 1880* (New York: Oxford University Press, 1987).

15. Sheila M. Rothman, *Living in the Shadow of Death: Tuberculosis and the Social Experience of Illness in American History* (New York: Basic Books, 1994).

16. Thomas B. Stoddard and Walter Rieman, "AIDS and the Rights of the Individual: Toward a More Sophisticated Analysis," *Milbank Quarterly* 68, supp. 1 (1990): 143–74.

17. UNAIDS and OHCHR, *HIV/AIDS and Human Rights: International Guidelines* (Geneva: UNAIDS and OHCHR, 1998, updated 2002); Joint UNAIDS/OHCHR Press Release, "United Nations Entrenches Human Rights Principles in AIDS Response" (Geneva: UNAIDS and OHCHR, September 10, 2002).

18. Sofia Gruskin and Bebe Loff, "Do Human Rights Have a Role in Public Health Work?" *Lancet* 360 (December 7, 2002): 1880; Lawrence O. Gostin and Zita Lazzarini, *Public Health and Human Rights in the HIV Pandemic* (New York: Oxford University Press, 1997).

19. UNAIDS, *Fact Sheet: An Overview of HIV/AIDS-Related Stigma and Discrimination* (Geneva: UNAIDS, 2002).

20. Lawrence O. Gostin, *Confidentiality, Privacy, and the "Right to Know"* (Chicago: HIV/AIDS Resource Center, *JAMA*, April 1996), ‹http://www.ama-assn.org/special/hiv/policy/confide.htm›.

21. Lawrence O. Gostin, Zita Lazzarini, Verla S. Neslund, and Michael T. Osterholm, "The Public Health Information Infrastructure: A National Review of the Law on Health Information Privacy," *JAMA* 275 (June 26, 1996): 1921–27.

22. HHS, Standards for Privacy of Individually Identifiable Health Information, 67 Fed. Reg. 53181 (August 14, 2002); Gostin, James G. Hodge Jr., and Mira S. Burghardt, "Balancing Communal Goods and Personal Privacy under a National Health Information Privacy Rule," *Saint Louis University Law Journal* 46 (Winter 2002): 5–35.

23. Lawrence O. Gostin and James G. Hodge Jr., "Model State Public Health Privacy Act" (1999), ‹http://www.publichealthlaw.net/Resources/Modellaws.htm›; Gostin, Hodge, and Ronald O. Valdiserri, "Informational Privacy and the Public's Health: The Model State Public Health Privacy Act," *AJPH* 91 (September 2001): 1388–92.

24. CDC, "CDC Guidelines for National Human Immunodeficiency Virus Case Surveillance, Including Monitoring for Human Immunodeficiency Virus Infection and Acquired Immunodeficiency Syndrome," *MMWR* 48 (December 10, 1999): 1–28.

25. Lawrence O. Gostin, Chai R. Feldblum, and David W. Webber, "Disability Discrimination in America: HIV/AIDS and Other Health Conditions," *JAMA* 281 (February 24, 1999): 745–52. In 2002 UNAIDS amended the International Guidelines on HIV/AIDS and Human Rights to encompass a right to treatment and care. OHCHR and UNAIDS, *HIV/AIDS and Human Rights International Guidelines*, Third International Consultation on HIV/AIDS and Human Rights, Geneva, July 25–26, 2002, HR/PUB/2002/1 (New York: United Nations, 2002).

26. Albert R. Jonsen, "The Duty to Treat Patients with AIDS and HIV Infection," in *AIDS and the Health Care System*, edited by Lawrence O. Gostin (New Haven: Yale University Press, 1990), 155–68.

27. Chai R. Feldblum, "Medical Examinations and Inquiries under the Americans with Disabilities Act: A View from the Inside," *Temple Law Review* 64 (Summer 1991): 521–49.

28. *Bragdon v. Abbott*, 524 U.S. 624 (1998).

29. Chai R. Feldblum, "Definition of Disability under Federal Anti-Discrimination Law: What Happened? Why? And What Can We Do about It?," *Berkeley Journal of Employment and Labor Law* 21 (2000): 91–147.

30. Ruth Colker, "Winning and Losing under the Americans with Disabilities Act," *Ohio State Law Journal* 62 (2001): 239–83.

31. *Albertsons v. Kirkinburg*, 527 U.S. 555 (1999).

32. *Toyota Motor Mfg. Ky Inc. v. Williams*, 534 U.S. 184 (2002).

33. *Murphy v. United Parcel Service, Inc.*, 527 U.S. 516 (1999); *Sutton v. United Airlines, Inc.*, 527 U.S. 471 (1999) (holding that severely myopic job applicants for airline pilot positions are not disabled because eyeglasses mitigate their impairment).

34. *Chevron USA Inc. v. Echazabal*, 122 S. Ct. 2045 (2002).

35. *Toyota Motor Mfg.*, 534 U.S. at 184.

36. Lawrence O. Gostin, *Public Health Law: Power, Duty, Restraint* (Berkeley: Milbank Memorial Fund and University of California Press, 2000).

37. Ronald Bayer, "Public Health Policy and the AIDS Epidemic: An End to HIV Exceptionalism," *NEJM* 324 (May 23, 1991): 1500–1504.

38. David I. Schulman, "AIDS Discrimination: Its Nature, Meaning, and Function," *Nova Law Review* 12 (Spring 1998): 1113–46.

39. Sten H. Vermund and Craig M. Wilson, "Barriers to HIV Testing—Where Next?," *Lancet* 360 (October 19, 2002): 1186–87.

40. CDC, "Approval of a New Rapid Test for HIV Antibody," *MMWR* 46 (November 22, 2002): 1051–52.

41. William J. Kassler, "Advances in HIV Testing Technology and Their Potential Impact on Prevention," *AIDS Education and Prevention* 9, supp. B (June 1997): 27–40.

42. CDC, "Advancing HIV Prevention: New Strategies for a Changing Epidemic," *MMWR* 52 (April 18, 2003): 329-32.

43. Center for Biologics Evaluation and Research, *Testing Yourself for HIV-1, the Virus That Causes AIDS* (Rockville, Md.: FDA, 2001), ‹http://www.fda.gov/cber/infosheets/hiv-home2.htm›.

44. CDC, "CDC Guidelines for National Human Immunodeficiency Virus Case Surveillance."

45. ACLU, *HIV Partner Notification: Why Coercion Won't Work* (New York: ACLU, March 1998).

46. Karen H. Rothenberg and Stephen J. Paskey, "The Risk of Domestic Violence and Women with HIV Infection: Implications for Partner Notification, Public Policy, and the Law," *AJPH* 85 (November 1995): 1569–76.

47. Ronald Bayer and Kathleen E. Toomey, "HIV Prevention and the Two Faces of Partner Notification," *AJPH* 82 (August 1992): 1158–64.

48. CDC, "Revised Guidelines for HIV Counseling, Testing, and Referral," *MMWR* 50 (November 9, 2001): 1–58.

49. Lawrence O. Gostin and James G. Hodge Jr., "Piercing the Veil of Secrecy in HIV/AIDS and Other Sexually Transmitted Diseases: Theories of Privacy and Disclosure in Partner Notification," *Duke Journal of Gender Law and Policy* 5 (Spring 1998): 9–88.

50. Jane Durch, Linda A. Bailey, and Michael A. Stoto, *Improving Health in the Community: A Role for Performance Monitoring* (Washington, D.C.: National Academy Press, 1997).

51. Carol Ciesielski, Donal W. Marianos, Gerald Schochetman, John J. Witte, and Harold W. Jaffe, "The 1990 Florida Dental Investigation: The Press and the Science," *Annals of Internal Medicine* 121 (December 1, 1994): 886–88.

52. David I. Schulman, "HIV-infected Health Care Providers: Legal Rights and Protections," *Annals of Emergency Medicine* 20 (December 1991): 1379–80.

53. CDC, "Recommendations for Preventing Transmission of Human Immunodeficiency Virus and Hepatitis B Virus to Patients during Exposure-prone Invasive Procedures," *MMWR* 40 (July 12, 1991): 1–9.

54. P.L. 102–141, Title VI, § 663, 42 U.S.C. § 300ee-2 (2001).

55. Lawrence O. Gostin, "HIV-infected Physicians and the Practice of Seriously Invasive Procedures," *Hastings Center Report* 19 (January–February 1989): 32–39.

56. Lawrence O. Gostin and David W. Webber, "The AIDS Litigation Project, Part 1: HIV/AIDS in the Courts in the 1990s," *APPJ* 12 (Winter 1997): 105–21.

57. Julie Gerberding, "Provider-to-Patient HIV Transmission: How to Keep It Exceedingly Rare," *Annals of Internal Medicine* 130 (January 5, 1999): 64–65; Gerberding, "The Infected Health Care Provider," *NEJM* 334 (February 29, 1996): 594–95.

58. Edward M. Connor et al., "Reduction of Maternal-Infant Transmission of Human Immunodeficiency Virus Type 1 with Zidovudine Treatment," *NEJM* 331 (November 3, 1994): 1173–80.

59. USPHS, "Recommendations of the U.S. Public Health Service Task Force on the Use of Zidovudine to Reduce Perinatal Transmission of Human Immunodeficiency Virus," *MMWR* 43 (August 5, 1994): 1–20.

60. USPHS, "United States Public Health Service Recommendations for Human

Immunodeficiency Virus Counseling and Voluntary Testing for Pregnant Women," *MMWR* 44 (July 7, 1995): 1–15.

61. Lynne M. Mofenson, "U.S. Public Health Service Task Force Recommendations for Use of Antiretroviral Drugs in Pregnant HIV-1 Infected Women for Maternal Health and Interventions to Reduce Perinatal HIV-1 Transmission in the United States," *MMWR* 51 (November 22, 2002): 1–38.

62. CARE Amendments of 1996, PL 104–146, 42 USC 300ff-34 (1994).

63. Secretary of Health Determines Required Newborn HIV Testing Not Routine Practice, 65 Fed. Reg. 3367–3374 (Washington, D.C.: HHS, January 20, 2000).

64. Miriam Davis, "Workshop I Summary," in *Reducing the Odds: Preventing Perinatal Transmission of HIV in the United States*, edited by Michael A. Stoto, Donna A. Almario, and Marie C. McCormick (Washington, D.C.: National Academy Press, 1999).

65. CDC, "HIV Testing among Pregnant Women—United States and Canada, 1998–2001," *MMWR* 51 (November 15, 2002): 1013–16.

66. Michael A. Stoto, Donna A. Almario, and Marie C. McCormick, eds., *Reducing the Odds: Preventing Perinatal Transmission of HIV in the United States* (Washington, D.C.: National Academy Press, 1999).

67. CDC, "Revised Guidelines for HIV Counseling, Testing, and Referral and Revised Recommendations for HIV Screening of Pregnant Women," *MMWR* 50 (November 9, 2001): 59–86.

68. CDC, "Advancing HIV Prevention: New Strategies for a Changing Epidemic," *MMWR* 52 (April 18, 2003): 329–32.

69. CDC, *H/AR* 13 (Atlanta: CDC, December 2001): 14, ⟨http://www.cdc.gov/hiv/stats/hasr1302.pdf⟩.

70. Jonathan A. Cohn, "HIV-1 Infection in Injection Drug Users," *Infectious Disease Clinics of North America* 16 (September 2002): 745–70.

71. Dawn Day, *Health Emergency 2003: The Spread of Drug-Related AIDS and Hepatitis C among African Americans and Latinos* (Princeton, N.J.: Dogwood Center, 2003).

72. Don C. Des Jarlais and Samuel R. Friedman, "The Psychology of Preventing AIDS among Intravenous Drug Users: A Social Learning Conceptualization," *American Psychologist* 43 (November 1988): 865–70.

73. Stephen K. Koester, "Copping, Running, and Paraphernalia Laws: Contextual Variables and Needle Risk Behavior among Injection Drug Users in Denver," *Human Organization* 53 (Fall 1994): 287–95.

74. Jacques Normand, David Vlahov, and Lincoln E. Moses, eds., *Preventing HIV Transmission: The Role of Sterile Needles and Bleach* (Washington, D.C.: National Academy Press, 1995).

75. Donna E. Shalala, *Report to the Committee on Appropriations for the Departments of Labor, Health and Human Services, and Education and Related Agencies: Needle Exchange Programs in America: Review of Published Studies and Ongoing Research* (Washington, D.C.: HHS, February 18, 1997).

76. Howard Markel and Alexandra Minna Stern, "The Foreignness of Germs: The Persistent Association of Immigrants and Disease in American Society," *Milbank Quarterly* 80 (2002): 757–88; David F. Musto, "Quarantine and the Problem of AIDS," *Milbank Quarterly* 64, supp. 1 (1986): 97–117.

77. Bureau of Consular Affairs, *Human Immunodeficiency Virus (HIV) Testing Requirements for Entry into Foreign Countries* (Washington, D.C.: DOS, February 2002), ⟨http://travel.state.gov/HIVtestingreqs.html⟩.

78. Alana Klein, *HIV and Immigration: Final Report* (Montreal: Canadian HIV/AIDS Legal Network, 2001), ⟨http://www.aidslaw.ca/Maincontent/issues/Immigration/finalreport/Immigration2001E.pdf⟩.

79. National Commission on AIDS, *Resolution on U.S. Visa and Immigration Policy* (Washington, D.C.: National Commission on AIDS, December 1989).

80. Amnesty International, *Crimes of Hate, Conspiracy of Silence, Torture, and Ill-treatment Based on Sexual Identity* (London: Amnesty International Publications, 2001), 49–52.

81. Immigration and Nationality Act § 212(a)(1)(A)(i) (2003).

82. Supplemental Appropriations Act of 1987, S.518, P.L. 100–71, HR 1827 (July 11, 1987) (Helms Amendment).

83. 51 Fed. Reg. 32, 540–44 (1987); 52 Fed. Reg. 21, 607 (effective Dec. 1, 1987).

84. This is subject to certain waivers that may be granted. "Immigration and Naturalization Service," press release, *In re Hans Paul Verhoef* (Washington, D.C.: INS, April 7, 1989).

85. INS, *Medical Examination of Aliens Seeking Adjustment of Status* (Washington, D.C.: U.S. Department of Justice, September 1, 1987), ⟨http://www.ins.usdoj.gov/graphics/formsfee/forms/files/I-693.pdf⟩.

86. UNAIDS, "Migration and HIV/AIDS," Second Ad Hoc Thematic Meeting, New Delhi, December 9–11, 1998 (Geneva: UNAIDS Programme Coordinating Board, October 28, 1998), UNAIDS/PCB(7)98.5.

87. World Health Assembly, *International Health Regulations, 1969*, 3d annotated ed. (Geneva: WHO, 1983), art. 81.

88. WHO, "International Health Regulations, 1969," *Weekly Epidemiological Record* 60 (October 4, 1985): 311.

89. UNAIDS and WHO, *AIDS Epidemic Update* (Geneva: UNAIDS and WHO, December 2002), ⟨http://www.unaids.org/worldaidsday/2002/press/Epiupdate.html⟩.

90. *Treatment Action Campaign v. Minister of Health and Others*, (2002)(4) BCLR 356.

91. Editorial, "A Global Medicine Deal," *NYT*, January 5, 2003.

Chapter 2

This chapter is based on Lawrence O. Gostin, Chai Feldblum, and David W. Webber, "Disability Discrimination in America: HIV/AIDS and Other Health Conditions," *JAMA* 281 (February 24, 1999): 745–52; Gostin and Webber, "HIV Infection and AIDS in the Public Health and Health Care Systems: The Role of Law and Litigation," *JAMA* 279 (April 8, 1998): 1108–13; Gostin and Webber, "The AIDS Litigation Project: HIV/AIDS in the Courts in the 1990s, Part 1," *APPJ* 12 (Winter 1997): 105–21; Gostin and Webber, "The AIDS Litigation Project: HIV/AIDS in the Courts in the 1990s, Part 2," *APPJ* 13 (Spring 1998): 3–19; and Gostin, "The AIDS Litigation Project: A National Review of Court and Human Rights Commission Decisions, Part I: The Social Impact of AIDS," *JAMA* 263 (April 11, 1990): 1961–70; and Gostin, "The

AIDS Litigation Project: A National Review of Court and Human Rights Commission Decisions, Part II: Discrimination in Education, Employment, Housing, Insurance, and Health Care," *JAMA* 263 (April 18, 1990): 2086–93. I am indebted to Chai Feldblum, Kathleen Flaherty, Zita Lazzarini, Lane Porter, Hazel Sandomire, Robert Scherer, and David W. Webber who coauthored various aspects of the AIDS Litigation Project with me. I am also indebted to the many litigators and community-based organizations that provided case materials. The ALP was supported by the National AIDS Program Office in the Department of Health and Human Services and by the Henry J. Kaiser Family Foundation.

1. Lawrence O. Gostin, Lane Porter, and Hazel Sandomire, *U.S. AIDS Litigation Project I: A National Survey of Federal, State, and Local Cases before Courts and Human Rights Commissions*, vol. 1 (Washington, D.C.: GPO, 1990); Gostin, Porter, and Sandomire, *U.S. AIDS Litigation Project: Objective Description of Trends in AIDS Litigation*, vol. 2 (Washington, D.C.: GPO, 1990); Gostin, Zita Lazzarini, Kathleen Flaherty, and Robert Scherer, *The AIDS Litigation Project III: A Look at HIV/AIDS in the Courts in the 1990s* (Menlo Park, Calif.: Henry J. Kaiser Family Foundation, 1996).

2. David W. Webber, ed., *AIDS and the Law*, 3d ed. (New York: John Wiley and Sons, 1997, with 2000 Supp.).

3. William E. Dannemeyer, "Proposed 'Sex Survey,'" *Science* 244 (1989): 1530; Mark Barnes, "Towards Ghastly Death: The Censorship of AIDS Education," *Columbia Law Review* 89 (April 1989): 698–724.

4. HOPE Act of 1988, P.L. 100–607, 102 Stat. 3048 (codified as amended in scattered sections of 42 U.S.C.).

5. Memorandum from the AIDS Material Review Committee to AIDS Community Education Contractors, California Department of Health Services, December 18, 1985, cited in Barnes, "Towards Ghastly Death," 708–9.

6. Ronald Bayer, *Private Acts, Social Consequences: AIDS and the Politics of Public Health* (New York: Free Press, 1989), 215–16; Leslie Maitland Werner, "Reagan Officials Debate AIDS Education Policy," *NYT*, January 24, 1987.

7. HHS, *Surgeon General's Report on Acquired Immune Deficiency Syndrome* (Rockville, Md.: Office of the Surgeon General, 1986), 17–19.

8. *Reno v. Am. Civil Liberties Union*, 521 U.S. 844 (1997); *Ashcroft v. Am. Civil Liberties Union*, 535 U.S. 564 (2002) (holding that the Child Online Protection Act, which was limited to communications with commercial intent, was not overbroad due to its reliance on "community standards").

9. *Gay Men's Health Crisis v. Sullivan*, 792 F. Supp. 278 (S.D.N.Y. 1992).

10. For the right to distribute HIV-related information on college campuses, see *Gay Lesbian Bisexual Alliance v. Pryor*, 110 F.3d 1543 (11th Cir. 1997).

11. *AIDS Action Comm. v. Mass. Bay Transp. Auth.*, 42 F.3d 1 (1st Cir. 1994).

12. Sarah E. Samuels and Mark D. Smith, eds., *Condoms in the Schools* (Menlo Park, Calif.: Henry J. Kaiser Family Foundation, 1993).

13. *Brown v. Hot, Sexy & Safer Prods.*, 68 F.3d 525 (1st Cir. 1995), *cert. denied*, 516 U.S. 1159 (1996).

14. *Parents United For Better Schools, Inc. v. School Dist. of Philadelphia Bd. of Educ.*, 148 F.3d 260 (3d Cir. 1998); *Curtis v. School Comm.*, 652 N.E.2d 580 (Mass. 1995), *cert. denied*, 516 U.S. 1067 (1996).

15. CDC, "Epidemiologic Notes and Reports: *Pneumocystis carinii* Pneumonia among Persons with Hemophilia A," *MMWR* 31 (July 16, 1982): 365–67.

16. CDC, "Epidemiologic Notes and Reports: Possible Transfusion-Associated Acquired Immune Deficiency Syndrome (AIDS)—California," *MMWR* 31 (December 10, 1982): 652–54.

17. Lauren B. Levton, Harold C. Sox Jr., and Michael A. Stoto, eds., *HIV and the Blood Supply: An Analysis of Crisis Decisionmaking* (Washington, D.C.: National Academy Press, 1995).

18. Verla S. Neslund, Eugene W. Matthews, and William J. Curran, "The Role of CDC in the Development of AIDS Recommendations and Guidelines," *Law, Medicine, and Health Care* 15 (Summer 1987): 73–79.

19. CDC, "Acquired Immunodeficiency Syndrome—United States, 1992," *MMWR* 42 (July 23, 1993): 547–51, 557.

20. George W. Conk, "Is There a Design Defect in the Restatement (Third) of Torts: Products Liability?," *Yale Law Journal* 109 (March 2000): 1087.

21. *Rogers v. Miles Lab., Inc.*, 802 P.2d 1346 (Wash. 1991); *Spence v. Miles Lab., Inc.*, 37 F.3d 1185 (6th Cir. 1994).

22. *Johnson v. Am. Nat'l Red Cross*, 569 S.E.2d 242, 248 (Ga. Ct. App. 2002); *Pettigrew v. Putterman*, 711 N.E.2d 1008 (Ill. App. Ct. 2002); *Otero v. Presbyterian Hosp.*, 659 N.Y.S.2d 743 (App. Div. 1997) (mem.), *aff'g*, 653 N.Y.S.2d 21 (App. Div. 1997), *prior opinion* 658 N.Y.S.2d 624 (App. Div. 1997); *Weiner v. Lenox Hill Hosp.*, 673 N.E.2d 914 (N.Y. 1996); Robert K. Jenner, *Transfusion-Associated AIDS* (Washington, D.C.: Lawyers and Judges, 1995).

23. *N. N. V. v. American Assn. of Blood Banks*, 89 Cal. Rptr. 2d 885 (Cal. Ct. App. 1999); *Spann v. Irwin Mem'l Blood Ctrs.*, 40 Cal. Rptr. 2d 360 (Cal. Ct. App. 1995).

24. *Estate of Doe v. Vanderbilt Univ., Inc.*, 958 S.W.2d 117 (Tenn. Ct. App. 1997); *Reisner v. Regents of Univ. of Cal.*, 37 Cal. Rptr. 2d 518 (Cal. Ct. App. 1995).

25. *Watson v. Lowcountry Red Cross*, 974 F.2d 482 (4th Cir. 1992).

26. *Doe v. American Nat'l Red Cross*, 34 F.3d 231 (4th Cir. 1994); *Doe v. Puget Sound Blood Ctr.*, 819 P.2d 370 (Wash. 1991) (en banc); *Arnold v. Am. Nat'l Red Cross*, 639 N.E.2d 484 (Ohio Ct. App. 1994).

27. *Marcella v. Brandywine Hosp.*, 47 F.3d 618 (3d Cir. 1995), *aff'g in part & rev'g in part*, 838 F. Supp. 1004 (E.D. Pa. 1993).

28. *Herring v. Keenan*, 218 F.3d 1171 (10th Cir. 2000); *Doe v. American Nat'l Red Cross*, 34 F.3d at 231.

29. *New v. Armour Pharmaceutical Co.*, 67 F.3d 716 (9th Cir. 1995); *Erickson v. Baxter Healthcare, Inc.*, 131 F. Supp. 2d 995 (N.D. Ill. 2001).

30. *King v. Cutter Laboratories, Division of Miles, Inc.*, 714 So. 2d 351 (Fla. 1998).

31. *Doe v. Alpha Therapeutic Corp.*, 3 S.W.3d 404 (Mo. Ct. App. 1999).

32. *Wadleigh v. Rhone-Poulenc Rorer, Inc.*, 157 F.R.D. 410 (N.D. Ill. 1994), *rev'd sub nom. In re Rhone-Poulenc Rorer Inc.*, 51 F.3d 1293 (7th Cir. 1995), *cert. denied*, 516 U.S. 867 (1995), *on*

remand sub nom. *In re Factor VII or IX Concentrate Blood Prods. Litig.*, 169 F.R.D. 632 (N.D. Ill. 1996).

33. Ricky Ray Hemophilia Relief Fund Act, 42 U.S.C. § 300c-22 (1998).

34. Ronald Bayer, "Public Health Policy and the AIDS Epidemic: An End to HIV Exceptionalism," *NEJM* 324 (May 23, 1991): 1500–1504; Michael T. Isbell, "AIDS and Public Health: The Enduring Relevance of a Communitarian Approach to Disease Prevention," *APPJ* 4 (Winter 1993): 157–77.

35. *New York State Soc'y of Surgeons v. Axelrod*, 572 N.E.2d 605 (N.Y. 1991).

36. *Anonymous Fireman v. City of Willoughby*, 779 F. Supp. 402 (N.D. Ohio 1991) (upholding mandatory HIV testing for firefighters and paramedics because they are "high risk" employees).

37. *Plowman v. United States Dep't of Army*, 698 F. Supp. 627 (E.D. Va. 1988) (upholding HIV testing of federal civilian employees).

38. *Local 1812, Am. Fed'n of Gov't Employees v. United States Dep't of State*, 662 F. Supp. 50 (D.D.C. 1987) (upholding HIV testing of foreign service employees).

39. *Haitian Ctrs. Council v. Sale*, 823 F. Supp 1028 (E.D.N.Y. 1993) (upholding HIV screening of immigrants).

40. *In re Juveniles A,B,C,D,E*, 847 P.2d 455 (Wash. 1993) (upholding mandatory HIV testing for juveniles convicted of sexual offenses); *Adams v. State*, 498 S.E.2d 268 (Ga. 1998) (upholding statute permitting victim of crime involving significant risk of exposure to HIV to request HIV blood test from defendant).

41. *Adams v. State*, 498 S.E.2d 268 (Ga. 1998); *Glover v. E. Neb. Cmty. Office of Retardation*, 867 F.2d 461 (8th Cir. 1989), *cert. denied*, 493 U.S. 932 (1989).

42. *Skinner v. Railway Labor Executives' Ass'n*, 489 U.S. 602, 613–14 (1989) (upholding drug tests following major train accidents for employees who violate safety rules, even without reasonable suspicion of impairment); *Nat'l Treasury Employees Union v. Von Raab*, 489 U.S. 656 (1989) (upholding suspicionless drug testing by U.S. Customs Service due to government's "compelling" interest in safeguarding borders and public safety); Diana Chapman Walsh, Lynn Elinson, and Lawrence O. Gostin, "Worksite Drug Testing," *Annual Review of Public Health* 13 (1992): 197–221.

43. *Ferguson v. City of Charleston*, 532 U.S. 67 (2001).

44. *Skinner*, 489 U.S. at 625.

45. *Board of Educ. v. Earls*, 122 S. Ct. 2559 (2002) (extending the authority of public schools to conduct random drug tests among students as a "special needs" situation); *Vernonia School Dist. 47J v. Acton*, 515 U.S. 646 (1995) (upholding random urinalysis for participation in interscholastic athletics).

46. *Hill v. Evans*, No. 91-A-626-N, 1993 WL 595676 (M.D. Ala. Oct. 7, 1993).

47. *ACT-UP Triangle v. Comm'n for Health Servs.*, 472 S.E.2d 605 (N.C. Ct. App. 1996), *rev'd*, 483 S.E.2d 388 (N.C. 1997).

48. *Marsoner v. Pima County*, 803 P.2d 897 (Ariz. 1991); *New York v. New St. Mark's Baths*, 497 N.Y.S.2d 979 (N.Y. Sup. Ct. 1986).

49. *Blue Moon Enters. v. Pinellas County Dept. of Consumer Prot. ex rel.* Pinellas County, 97 F. Supp. 2d 1134 (M.D. Fla. 2000); *City of New York v. Capri Cinema, Inc.*, 641 N.Y.S.2d 969 (N.Y. County Ct. 1995).

50. *University Books and Videos, Inc. v. Metropolitan Dade County*, 78 F. Supp. 2d 1327 (S.D. Fla. 1999); *Scope Pictures of Missouri, Inc. v. City of Kansas City*, 140 F.3d 1201 (8th Cir. 1998).

51. Ralph Bolton et al., "Gay Baths Revisited: An Empirical Analysis," *Journal of Gay and Lesbian Studies* 1 (1994): 255 (arguing that bathhouses could serve as a focal point in which gay men could be educated about AIDS).

52. *New York v. New St. Mark's Baths*, 497 N.Y.S.2d 979.

53. *Scope Pictures*, 140 F.3d at 1201; *Ben Rich Trading v. City of Vineland*, 126 F.3d 155 (3d Cir. 1997).

54. *Scope Pictures*, 140 F.3d at 1203; *Matney v. County of Kenosha*, 86 F.3d at 692–95 (7th Cir. 1996).

55. *Scope Pictures*, 140 F.3d at 1204; *Matney*, 86 F.3d at 696–98.

56. *R. J. v. Humana of Florida, Inc.*, 652 So. 2d 360 (Fla. 1995); *Doe v. Philadelphia Cmty. Health Alternatives AIDS Task Force*, 745 A.2d 25 (Pa. Super. Ct. 2000).

57. *M. M. H. v. United States*, 966 F.2d 285 (7th Cir. 1992); *Mackie v. Chizmar*, 965 P.2d 1202 (Alaska 1998).

58. *Baker v. Dorfman*, 239 F.3d 415 (2d Cir. 2000); *Bramer v. Dotson*, 437 S.E.2d 773 (W.Va. 1993).

59. *Doe v. McNulty*, 630 So. 2d 825 (La. Ct. App. 1993), *cert. denied*, 631 So. 2d 1167 (La. 1994).

60. *Mixon v. Cason*, 622 So. 2d 918 (Ala. 1993), *but see*, *Eaton v. Cont'l Gen. Ins. Co.*, 147 F. Supp. 2d 829 (N.D. Ohio 2001).

61. *Reisner v. Regents of Univ. of Cal.*, 37 Cal. Rptr. 2d 518 (Ct. App. 1995).

62. *Baker v. English*, 894 P.2d 505 (Or. Ct. App. 1995), *aff'd in part & rev'd in part*, 932 P.2d 57 (Or. 1997); *Morton v. Mutchnick*, 904 S.W.2d 14 (Mo. Ct. App. 1995).

63. Laurent Mandelbrot et al., "Lamivudine-Zidovudine Combination for Prevention of Maternal-Infant Transmission of HIV-1," *JAMA* 285 (April 25, 2001): 2083–93.

64. Michael A. Stoto, Donna A. Almario, and Marie C. McCormick, eds., *Reducing the Odds: Preventing Perinatal Transmission of HIV in the United States* (Washington, D.C.: National Academy Press, 1999).

65. USPHS, "Recommendations for HIV Screening of Pregnant Women," *MMWR* 50 (November 9, 2001): 59–86.

66. CARE, P.L. 101–381, 104 Stat. 576 (codified as amended in scattered sections of 42 U.S.C.).

67. *Anastosopoulos v. Perakis*, 644 A.2d 480 (Me. 1994).

68. *Ruch v. Conrad*, 526 N.W.2d 653 (Neb. 1995).

69. *Coca-Cola Bottling Co. v. Hagan*, 813 So. 2d 167, 169 (Fla. Dist. Ct. App. 2002).

70. *Bussell v. W. Calcasieu Cameron Hosp.*, 774 So. 2d 83 (La. 2000); *Natale v. Gottlieb Mem'l Hosp.*, 733 N.E.2d 380 (Ill. App. Ct. 2000).

71. *Ordway v. County of Suffolk*, 583 N.Y.S.2d 1014 (N.Y. Sup. Ct. 1992).

72. *Funeral Servs. by Gregory, Inc. v. Bluefield Community Hosp.*, 413 S.E.2d 79 (W.Va. 1991), *overruled in part by Courtney v. Courtney*, 437 S.E.2d 436 (W.Va. 1993).

73. *Wilson-Watson v. Dax Arthritis Clinic, Inc.*, 766 So. 2d 1135 (Fla. App. 2000); *McLarney v. Cmty. Health Plan*, 680 N.Y.S.2d 281 (N.Y. App. Div. 1998).

74. *O'Neill v. O'Neill*, 694 N.Y.S.2d 772 (N.Y. App. Div. 1999); *In re Marriage of J. T.*, 891 P.2d 729 (Wash. Ct. App. 1995).

75. *Johnson v. West Virginia Hosps.*, 413 S.E.2d 889 (W.Va. 1991); *South Cent. Reg'l Med. Ctr. v. Pickering*, 749 So. 2d 95 (Miss. 1999). One court has held that the risk of developing AIDS must be significant. *In re Needles Cases*, No. H023692, 2003 WL 133460, at *7 (Cal. Ct. App. Jan. 16, 2003).

76. *Bussell v. W. Calcasieu Cameron Hosp.*, 774 So. 2d 83, 84 (La. 2000); *Majca v. Beekil*, 701 N.E.2d 1084 (Ill. 1998).

77. *Pickering*, 749 So. 2d at 103; *Bain v. Wells*, 936 S.W.2d 618, 624 (Tenn. 1997).

78. *Syring v. Tucker*, 498 N.W.2d 370 (Wis. 1993), *reconsideration denied*, 505 N.W.2d 142 (Wis. 1993).

79. *Doe v. Burgos*, 638 N.E.2d 701 (Ill. App. Ct. 1994).

80. *Madrid v. Lincoln County Med. Ctr.*, 923 P.2d 1154 (N.M. 1996).

81. OSHA, *Bloodborne Pathogens*, 29 C.F.R. § 1910.1030 (1997).

82. *Am. Dental Ass'n v. Martin*, 984 F.2d 823 (7th Cir. 1993).

83. *Armstrong v. Flowers Hosp.*, 33 F.3d 1308 (11th Cir. 1994).

84. *EBI/Orion Group v. Blythe*, 931 P.2d 38 (Mont. 1997).

85. *New York State Court Guidelines* (Albany, January 1988).

86. *Wiggins v. Maryland*, 554 A.2d 356 (Md. 1989).

87. *In re Peacock*, 59 B.R. 568 (Bnkr. S.D. Fla. 1986).

88. *Doe v. Philadelphia Sheriff's Office*, press release, February 23, 1988, from the Philadelphia AIDS Task Force.

89. "Re: Jefferson County District Court Judges," *AIDS Litigation Reporter*, January 1989.

90. *Commonwealth v. Martin*, 676 N.E.2d 451 (Mass. 1997), *rev'g*, 660 N.E.2d 670 (Mass. App. Ct. 1996).

91. *People v. Parker*, 522 N.E.2d 1063 (N.Y. 1988); *Scroggins v. State*, 401 S.E.2d 13 (Ga. App. 1990).

92. *State v. Van Straten*, 409 N.W.2d 448 (Wis. Ct. App. 1987), *cert. denied*, 484 U.S. 932 (1987).

93. *State v. Mercer*, 544 A.2d 611 (Conn. 1988).

94. *State v. Mahan*, 971 S.W.2d 1202 (Alaska 1998); *State v. Tokar*, 918 S.W.2d 753 (Mo. 1996).

95. *Santelli v. Electro-Motive*, 188 F.R.D. 306, 310 (N.D. Ill. 1999); *Adams v. State*, 927 P.2d 751 (Alaska Co. App. 1996).

96. *State v. Pinkal*, 2001 WL 55463 (Minn. App., 2001); *U.S. v. Whalen*, 940 F.2d 1027 (7th Cir.), *cert. denied*, 502 U.S. 951 (1991).

97. *Sanfilippo v. Carrington's of Melville, Inc.*, 601 N.Y.S.2d 663 (N.Y. Sup. Ct. 1993).

98. *Doe v. Tris Comprehensive Mental Health, Inc.*, 690 A.2d 160 (N.J. Super. Ct. Law Div. 1996).

99. *Roe v. City of Milwaukee*, 37 F. Supp. 2d 1127 (E.D. Wis. 1999); *In re Marriage of R. E. G.*, 571 N.E.2d 298 (Ind. Ct. App. 1991).

100. *Doe v. Alexian Bros. Med. Ctr.*, No. 96 C 242, 1996 WL 210074 (N.D. Ill. 1996); *Doe v. Shapiro*, 852 F. Supp. 1256 (E.D. Pa. 1994).

101. *Doe v. Bell Atlantic Business Sys. Servs., Inc.*, Civ. A. No. 95-40057-NMG, 1995 U.S. Dist. LEXIS 11030 (D. Mass. 1995); *Mateer v. Ross, Suchoff, Egert, Hankin, Maidenbaum & Mazel, P.C., No. 96 Civ. 1756 (LAP)*, 1997 U.S. Dist. LEXIS 4517 (S.D.N.Y. Apr. 10, 1997).

102. *Delay v. Delay*, 707 So. 2d 400 (Fla. App. 1998); *Maraham v. Maraham*, 123 A.D.2d 165 (N.Y. 1986)

103. *Doe v. Estate of Frank W. Silva*, 2d Jud. Dist. Ct., Nev., *AIDS Litigation Reporter*, January 27, 1989.

104. *Doe v. Doe*, 519 N.Y.S.2d 595 (N.Y. Sup. Ct. 1987).

105. *Newton v. Riley*, 899 S.W.2d 509 (Ky. Ct. App. 1995); *D v. K*, 917 S.W.2d 682 (Tenn. Ct. App. 1995), *appeal denied*, 1996 Tenn. LEXIS 91 (Tenn. Feb. 5, 1996); Andrew Schepard, "AIDS and Divorce," *Family Law Quarterly* 23 (Spring 1989): 1–42.

106. *Michael M. v. Tanya E.*, 256 A.D.2d 1137 (N.Y.A.D. 1998); *Anonymous v. Anonymous*, 617 So. 2d 694 (Ala. Civ. App. 1993), *aff'd*, 631 So. 2d 1030 (Ala. Civ. App. 1993).

107. *In re Interest of John T.*, 538 N.W.2d 761, 772 (Neb. Ct. App. 1995).

108. Lawrence O. Gostin, "Public Health Strategies for Confronting AIDS: Legislative and Regulatory Policy in the United States," *JAMA* 261 (March 17, 1989): 1621–30.

Chapter 3

This chapter is based on Lawrence O. Gostin, Chai Feldblum, and David W. Webber, "Disability Discrimination in America: HIV/AIDS and Other Health Conditions," *JAMA* 281 (February 24, 1999): 745–52; Gostin and Webber, "HIV Infection and AIDS in the Public Health and Health Care Systems: The Role of Law and Litigation," *JAMA* 279 (April 8, 1998): 1108–13; Gostin and Webber, "The AIDS Litigation Project: HIV/AIDS in the Courts in the 1990s, Part 1," *APPJ* 12 (Winter 1997): 105–21; Gostin and Webber, "The AIDS Litigation Project: HIV/AIDS in the Courts in the 1990s, Part 2," *APPJ* 13 (Spring 1998): 3–19; Gostin, "The AIDS Litigation Project: A National Review of Court and Human Rights Commission Decisions, Part I: The Social Impact of AIDS," *JAMA* 263 (April 11, 1990): 1961–70; and Gostin, "The AIDS Litigation Project: A National Review of Court and Human Rights Commission Decisions, Part II: Discrimination in Education, Employment, Housing, Insurance, and Health Care," *JAMA* 263 (April 18, 1990): 2086–93.

I am indebted to Chai Feldblum, Kathleen Flaherty, Zita Lazzarini, Lane Porter, Hazel Sandomire, Robert Scherer, and David Webber, all of whom coauthored various aspects of the AIDS Litigation Project with me. I am also indebted to the many litigators and community-based organizations that provided case materials. The ALP was supported by the National AIDS Program Office in the Department of Health and Human Services and the Henry J. Kaiser Family Foundation.

1. CDC, "Revised Guidelines for HIV Counseling, Testing, and Referral," *MMWR* 50 (November 9, 2001): 1–57. ("Clients who test positive should be referred to legal services as soon as possible after learning their test result for counseling on how to prevent discrimination in employment, housing, and public accommodation by only dis-

closing their status to those who have a legal need to know.") See David I. Schulman, Supervising Attorney, AIDS/HIV Discrimination Unit, Los Angeles City Attorney's Office, "Letter to U.S. Centers for Disease Control and Prevention, Re: Public Comments, 10/17/00, Draft Revised Guidelines for HIV Counseling Testing and Referral," November 26, 2000, 4. ("It is not enough for the CDC to insist that counseling and testing programs protect confidentiality. AIDS happens in a profoundly volatile social field, and public health must account for that volatility. Public health must refer newly diagnosed HIV positive persons to legal counsel to learn to protect their privacy outside the test site.")

2. "Proposal Seeks to Extend 'Legal Checkups' Nationwide," *AIDS Policy and Law* 16 (February 16, 2001): 1; "Legal Checkups: How They Work," *AIDS Policy and Law* 16 (February 16, 2001): 7; "Legal Checkups: A Sample Form," *AIDS Policy and Law* 16 (February 16, 2001): 8–9.

3. Lawrence O. Gostin, "Health Information Privacy," *Cornell Law Review* 80 (March 1995): 101–84.

4. James G. Hodge Jr., Lawrence O. Gostin, and Peter D. Jacobson, "Legal Issues concerning Electronic Health Information: Privacy, Quality, and Liability," *JAMA* 282 (October 20, 1999): 1466–71.

5. *Crumrine v. Harte-Hanks Television*, 37 S.W.2d 124 (Tex. App. 2001).

6. Ibid., 127.

7. *Dinkel v. Lincoln Publ'g*, 638 N.E.2d 611 (Ohio Ct. App. 1994).

8. *McCormack v. County of Westchester*, 731 N.Y.S.2d 5 (N.Y. App. Div. 2001).

9. *Woody v. West Publishing Co.*, No. Civ.A.95-C-5247, 1995 WL 686028 (N.D. Ill. Nov. 13, 1995).

10. *In re Multimedia KSDK*, 581 N.E.2d 911 (Ill. App. 1991).

11. *Chapman v. Byrd*, 475 S.E.2d 734 (N.C. Ct. App. 1996); *Retterer v. Whirlpool Corp.*, 677 N.E.2d 417 (Ohio Ct. App. 1996).

12. *Dorsey v. National Enquirer*, 952 F.2d 250 (9th Cir. 1991).

13. *Ackerman v. Med. College of Ohio Hosp.*, 680 N.E.2d 1309 (Ohio App. 1996).

14. *Waddell v. Bhat*, 571 S.E.2d 565 (Ga. Ct. App. 2002); *Doe v. Div. of Youth and Family Servs.*, F. Supp. 2d 462 (D.N.J. 2001); *Doe v. Marselle*, 675 A.2d 835 (Conn. 1996); *Doe v. Roe*, 659 N.Y.S.2d 671 (N.Y. App. Div. 1997).

15. *Doe v. American Stores Co.*, 74 F. Supp. 2d 855 (E.D. Wis. 1999).

16. *Doe v. Marsh*, 899 F. Supp. 933 (N.D.N.Y. 1995); *Doe v. Archdiocese of the Catholic Church of Miami*, 721 So. 2d 428 (Fla. Dist. Ct. App. 1998).

17. *Herring v. Keenan*, 218 F.3d 1171 (10th Cir. 2000); *Doe v. Township of Robinson*, 637 A.2d 764 (Pa. Commw. Ct. 1994).

18. *Devilla v. Schriver*, 245 F.3d 192 (2d Cir. 2001); *Davis v. District of Columbia*, 158 F.3d 1342 (D.C. Cir. 1998); *Roe v. City of Milwaukee*, 26 F. Supp. 2d 1119 (E.D. Wis. 1998).

19. *Ex parte Dep't of Health and Environmental Control v. Doe*, 529 S.E.2d 290 (S.C. Ct. App. 2000); *Texas Dep't of Health v. Doe*, 994 S.W.2d 890 (Tex. App. 1999).

20. *P. F. v. Mendres*, 21 F. Supp. 476 (D.N.J. 1998); *Ramirez v. Brooklyn AIDS Task Force*, 175 F.R.D. 423 (E.D.N.Y. 1997), aff'd, 164 F.3d 619 (2d Cir. 1998).

21. *Tolman v. Doe*, 988 F. Supp. 582 (E.D. Va.1997); *Doe v. Methodist Hosp.*, 690 N.E.2d 681 (Ind. 1997); *Goins v. Mercy Ctr.*, 667 N.E.2d 652 (Ill. App. Ct. 1996).

22. *Rivera v. Heyman*, 982 F. Supp. 932 (S.D.N.Y. 1997), *aff'd in part, rev'd in part*, 157 F.3d 101 (2d Cir. 1998); *Poveromo-Spring v. Exxon Corp.*, 968 F. Supp. 219 (D.N.J. 1997); *Doe v. Southeastern Pa. Transp. Auth.*, 72 F.3d 1133 (3d Cir. 1995).

23. *Jeffrey H. v. Imai, Tadlock and Keeney*, 101 Cal. Rptr. 2d 916 (Cal. Ct. App. 2001).

24. *Faison v. Parker*, 823 F. Supp. 1198 (E.D. Pa. 1993); *Barese v. Clark*, 773 A.2d 946 (Conn. App. Ct. 2001); *State ex rel. Callahan v. Kinder*, 879 S.W.2d 677 (Mo. Ct. App. 1994).

25. *Doe v. City of New York*, 15 F.3d 264 (2d Cir. 1994).

26. *Estate of Behringer v. Medical Ctr.*, 592 A.2d 1251 (N.J. Super. Ct. Law Div. 1991).

27. *Hirschfield v. Stone*, 193 F.R.D. 175 (S.D.N.Y. 2000).

28. *Biddle v. Warren Gen. Hosp.*, 715 N.E.2d 518 (Ohio 1999).

29. *Lee v. Calhoun*, 948 F.2d 1162 (10th Cir. 1991); *but cf. In re Marriage of Bonneau*, 691 N.E.2d 123 (Ill. App. 1998) (stating that in property distribution phase of a divorce case, husband had not put his health status at issue; thus wife could not seek to discover husband's HIV status).

30. *State v. Stark*, 832 P.2d 109 (Wash. Ct. App. 1992); *Ex parte Dep't of Health and Environmental Control v. Doe*, 529 S.E.2d 290 (S.C. Ct. App. 2000) (ordering the health department to release suspect's HIV test results and information about when suspect learned that he was HIV positive in order to aid in criminal prosecution).

31. *Bitner v. Pekin Memorial Hosp.*, 741 N.E.2d 1075 (Ill. App. 2000); *State v. J. E.*, 606 A.2d 1160 (N.J. Super. Ct. Law Div. 1992).

32. *Yoder v. Ingersoll-Rand Co.*, 31 F. Supp. 2d 565 (N.D. Ohio 1997), *aff'd*, 172 F.3d 51 (6th Cir. 1998).

33. *Doe v. Township of Robinson*, 637 A.2d 764 (Pa. Commw. Ct. 1994).

34. *Washington v. Meachum*, 680 A.2d 262 (Conn. 1996).

35. *A. L. A. v. West Valley City*, 26 F.3d 989 (10th Cir. 1994), *but see Herring v. Keenan*, 218 F.3d 1171 (10th Cir. 2000) (finding that although probationer had a right to privacy in his HIV status, defendant probation officer was not liable for disclosing the probationer's HIV status to the probationer's sister and employer because the right was not clearly established when disclosure occurred), December 31, 2002.

36. *Middlebrooks v. State Bd. of Health*, 710 So. 2d 891–893 (Ala. 1998) (finding that state could compel physician to release information about HIV-infected patients to the health department and stating, "prevention of the spread of HIV and AIDS is a legitimate governmental interest, and that, even in regard to HIV and AIDS, where, in some situations, the disclosure may reflect unfavorably on the character of the patient, the State can require disclosure to representatives of the State having responsibility for the health of the community").

37. *In re Gribetz*, 605 N.Y.S.2d 834 (Rockland County Ct. 1993).

38. *McBarnette v. Feldman*, 582 N.Y.S.2d 900 (Suffolk County Sup. Ct. 1992).

39. Ibid. at 905.

40. *Mussivand v. David*, 544 N.E.2d 265 (Ohio 1989); *O'Neill v. O'Neill*, 694 N.Y.S.2d 772 (N.Y. App. Div. 1999).

41. *Tischler v. Dimenna*, 609 N.Y.S.2d 1002 (N.Y. Sup. Ct. 1994).

42. *Doe v. Johnson*, 817 F. Supp. 1382 (W.D. Mich. 1993), *subsequent opinion sub nom Moore v. Johnson*, 826 F. Supp. 1106 (W.D. Mich. 1993); *O'Neill v. O'Neill*, 694 N.Y.S.2d 772 (N.Y. App. Div. 1999).

43. *Reisner v. Regents of Univ. of Cal.*, 37 Cal. Rptr. 2d 518 (Cal. Ct. App. 1995); *but see Santa Rosa Health Care Corp. v. Garcia*, 964 S.W.2d 940 (Tex. 1998) (holding that hospital had no duty to inform a patient's spouse of the patient's possible exposure to HIV as a result of a transfusion, and stating that in fact the hospital was barred from informing the spouse about the possible exposure until the patient tested positive for HIV).

44. *Estate of Amos v. Vanderbilt University*, 2001 WL 1635476 (Tenn. 2001).

45. *Funeral Servs. by Gregory, Inc. v. Bluefield Community Hosp.*, 413 S.E.2d 79 (W.Va. 1991), *overruled in part by Courtney v. Courtney*, 437 S.E.2d 436 (W.Va. 1993).

46. *Gilkes v. Warren Gen. Hosp.*, 628 N.E.2d 157 (Ohio Ct. App. 1993).

47. 42 U.S.C.A. §§ 300-ff-83-300-ff-85 (2001).

48. Lawrence O. Gostin and James G. Hodge Jr., "Piercing the Veil of Secrecy in HIV/AIDS and Other Sexually Transmitted Diseases: Theories of Privacy and Disclosure in Partner Notification," *Duke Journal of Gender Law and Policy* 5 (Spring 1998): 9–88.

49. Ibid., 41–44.

50. *Chizmar v. Mackie*, 896 P.2d 196 (Alaska 1995).

51. *J. B. v. Sacred Heart Hospital*, 996 F.2d 276, 278 (11th Cir.1993), *certifying question to* 635 So. 2d 945 (Fla. 1994), *conformed answer*, 27 F.3d 506 (11th Cir. 1994).

52. *Waddell v. Bhat*, 571 S.E.2d 565, 568 (Ga. Ct. App. 2002).

53. *N. O. L. v. District of Columbia*, 674 A.2d 498 (D.C. 1998).

54. *Chizmar*, 896 P.2d 196.

55. *Bain v. Wells*, 936 S.W.2d 618 (Tenn. 1997).

56. *Greer v. Shoop*, 141 F.3d 824 (8th Cir. 1998).

57. *Haybeck v. Prodigy Servs. Co.*, 944 F. Supp. 326 (S.D.N.Y. 1996).

58. *Report of the Presidential Commission on the Human Immunodeficiency Virus Epidemic* (Washington, D.C.: GPO, 1988); CDC, *Recommended Additional Guidelines for HIV Antibody Counseling and Testing in the Prevention of HIV Infection and AIDS* (Washington, D.C.: USPHS, 1987).

59. IOM, *Confronting AIDS: Directions for Public Health Care and Research* (Washington, D.C.: National Academy Press, 1986) (1988 update); American Medical Association Board of Trustees, "Prevention and Control of Acquired Immunodeficiency Syndrome: An Interim Report," *JAMA* 258 (October 16, 1987): 2097–2103.

60. ASTHO, *Guide to Public Health Practice: AIDS Confidentiality and Anti-discrimination Principle: Interim Report* (Washington, D.C.: ASTHO, 1987).

61. ABA AIDS Coordinating Committee, *AIDS: The Legal Issues* (Washington, D.C.: ABA, 1988), and *Policy on AIDS* (Chicago: ABA, 1989) (adopted by the House of Delegates in August 1989).

62. David W. Webber, ed., *AIDS and the Law*, 3d. ed. (New York: John Wiley and Sons, 1997, with 2000 Supp.).

63. David W. Webber and Lawrence O. Gostin, "Discrimination Based on HIV/ AIDS and Other Health Conditions: 'Disability' as Defined under Federal and State Law," *Journal of Health Care Law and Policy* 3 (2000): 266–329.

64. 42 U.S.C. §§ 12101 *et seq.* (2001).

65. 42 U.S.C. § 12111(8) (2001).

66. *EEOC v. Yellow Freight System, Inc.*, 253 F.3d 943 (7th Cir. 2000); *Hilton v. Southwest-*

ern Bell Tel. Co., 936 F.2d 823 (5th Cir. 1991); *Severino v. North Fort Myers Fire Control Dist.*, 935 F.2d 1179 (11th Cir. 1991).

67. *McNemar v. Disney Stores, Inc.*, 91 F.3d 610 (3d Cir. 1996); *Reigel v. Kaiser Found. Health Plan*, 859 F. Supp. 963 (E.D.N.C. 1994).

68. *Cleveland v. Policy Mgmt. Sys. Corp.*, 526 U.S. 795 (1999).

69. *Holiday v. City of Chattanooga*, 206 F.3d 637 (6th Cir. 1999); *Ihekwu v. City of Durham*, 129 F. Supp. 2d 870 (M.D.N.C. 2000) (granting summary judgment to employer because employee failed to show that he was discriminated against because of his HIV status); *Wallengren v. French, Inc.*, 39 F. Supp. 2d 343 (S.D.N.Y. 1999); *Gilbert v. Related Mgmt. Co.*, 678 N.Y.S.2d 326 (N.Y. App. Div. 1998).

70. 42 U.S.C. § 12112(a) (2001); *Flowers v. Southern Regional Physician Servs., Inc.*, 247 F.3d 229; *Dollinger v. State Insurance Fund*, 44 F. Supp. 2d 467 (N.D.N.Y. 1999); *but see Ballard v. Healthsouth Corp.*, 147 F. Supp. 2d 529 (N.D. Tex. 2001).

71. *Phelps v. Field Real Estate Co.*, 991 F.2d 645 (10th Cir. 1993); *Cruz Carrillo v. AMR Eagle, Inc.*, F. Supp. 2d 142 (D.P.R. 2001); *Velez Cajigas v. Order of St. Benedict*, 115 F. Supp. 246 (D.P.R. 2000); *Chockla v. Celebrity Cruise Lines*, 47 F. Supp. 2d 1365 (S.D. Fla. 1999).

72. *Buckingham v. U.S.*, 998 F.2d 735 (9th Cir. 1993); *Parks v. Female Health Care Assocs., NO. 96 C 7133*, 1997 WL 285870 (N.D. Ill. May 23, 1997); *Prilliman v. United Air Lines*, 62 Cal. Rptr. 2d 142 (Cal. Ct. App. 1997).

73. *School Bd. v. Arline*, 480 U.S. 273, 287 n. 16 (1987); *EEOC v. Prevo's Family Market*, 135 F.3d 1089 (6th Cir. 1998); *Sanchez v. Lagoudakis*, 581 N.W.2d 257 (Mich. 1998).

74. *Chevron U.S.A., Inc. v. Echazabal*, 122 S. Ct. 2045 (2002).

75. 42 U.S.C. § 12112(b)(4) (2001) (prohibiting, "excluding or otherwise denying equal jobs or benefits to a qualified individual because of the known disability of an individual with whom the qualified individual is known to have a relationship or association").

76. *Mora v. Chem-tronics, Inc.*, 16 F. Supp. 2d 1192 (S.D. Cal. 1998).

77. *In re New York State Div. of Human Rights v. Marcus Garvey Nursing Home*, 672 N.Y.S.2d 130 (N.Y. App. Div. 1998).

78. 42 U.S.C. § 12182(a) (2001).

79. 42 U.S.C. § 12181(7) (2001).

80. *Merchant v. Kring*, 50 F. Supp. 2d 433 (W.D. Pa. 1999); *A. R. v. Kogan*, 964 F. Supp. 269 (N.D. Ill. 1997).

81. *Lasser v. Rosa*, 654 N.Y.S.2d 822 (N.Y. App. Div. 1997); *Fiske v. Rooney*, 663 N.E.2d 1014 (Ohio Ct. App. 1995).

82. *Cahill v. Rosa*, 674 N.E.2d 274 (N.Y. 1996); *but see Baksh v. Human Rights Comm'n*, 711 N.E. 416 (Ill. App. Ct. 1999) (holding that dental office was not a place of public accommodation under the Illinois Human Rights Acts; thus a dentist who refused to treat an HIV-infected patient was not liable to the patient for discrimination).

83. *Phillips v. Mufleh*, 642 N.E.2d 411 (Ohio Ct. App. 1994).

84. *Cheung v. Merrill Lynch, Pierce, Fenner & Smith Inc.*, 913 F. Supp. 248 (S.D.N.Y. 1996).

85. *Hamlyn v. Rock Island County Metro. Mass Transit Dist.*, 986 F. Supp. 1126 (C.D. Ill. 1997).

86. *Montalvo v. Radcliffe*, 167 F.3d 873 (4th Cir. 1999).

87. *United States v. Happy Time Day Care Ctr.*, 6 F. Supp. 2d 1073 (W.D. Wis. 1998).

88. *Doe v. Dep't Corr.*, 611 N.W.2d 1 (Mich. Ct. App. 2000).

89. *Palmer v. City of Yonkers*, 22 F. Supp. 2d 283 (S.D.N.Y. 1998).

90. *Doe v. Div. Youth and Family Servs.*, 148 F. Supp. 2d 462 (D.N.J. 2001); *Merchant v. Kring*, 50 F. Supp. 2d 433 (W.D. Pa. 1999); *Fiske v. Rooney*, 663 N.E.2d 1014 (Ohio Ct. App. 1995).

91. *Lesley v. Chie*, 250 F.3d 47 (1st Cir. 2001); *Schulman v. State Div. of Human Rights*, 658 N.Y.S.2d 70 (N.Y. App. Div. 1997).

92. *Bragdon v. Abbott*, 524 U.S. 624 (1998).

93. *Syracuse Community Health Ctr. v. Wendi A.M.*, 659 N.E.2d 760 (N.Y. 1995); *Cerio v. New York State Div. of Human Rights*, 684 N.Y.S.2d 738 (N.Y. App. Div. 1999); *North Shore Univ. Hosp. v. Rosa*, 657 N.E.2d 483 (N.Y. 1995).

94. *Doe v. Kahala Dental Group*, 808 P.2d 1276 (Hawaii 1991).

95. *Sharrow v. Bailey*, 910 F. Supp. 187 (M.D. Pa. 1995).

96. *Hill v. Community of Damien of Molokai*, 911 P.2d 861 (N.M. 1996); *Eichlin v. Zoning Hearing Bd. of New Hope Borough*, 671 A.2d 1173 (Pa. Commw. Ct. 1996).

97. *Neithamer v. Brenneman Prop. Servs.*, 81 F. Supp. 2d 1 (D.D.C. 1999); *Ryan v. Ramsey*, 936 F. Supp. 417 (S.D. Tex. 1996); *Hill*, 911 P.2d 861.

98. *Joel Truitt Mgmt., Inc. v. District of Columbia Comm'n on Human Rights*, 646 A.2d 1007 (D.C. 1994); *119–121 East 97th St. Corp. v. New York City Comm'n on Human Rights*, 642 N.Y.S.2d 638 (App. Div. 1996).

99. *Joel Truitt Mgmt.*, 646 A.2d 1007.

100. *119–121 East 97th St. Corp.*, 642 N.Y.S.2d 638.

101. *Charles v. Rice*, 28 F.3d 1312 (1st Cir. 1994).

102. *Steffan v. Aspin*, 780 F. Supp. 1 (D.D.C. 1991), *rev'd*, 8 F.3d 57 (D.C. Cir. 1994), *subsequent opinion sub nom. Steffan v. Perry*, 41 F.3d 677, 720 (D.C. Cir. 1994) (en banc).

103. *Doe v. Mut. of Omaha Ins.*, 179 F.3d 557 (7th Cir. 1999); *World Ins. Co. v. Branch*, 966 F. Supp. 1203 (N.D. Ga. 1997); *Doukas v. Metropolitan Life Ins. Co.*, 950 F. Supp. 422 (D.N.H. 1996).

104. *Shaw v. PACC Health Plan, Inc.*, 908 P.2d 308 (Oreg. 1995).

105. *DeSimone v. Transprint USA, Inc.*, No. 94 CIV.3130 (JFK), 1996 WL 209951 (S.D.N.Y. 1996).

106. *McGann v. H & H Music Co.*, 946 F.2d 401 (5th Cir. 1991); Lawrence O. Gostin and Alan I. Widiss, "What's Wrong with the ERISA Vacuum?," *JAMA* 269 (May 19, 1993): 2527–32.

107. EEOC, *Interim Enforcement Guidance on the Application of the Americans with Disabilities Act of 1990 to Disability-Based Distinctions in Employer-Provided Health Insurance* (Washington, D.C.: GPO, June 8, 1993).

108. *Anderson v. Gus Mayer Boston Store*, 924 F. Supp. 763 (E.D. Tex. 1996).

109. *Fioretti v. Massachusetts Gen. Life Ins. Co.*, 53 F.3d 1228 (11th Cir. 1995); *New York Life Ins. Co. v. Johnson*, 923 F.2d 279 (3d Cir. 1991); *Kieser v. Old Line Life Ins. Co. of Am.*, 712 So. 2d 1261 (Fla. Dist. Ct. App. 1998).

110. *Galanty v. Paul Revere Life Ins.*, 1 P.3d 658 (Cal. 2000); *New England Mut. Life Ins. v. Doe*, 710 N.E.2d 1060 (N.Y. 1999); *Amex Life Assur. Co. v. Superior Court*, 930 P.2d 1264 (Cal. 1997); *Blue Cross & Blue Shield v. Sheehan*, 450 S.E.2d 228 (Ga. Ct. App. 1994).

111. *Waxse v. Reserve Life Ins. Co.*, 809 P.2d 533 (Kans. 1991).

112. *Krakowiak v. Paul Revere Life Ins. Co.*, App. No. 01-A-01-9511-CH-00541, 1996 Tenn. App. LEXIS 346 (Tenn. Ct. App. 1996).

113. *McNeil v. Time Ins.*, 205 F.3d 179 (5th Cir. 2000); *Doe v. Mut. of Omaha Ins.*, 179 F.3d 557 (7th Cir. 1999); *Gonzales v. Garner Food Servs.*, 89 F.3d 1523 (11th Cir. 1996).

114. *Cloutier v. Prudential Ins. Co.*, 964 F. Supp. 299 (N.D. Cal. 1997); *Kotev v. First Colony Life Ins. Co.*, 927 F. Supp. 1316 (C.D. Cal. 1996).

115. *Florence Nightingale Nursing Serv. v. Blue Cross & Blue Shield*, 832 F. Supp. 1456 (N.D. Ala. 1993), *aff'd*, 41 F.3d 1476 (11th Cir. 1995).

116. *Rosetti v. Shalala*, 12 F.3d 1216 (3d Cir. 1993).

117. 20 C.F.R. Part 404, Subpart P, App. 1, Listing 14.08 (1996).

118. *Hamilton v. Chater*, 942 F. Supp. 1354 (D. Oreg. 1996); William B. Rubenstein, Ruth Eisenberg, and Lawrence O. Gostin, *Rights of Persons Who Are HIV Positive: The Authoritative ACLU Guide to the Rights of People Living with HIV Disease and AIDS* (Carbondale: Southern Illinois University Press, 1996).

119. *Pratts v. Chater*, 94 F.3d 34 (2d Cir. 1996); *Rodriguez v. Chater*, 962 F. Supp. 298 (D. Conn. 1997).

120. *Saathoff v. Gober*, 10 Vet. App. 326 (1997); *ZN v. Brown*, 6 Vet. App. 183 (1994).

121. *Wright v. Giuliani*, 230 F.3d 543 (2d Cir. 2000); *Mixon v. Grinker*, 627 N.Y.S.2d 668 (App. Div. 1995) (per curiam), *rev'd*, 669 N.E.2d 819 (N.Y. 1996).

122. *Holder v. Harlem Men's Shelter*, 613 N.Y.S.2d 899 (App. Div. 1994); Lawrence O. Gostin, "The Resurgent Tuberculosis Epidemic in the Era of AIDS," *Maryland Law Review* 54 (1995): 1–131.

123. *Henrietta D. v. Giuliani*, 119 F. Supp. 2d 181 (E.D.N.Y. 2000), *appeal dismissed*, 246 F.3d 176 (2d Cir. 2001); *Salazar v. District of Columbia*, 954 F. Supp. 278 (D.D.C. 1996).

124. *Hines v. Sheehan*, Civil No. 94-326-P-H, 1995 U.S. Dist. LEXIS 11031 (D. Me. 1995).

125. U.S. Const. amend. VIII.

126. *Farmer v. Brennan*, 511 U.S. 825 (1994); *Wilson v. Seiter*, 501 U.S. 294 (1991); *Estelle v. Gamble*, 429 U.S. 97, 103 (1976).

127. *Billman v. Indiana Dep't of Corrs.*, 56 F.3d 785 (7th Cir. 1995); *Claude H. v. County of Oneida*, 626 N.Y.S.2d 933 (App. Div. 1995); *Whitfield v. Scully*, No. 94 Civ. 3290 (DC), 1996 WL 706932 (S.D.N.Y. Dec. 6, 1996).

128. *Charowsky v. Wapinsky*, No. 95-CV-4481, 1996 WL 165521 (E.D. Pa. 1996); *Randles v. Moore*, 780 So. 2d 158 (Fla. Dist. Ct. App. 2001) (refusing to dismiss complaint by inmate who brought action under state law after being infected with HIV while cleaning blood spills in medical/psychiatric ward).

129. *Oladipupo v. Austin*, 104 F. Supp. 2d 626 (W.D. La. 2000).

130. *Zaczek v. Murray*, 983 F.2d 1059 (4th Cir. 1992).

131. *Canell v. Multnomah County*, 141 F. Supp. 2d 1046 (D. Oreg. 2001); *Bolton v. Goord*, 992 F. Supp. 604 (S.D.N.Y. 1998).

132. *Robbins v. Clarke*, 946 F.2d 1331 (8th Cir. 1991); *Hoover v. Watson*, 886 F. Supp. 410 (D. Del. 1995).

133. *Powell v. Schriver*, 175 F.3d 107 (2d Cir. 1999); *Leon v. Johnson*, 96 F. Supp. 2d 244 (W.D.N.Y. 2000); *Hillman v. Columbia County*, 474 N.W.2d 913 (Wis. Ct. App. 1991).

134. *Herring v. Keenan*, 218 F.3d 117 (10th Cir. 2000); *Tokar v. Armontrout*, 97 F.3d 1078 (8th Cir. 1996); *Anderson v. Romero*, 72 F.3d 518 (7th Cir. 1995); *Quinones v. Howard*, 948 F. Supp. 251 (W.D.N.Y. 1996).

135. *Leon v. Johnson*, 96 F. Supp. 2d 244 (W.D.N.Y. 2000).

136. *Roe v. City of Milwaukee*, 26 F. Supp. 2d 1119 (E.D. Wis. 1998).

137. *Camarillo v. McCarthy*, 998 F.2d 638 (9th Cir. 1993).

138. *Paramo v. Matthew*, No. 92–3144, 1992 U.S. App. LEXIS 26256 (10th Cir. Oct. 9, 1992); *Turner v. Masters*, No. 01-91-01020-CV, 1992 WL 190964 (Tex. Ct. App. Aug. 13, 1992).

139. *Stanley v. Swinson*, 47 F.3d 1176 (table), *reported in full*, 1995 U.S. App. LEXIS 2262 (9th Cir. 1995).

140. *Murdock v. Washington*, 193 F.3d 510 (7th Cir. 1999); *Gates v. Rowland*, 39 F.3d 1439 (9th Cir. 1994).

141. *Gates v. Rowland*, 39 F.3d at 1447–48 (9th Cir. 1994).

142. *Perkins v. Kansas Dep't of Corrs.*, 165 F.3d 803 (10th Cir. 1999).

143. *Meneweather v. Ylst*, 19 F.3d 28 (table), *reported in full*, 1994 U.S. App. LEXIS 6097 (9th Cir. 1994); *Moore v. Mabus*, 976 F.2d 268 (5th Cir. 1992); *Camarillo v. McCarthy*, 998 F.2d 638 (9th Cir. 1993); *Harris v. Thigpen*, 941 F.2d 1495 (11th Cir. 1991); *Timmons v. New York State Dep't of Corr. Servs.*, 887 F. Supp. 576 (S.D.N.Y. 1995).

144. *Oneishea v. Hopper*, 171 F.3d 1289 (11th Cir. 1999), *cert. denied sub. nom Davis v. Hopper*, 528 U.S. 1114 (2000).

145. Ibid.

146. *Farmer v. Hawk*, NO. 94-CV-2274(GK) 1996 WL 525321 (D.D.C. Sept. 5, 1996).

147. *Hallett v. New York State Dep't of Corr. Servs.*, 109 F. Supp. 2d 190 (S.D.N.Y. 2000); *Taylor v. Barnett*, 105 F. Supp. 2d 483 (E.D. Va. 2000); *Rivera v. Sheahan*, No. 97 C 2735, 1998 WL 531875 (N.D. Ill. Aug. 14, 1998); *Hetzel v. Swartz*, 31 F. Supp. 2d 444 (M.D. Pa. 1998).

148. *Inmates of N.Y. State with HIV v. Cuomo*, No. 90-CV-252, 1991 U.S. Dist. LEXIS 1488 (N.D.N.Y. Feb. 7, 1991).

149. *Madrid v. Gomez*, 889 F. Supp. 1146 (N.D. Cal. 1995).

150. *Walker v. Peters*, 233 F.3d 494 (7th Cir. 2000); *Leon v. Johnson*, 96 F. Supp. 2d 244 (W.D.N.Y. 2000); *Taylor v. Barnett*, 105 F. Supp. 2d 483 (E.D. Va. 2000); *State ex rel. Peeples v. Anderson*, 653 N.E.2d 371 (Ohio 1995).

151. 8 U.S.C. § 1182(a)(1)(A)(I) (2000); Jeremy R. Tarwate, "The Tuberculosis and HIV Debate in Immigration Law: Critical Flaws in United States Academic and Anti-exclusion Arguments," *Georgetown Immigration Law Journal* 15 (Winter 2001): 357–79.

152. Lynne Duke, "U.S. Ordered to Free HIV-infected Haitians, Judge Cites 'Abuse of Discretion' Regarding Refugees at Guantánamo," *Washington Post*, June 9, 1993.

153. *Haitian Ctrs. Council, Inc. v. Sale*, 823 F. Supp. 1028 (E.D.N.Y. 1993).

154. Webber, *AIDS and the Law*, 477–79.

155. John M. Karon, Patricia L. Fleming, Richard W. Steketee, and Kevin M. De-Cock, "HIV in the United States at the Turn of the Century: An Epidemic in Transition," *AJPH* 91 (July 2001): 1060–68.

156. Ibid.

157. Richard J. Wolitski, Ronald O. Valdiserri, P. H. Denning, and W. C. Levine, "Are We Headed for a Resurgence in the HIV Epidemic among Men Who Have Sex with Men?," *AJPH* 91 (June 2001): 883–88.

Chapter 4

This chapter is based on Lawrence O. Gostin and Zita Lazzarini, *Public Health and Human Rights in the HIV Pandemic* (Oxford: Oxford University Press, 1997); Gostin and Jonathan Mann, "Towards the Development of a Human Rights Impact Assessment for the Formulation and Evaluation of Health Policies," *JHHR* 1 (1994): 58–81; Mann, Gostin, Sofia Gruskin, Troyen Brennan, Lazzarini, and Harvey V. Fineberg, "Health and Human Rights," *JHHR* 1 (1994): 6–22; Gostin, "Human Rights of Persons with Mental Disabilities: The European Convention of Human Rights," *International Journal of Law and Psychiatry* 23 (2000): 125–59; Gostin, "Public Health, Ethics, and Human Rights: A Tribute to the Late Jonathan Mann," *Journal of Law, Medicine, and Ethics* 29 (2000): 121–30; and Gostin, "The Human Right to Health: A Right to the Highest Attainable Standard of Health," *Hastings Center Report* 31 (March–April 2001): 29–30.

1. Louis Henkin, *How Nations Behave* (New York: Columbia University Press, 1979), 320.

2. Stanley H. Herr, Lawrence O. Gostin, and Harold Hongju Koh, *Equal but Different: The Rights of Persons with Mental Disabilities* (Oxford: Oxford University Press, 2003).

3. *Faccini-Dori v. Recreb* [1994] ECR I-3325.

4. Henry J. Steiner and Philip Alston, *International Human Rights in Context: Law, Politics, Morals*, 2d ed. (New York: Oxford University Press, 2000).

5. Jonathan Mann, Lawrence O. Gostin, Sofia Gruskin, Troyen Brennan, Zita Lazzarini, and Harvey V. Fineberg, "Health and Human Rights," *JHHR* 1 (1994): 6–22

6. CDC, *H/ASR* 13 (Atlanta: CDC, February 22, 2002), 15, ⟨http://www.cdc.gov/hiv/stats/hasr1301.pdf⟩.

7. U.S. Census Bureau, *U.S. Census, 2000* (August 2001), ⟨http://www.census.gov/prod/2001pubs/c2kbr01-5.pdf⟩.

8. By 2002 over 13 million children under the age of fifteen around the world lost one or both parents to AIDS. United Nations Children's Fund, *The State of the World's Children, 2002* (New York: UNICEF, 2001), 40; UNAIDS, *A Global Epidemic* (Geneva: UNAIDS and WHO, 2000).

9. Joanne Csete, "In the Shadow of Death: HIV/AIDS and Children's Rights in Kenya," *Human Rights Watch* 13 (June 2001).

10. Vincent Iacopino and Ronald J. Waldman, "War and Health: From Solferino to Kosovo—The Evolving Role of Physicians," *JAMA* 282 (August 4, 1999): 479–81.

11. The Supreme Court of India suspended the right of HIV-infected persons to marry in 1998. *Mr. X v. Hospital Y Authority*, 8 S.C.C. 296 (1998).

12. IOM, *The Future of the Public's Health in the Twenty-first Century* (Washington, D.C.: National Academy Press, 2002).

13. Norman Daniels, Bruce Kennedy, and Ichiro Kawachi, "Justice Is Good for Our Health," *Boston Review* (February–March 2000): 6–15.

14. Lisa F. Berkman and Ichiro Kawachi, eds., *Social Epidemiology* (New York: Oxford University Press, 2000).

15. Roman R. Gangakhedkar, Margaret E. Bentley, Anand D. Divekar, et al., "Spread of HIV Infection in Married Monogamous Women in India," *JAMA* 278 (December 17, 1997): 2090–92.

16. Janet Fleischman, "Fatal Vulnerabilities: Reducing the Acute Risk of HIV/AIDS among Women and Girls," CSIS, February 2003; Chalya Lar, "Combat AIDS in Africa with Sexual Equality," *Baltimore Sun*, July 11, 2002.

17. Janet Fleischman, "Suffering in Silence: The Links between Human Rights Abuses and HIV Transmission to Girls in Zambia," *Human Rights Watch* (November 2002).

18. WHO, "25 Questions and Answers on Health and Human Rights," Geneva, 2002; François-Xavier Bagnoud Center for Health and Human Rights, ⟨http://www.hsph.harvard.edu/fxbcenter/partners.htm⟩; University of Minnesota Human Rights Library, ⟨http://www1.umn.edu/humanrts/links/health.html⟩ (list of organizations involved in health and human rights activities).

19. Lawrence O. Gostin and Jonathan Mann, "Towards the Development of a Human Rights Impact Assessment for the Formulation and Evaluation of Public Health Policies," *JHHR* 1 (Fall 1994): 58.

20. United Nations Economics and Social Council (ECOSOC) (1985), "The Siracusa Principles on the Limitations and Derogation Provisions in the International Covenant on Civil and Political Rights," UN Doc. E/CN.4/1985/4, Annex. (Interference with a derogable right must be provided for and carried out in accordance with the law, be in the interest of a legitimate objective of general interest, not impair the democratic functioning of the society, and not be imposed arbitrarily or in a discriminatory manner. Government limitations must be the least restrictive means available to reach the stated goal).

21. Sofia Gruskin and Bebe Loff, "Do Human Rights Have a Role in Public Health Work?," *Lancet* 360 (December 7, 2002): 1880.

22. Allan M. Brandt, Paul D. Cleary, and Lawrence O. Gostin, "Routine Hospital Testing for HIV: Health Policy Considerations," in *AIDS and the Health Care System*, edited by Gostin (New Haven: Yale University Press, 1990), 125–39.

23. Paul Cleary, Michael Barry, Kenneth Mayer, Allan M. Brandt, Lawrence O. Gostin, and Harvey V. Fineberg, "Compulsory Premarital Screening for the Human Immunodeficiency Virus: Technical and Public Health Considerations," *JAMA* 258 (October 2, 1987): 1757–62.

24. The United States has ratified two health and human rights treaties: the ICCPR and the Convention on the Elimination of All Forms of Racial Discrimination. Several other treaties have been signed by the United States, but not ratified, including the ICESCR, the American Convention on Human Rights, the Convention on the Rights of the Child, the Convention on the Elimination of All Forms of Discrimination against Women, and the Kyoto Protocol.

25. Audrey R. Chapman, *Exploring a Human Rights Approach to Health Care Reform* (Washington, D.C.: American Association for the Advancement of Science, 1993).

26. Lawrence O. Gostin and Zita Lazzarini, *Public Health and Human Rights in the AIDS Pandemic* (New York: Oxford University Press, 1997).

27. United Nations Special Session on HIV/AIDS, *Global Crisis-Global Action: Declaration of Commitment on HIV/AIDS* (New York: United Nations, June 25–27, 2001).

28. Miriam Maluwa, Peter Aggleton, and Richard Parker, "HIV- and AIDS-Related Stigma, Discrimination, and Human Rights," *JHHR* 6 (2002): 1–18.

29. OHCHR and UNAIDS, *HIV/AIDS and Human Rights International Guidelines*, Third International Consultation on HIV/AIDS and Human Rights, Geneva, July 25–26, 2002, HR/PUB/2002/1 (New York: United Nations, 2002).

30. UNAIDS, *Report on HIV/AIDS and Human Rights: The Role of National Human Rights Institutions in the Asia Pacific* (Melbourne, Australia: UNAIDS, October 2001); *The Nairobi Declaration: An African Appeal for an AIDS Vaccine* (Nairobi, June 14, 2000); Kenneth Roth, "Human Rights and the AIDS Crisis: The Debate over Resources" (delivered at the plenary session of the Thirteenth International Conference on AIDS, Durban, South Africa: Human Rights Watch, July 11, 2000), ⟨http://www.hrw.org/editorials/2000/aids-p1.htm⟩; Getachew Gizaw, "Prevention, Care and Support, and the Promotion of Human Rights in the Context of HIV/AIDS" (delivered at the Fifty-fourth World Health Assembly, Geneva: International Federation of Red Cross and Red Crescent Societies, May 18, 2001), ⟨http://www.ifrc.org/Docs/News/speeches/gg180501.asp⟩; Lowenstein International Human Rights Clinic of Yale Law School, Center for Economic and Social Rights, Human Rights Watch, et al., *AIDS and Human Rights: A Call for Action* (New Haven: Yale Law School, June 26, 2001); Physicians for Human Rights, "Physicians for Human Rights Statement on HIV/AIDS and Human Rights," ⟨http://www.phrusa.org/campaigns/aids/bgrd_aids&hr.html⟩.

31. UNAIDS, *Handbook for Legislators on HIV/AIDS, Law, and Human Rights: Action to Combat HIV/AIDS in View of Its Devastating Human, Economic, and Social Impact* (Geneva: UNAIDS, 1999), ⟨http://www.unaids.org/publications/documents/human/law/ipue.pdf⟩.

32. OHCHR and UNAIDS, *HIV/AIDS and Human Rights International Guidelines*.

33. Rebecca J. Cook, *Women's Health and Human Rights* (Geneva: WHO, 1993).

34. Liz McGregor, "Botswana Battles against 'Extinction,'" *The Guardian*, July 8, 2002.

35. Steven D. Jamar, "The International Human Right to Health," *Southern University Law Review* 22 (Fall 1994): 1–68; Virginia A. Leary, "The Right to Health in International Human Rights Law," *JHHR* 1 (Fall 1994): 24–56; Paul Farmer, *Pathologies of Power* (Berkeley: University of California Press, 2003).

36. Eleanor D. Kinney, "The International Human Right to Health: What Does This Mean for Our Nation and World?," *Indiana Law Review* 34 (2001): 1457.

37. As cited in Gostin and Lazzarini, *Public Health and Human Rights*, 197; United Nations, *UDHR* (Geneva: United Nations, December 10, 1948), ⟨http://www.un.org/Overview/rights.html⟩.

38. American Convention on Human Rights, *opened for signatures* November 22, 1969, O.A.S. Official Records, OEA/Ser. K/XVI/II, doc. 65, rev. 1, corr. 2, 144 U.N.T.S. 123, 9 I.L.M. 673, 678 (1970) (Pact of San Jose).

39. Additional Protocol to the American Convention on Human Rights in the Area of Economic, Social, and Cultural Rights, November 14, 1988, O.A.S. T.S. 69 at art. 10 (1988), reprinted in David J. Harris and Stephen Livingstone, eds., *The Inter-American System of Human Rights* (Oxford: Clarendon Press, 1998), 500.

40. Kinney, "International Human Right to Health," 1457–75.

41. *Treatment Action Campaign v. Minister of Health and Others* (2002) (4) BCLR 356, ⟨http://www.concourt.gov.za/date2002.html⟩; Lawrence O. Gostin, "AIDS in Africa

among Women and Infants: A Human Rights Framework," *Hastings Center Report* 32 (September–October 2002): 9–10.

42. Michael Dynes, "HIV Drug Ruling Humiliates Mbeki," *The Times of London*, July 6, 2002.

43. *Treatment Action Campaign*, par. 72; George J. Annas, "The Right to Health and the Nevirapine Case in South Africa," *JAMA* 348 (February 20, 2003): 750–54.

44. WHO, Preamble to Constitution, Geneva, April 7, 1948, ⟨www.who.int.en⟩.

45. General Comment 14, E/C.12/2000/4 (July 4, 2000), ⟨www.unhchr.ch/tbs/doc.nsf⟩.

46. Lawrence O. Gostin, *Public Health Law: Power, Duty, Restraint* (New York: Milbank Memorial Fund and University of California Press, 2000).

47. United Nations Commission on Human Rights, Resolution 2002/31. Paul Hunt (New Zealand) was appointed in August 2002 for a three-year term.

48. Paul Hunt (2003), "The Right of Everyone to the Enjoyment of the Highest Attainable Standard of Physical and Mental Health," Commission on Human Rights, 59th sess., UN Doc. E/CN.4/2003/58.

Chapter 5

This chapter is based on Lawrence O. Gostin, James G. Hodge Jr., and Ronald O. Valdiserri, "Informational Privacy and the Public's Health," *AJPH* 91 (September 2001): 1388–92; Gostin, "National Health Information Privacy: Regulations under the Health Insurance Portability and Accountability Act," *JAMA* 285 (June 20, 2001): 3015–21; Gostin, "Personal Privacy in the Health Care System: Employer-Sponsored Insurance, Managed Care, and Integrated Delivery Systems," *Kennedy Institute of Ethics Journal* 7 (December 1997): 361–76; Gostin, Zita Lazzarini, Verla S. Neslund, and Michael T. Osterholm, "The Public Health Information Infrastructure: A National Review of the Law on Health Information Privacy," *JAMA* 275 (June 26, 1996): 1921–27; and Gostin, "Health Information Privacy," *Cornell Law Review* 80 (March 1995): 101–84. The survey of state privacy laws and the Model State Public Health Privacy Act were supported by the CDC and the Council of State and Territorial Epidemiologists, with the cooperation of the Association of State and Territorial Health Officials and the National Conference of State Legislatures.

1. Harris Equifax, *Health Information Privacy* (Atlanta: Equifax Inc., 1993), ⟨http://www.epic.org/privacy/medical/polls.html⟩.

2. William W. Lowrance, *Privacy and Health Research: A Report to the U.S. Secretary of Health and Human Services* (Washington, D.C.: HHS, 1997); National Research Council, *For the Record: Protecting Electronic Health Information* (Washington, D.C.: National Academy Press, 1997).

3. 5 U.S.C. § 552a(b) (1988).

4. 42 U.S.C. § 290dd-2 (Supp. V 1993).

5. Public Health Service Act, § 301(d), 42 U.S.C. § 241(d) (amended 1988); Office for Human Research Protections, *Privacy Protection for Research Subjects: Certificates of Confidentiality* (Washington, D.C.: HHS, 1978).

6. 42 U.S.C. § 299-c-3 (amended 1999).

7. Workgroup for Electronic Data Interchange, *Obstacles to EDI in the Current Health Care Infrastructure* (Washington, D.C.: HHS, 1992).

8. Institute for Health Care Research and Policy, *The State of Health Privacy: An Uneven Terrain* (Washington, D.C.: Georgetown University Press, 1999), ⟨http://www.healthprivacy.org⟩.

9. 18 U.S.C. § 24 (West 1994).

10. HHS, Standards for Privacy of Individually Identifiable Health Information, 64 Fed. Reg. 59918 (Nov. 3, 1999), to be codified, 45 C.F.R. §§ 160–164.

11. Ibid., Final Rule, 66 Fed. Reg. 12434 (Feb. 26, 2001), to be codified, 45 C.F.R. §§ 160–164.

12. HHS, Standards for Privacy of Individually Identifiable Health Information, 67 Fed. Reg. 14775 (Mar. 27, 2002), to be codified, 45 C.F.R. §§ 160–164, ⟨http://www.hhs.gov/ocr/hipaa/propmods.txb⟩; "HHS Proposes Changes That Protect Privacy," March 21, 2002, ⟨http://www.hhs.gov/news/press/2002pres/20020321.htmb⟩.

13. HHS, Standards for Privacy of Individually Identifiable Health Information, 67 Fed. Reg. 53181 (Aug. 14, 2002).

14. Norman Vieira, "Unwarranted Government Disclosures: Reflections on Privacy Rights, HIV, and Ad Hoc Balancing," *Wayne Law Review* 47 (Spring 2001): 173–99.

15. Lawrence O. Gostin and Alan Widiss, "What's Wrong with the ERISA Vacuum?: Employers' Freedom to Limit Health Care Coverage Provided by Risk Retention Plans," *JAMA* 269 (May 19, 1993): 2527–32.

16. *Doe v. City of New York*, 15 F.3d 264 (2d Cir. 1994) (finding that an individual revealing that she is HIV seropositive potentially exposes herself not to understanding or compassion but to discrimination and intolerance).

17. *Doe v. Borough of Barrington*, 729 F. Supp. 376 (D.N.J. 1999) (courts balance the need to investigate, record, and maintain HIV-related information against the risks of disclosure).

18. HHS Press Release, "Modifications to the Standards for Privacy of Individually Identifiable Health Information—Final Rule" (Washington, D.C.: HHS, August 9, 2002), ⟨http://www.hhs.gov/ocr/hipaa/whatsnew.htmb⟩.

19. Adam Butera, "HIPAA Preemption Implications for Covered Entities under State Law," *Connecticut Insurance Law Journal* 8 (2001–2): 363–99.

20. IOM, *The Future of Public Health* (Washington, D.C.: National Academy Press, 1988).

21. Daniel M. Fox, "From TB to AIDS: Value Conflicts in Reporting Disease," *Hastings Center Report* 16, supp. 1 (December 1986): 11–16.

22. Tom L. Beauchamp and James F. Childress, *Principles of Biomedical Ethics*, 4th ed. (New York: Oxford University Press, 1994).

23. Ronald Bayer, *Private Acts, Social Consequences: AIDS and the Politics of Public Health* (New York: Free Press, 1989).

24. South Dakota ST § 34-22—12.1.

25. Lawrence O. Gostin, Zita Lazzarini, Verla S. Neslund, and Michael T. Osterholm, "The Public Health Information Infrastructure: A National Review of the Law on Health Information Privacy," *JAMA* 275 (June 26, 1996): 1921–27.

26. Peter D. Jacobson, "National Health Information Privacy Regulations under HIPAA: Medical Records and HIPAA: Is It Too Late to Protect Privacy?," *Minnesota Law Review* 86 (June 2002): 1497–1514.

27. South Dakota ST § 34-22—12.1.

28. Lawrence O. Gostin and James G. Hodge Jr., *Model State Public Health Privacy Act* (Washington, D.C.: Georgetown University Press, 1999), ‹www.critpath.org/msphpa/privacy.htm›

29. CDC, "CDC Guidelines for National Human Immunodeficiency Virus Case Surveillance," *MMWR* 48 (December 10, 1999): 1–27.

Chapter 6

This chapter is based on Lawrence O. Gostin, Chai Feldblum, and David W. Webber, "Disability Discrimination in America: HIV/AIDS and Other Health Conditions," *JAMA* 281 (February 24, 1999): 745–52, and Webber and Gostin, "Discrimination Based on HIV/AIDS and Other Health Conditions: 'Disability' as Defined under Federal and State Law," *Journal of Health Care Law and Policy* 3 (2000): 266–329 (paper prepared for the HIV Law and Policy Study: A Project of the Federal Legislation Clinic, Georgetown University Law Center, supported by the Henry J. Kaiser Family Foundation).

1. CDC, *Recommended Additional Guidelines for HIV Antibody Counseling and Testing in the Prevention of HIV Infection and AIDS* (Washington, D.C.: GPO, 1987).

2. IOM, *Confronting AIDS: Directions for Public Health Care and Research* (Washington, D.C.: National Academy Press, 1986); American Medical Association Board of Trustees, "Prevention and Control of Acquired Immunodeficiency Syndrome: An Interim Report," *JAMA* 258 (October 16, 1987): 2097–103.

3. ASTHO, *Guide to Public Health Practice: AIDS Confidentiality and Anti-Discrimination Principles: Interim Report* (Washington, D.C.: ASTHO, 1987).

4. ABA, AIDS Coordinating Committee, *AIDS: The Legal Issues* (Washington, D.C.: ABA, 1988); ABA, *Policy on AIDS* (Chicago: ABA, 1989).

5. ACLU AIDS Project, *Epidemic of Fear: A Survey of AIDS Discrimination in the 1980s and Policy Recommendations for the 1990s* (New York: ACLU, 1990).

6. The concern about discrimination was not limited to the United States. See Council of Europe, *Comparative Study on Discrimination against Persons with HIV or AIDS* (Strasbourg: Council of Europe, 1993), and Canadian HIV/AIDS Legal Network, "HIV Related Stigma and Discrimination—The Epidemic Continues," *Canadian HIV/AIDS Policy and Law Review* 7 (July 2002): 8. In 2002–03 the World AIDS Campaign, launched on World AIDS Day, has as its theme "Stigma and Discrimination," ‹http://www.unaids.org/worldaidsday/2002/index.html›.

7. *School Board of Nassau County v. Arline*, 480 U.S. 273 (1987).

8. William B. Rubenstein, Ruth Eisenburg, and Lawrence O. Gostin, *The Rights of People Who Are HIV Positive: An American Civil Liberties Union Handbook* (Carbondale: Southern Illinois University Press, 1996).

9. CDC, "HIV-Related Knowledge and Stigma—United States," *MMWR* 49 (December 1, 2000): 1062–64; Scott Burris, "Studying the Legal Management of HIV-

Related Stigma," *American Behavioral Scientist* 42 (April 1999): 1229–43 (documenting the limits of our knowledge about HIV-related stigma and the need for more research on HIV-related discrimination to enable policymakers to more effectively address the public health consequences of the disease).

10. John Manuel Androte, *Victory Deferred: How AIDS Changed Gay Life in America* (Chicago: University of Chicago Press, 1999).

11. *Report of the Presidential Commission on the Human Immunodeficiency Virus Epidemic* (Washington, D.C.: GPO, 1988).

12. Richard A. Berk, ed., *The Social Impact of AIDS in the U.S.* (Cambridge, Mass.: Abt Books, 1988).

13. Chai Feldblum, "Medical Examinations and Inquiries under the Americans with Disabilities Act: A View from the Inside," *Temple Law Review* 64 (Summer 1991): 521–49; Feldblum, "The (R)evolution of Physical Disability Anti-Discrimination Law, 1976–96," *Mental and Physical Disability Law Reporter* (September–October 1996): 613–21.

14. National Commission on AIDS, *America Living with AIDS* (Washington, D.C.: National Commission on AIDS, 1991).

15. 29 U.S.C. 794 (1973).

16. Feldblum, "(R)evolution of Physical Disability Anti-Discrimination Law."

17. National Council on Disability, *Equality of Opportunity: The Making of the Americans with Disabilities Act* (Washington D.C.: National Council on Disability, 1997).

18. 42 U.S.C. § 12101(b)(1) (2001).

19. 42 U.S.C. §§ 12111–117 (2001).

20. 42 U.S.C. §§ 12131–165 (2001).

21. 42 U.S.C. §§ 12181–189 (2001).

22. 47 U.S.C. § 225 (2001); 47 U.S.C. § 611 (2001).

23. 42 U.S.C. § 12111(8) (2001); § 12112 (2001).

24. 42 U.S.C. § 12112 (2001).

25. 42 U.S.C. § 12102 (2001).

26. 45 C.F.R § 84.3(j)(2)(ii) (2001); 28 CFR § 41.31(b)(2) (2001).

27. 28 C.F.R § 36.104 (2001).

28. David W. Webber, ed., *AIDS and the Law*, 3d. ed. (New York: John Wiley and Sons, 1997, with 2000 Supp.), 121.

29. *Krocka v. City of Chicago*, 203 F.3d 507, 513–14 (7th Cir. 2000).

30. 42 U.S.C. § 12111(8) (2001).

31. Webber, *AIDS and the Law*, 124.

32. 42 U.S.C. 12111 (3) (2001); 42 U.S.C. 12182(b)(3) (2001); Joe Zopolsky, "HIV-infected Healthcare Workers and Practice Modification," *North Dakota Law Review* 78–98 (2002): 77 (summarizing state and federal case law for qualification standards of people with HIV under the ADA).

33. *School Board of Nassau County v. Arline*, 480 U.S. 273 (1987).

34. *Doe v. County of Centre*, 242 F.3d 437 (3d Cir. 2001).

35. *EEOC v. Prevo's Family Market*, 135 F.3d 1089, 1095 (6th Cir. 1998).

36. *Estate of Mauro v. Borgess Medical Center*, 137 F.3d 398, 407 (6th Cir. 1998).

37. Ibid.

38. *Chevron U.S.A. Inc. v. Echazabal*, 122 S. Ct. 2045 (2002).

39. 42 U.S.C. § 12113(b) (2001) (emphasis added).

40. Mark Barnes, Kimberlee A. Cleaveland, and Patrik S. Florencio, "Chevron v. Echazabal: Public Health Issues Raised by the 'Threat-to-Self' Defense to Adverse Employment Actions," *AJPH* 93 (April 2003): 536–39; Ronald Bayer, "Workers' Liberty, Workers' Welfare: The Supreme Court Speaks on the Rights of Disabled Employees," *AJPH* 93 (April 2003): 540–44; Norman Daniels, "Chevron v. Echazabal: Protection, Opportunity, and Paternalism," *AJPH* 93 (April 2003): 545–48.

41. 42 U.S.C. § 12111(9) (2001).

42. But see *U.S. Airways, Inc. v. Barnett*, 122 S. Ct. 1516 (2002) (holding that an employer's showing that a requested accommodation conflicts with seniority rules is ordinarily sufficient to show, as a matter of law, that an "accommodation" is not "reasonable"; however, the employee remains free to present evidence of special circumstances that makes a seniority rule exception reasonable in the particular case).

43. *Martin v. PGA*, 121 S. Ct. 1879 (2001).

44. 42 U.S.C. § 12112.

45. *Bragdon v. Abbott*, 524 U.S. 624 (1998); Wendy E. Parmet, "The Supreme Court Confronts HIV: Reflections on Bragdon v. Abbott," *Journal of Law, Medicine, and Ethics* 26 (Fall 1998): 225–40.

46. *Bragdon*, 524 U.S. at 639–40.

47. *Blanks v. Southwestern Bell Communications, Inc.*, 310 F.3d 398 (5th Cir. 2002).

48. Harry W. Haverkos and Robert J. Battjes, "Female-to-Male Transmission of HIV," *JAMA* 268 (October 14, 1992): 1855–59.

49. Catherine Peckham and Diana Gibb, "Mother-to-Child Transmission of the Human Immunodeficiency Virus," *NEJM* 333 (August 3, 1995): 298–302.

50. *Bragdon*, 524 U.S. at 640–41.

51. Ibid. at 637.

52. Ibid. at 656 (Ginsburg, J., concurring).

53. 42 U.S.C. § 122001(a) (1994).

54. Ruth Colker, "Winning and Losing under the Americans with Disabilities Act," *Ohio State Law Journal* 62 (2001): 239–83.

55. Thomas D'Agostino, "Defining 'Disability' under the ADA: 1997 Update," *National Disability Law Reporter—Special Report No. 3* (1997): 4–8.

56. *Toyota Motor Mfg. Ky Inc. v. Williams*, 534 U.S. 184, 197 (2002).

57. Ibid. at 184.

58. *Sutton v. United Air Lines, Inc.*, 527 U.S. 471, 492 (1999).

59. Lawrence O. Gostin, Chai Feldblum, and David W. Webber, "Disability Discrimination in America: HIV/AIDS and Other Health Conditions," *JAMA* 281 (1999): 745–52.

60. *Albertsons, Inc. v. Kirkingburg*, 527 U.S. 555 (1999).

61. *Sutton*, 527 U.S. at 471.

62. *Murphy v. United Parcel Service, Inc.*, 527 U.S. 516 (1999).

63. Katherine R. Annas, "Recent Development: Toyota Manufacturing, Kentucky, Inc. v. Williams: Part of an Emerging Trend of Supreme Court Cases Narrowing the Scope of the ADA," *North Carolina Law Review* 81 (January 2003): 835–52.

64. *Barnes v. Gorman*, 536 U.S. 181 (2002).

65. Lawrence O. Gostin, "The Supreme Court, Health Policy, and New Federalism," *Hastings Center Report* 30 (March–April 2000): 26–27.

66. *Board of Trustees of University of Alabama v. Garrett*, 531 U.S. 356 (2001).

67. *Medical Board of California v. Hason*, 2003 WL 1792116 (2003) (cert. dismissed); *Hason v. Medical Board of California*, 279 F.3d 1167 (9th Cir. 2002) (holding that Congress was within its constitutional authority in abrogating state sovereign immunity pursuant to Title II of the ADA).

68. 42 U.S.C. § 12201(b) (2001).

69. 775 Ill. Comp. Stat. 5/2-101 (B)(1)(b),(d),(e) (1993); Ky. Rev. Stat. Ann. § 344.030 (2) (1997); Md. Ann. Code art. 49B, § 43 (a) (1998).

70. 42 U.S.C. § 12111 (5) (A) (1990).

71. N.Y. City Adm. Code, tit. 8, § 102.16 (1991) (defining "disability" as any physical, medical, mental, or psychological impairment, or a history or record of such impairment, without regard to whether the impairment results in any limitation on any major life activity).

72. Los Angeles Municipal Code § 45.80 *et seq.* (1985).

73. San Francisco Police Code § 3813(a) (1985) (prohibiting discrimination based on "asymptomatic infection").

74. Arkansas, California, Florida, Hawaii, Kansas, Kentucky, Maine, Missouri, Montana, Nebraska, New Mexico, Ohio, Rhode Island, Texas, Vermont, Virginia, and Wisconsin.

75. Cal. Civ. Code § 51, 54 (1982).

76. Connecticut, Delaware, Illinois, Indiana, Maryland, Michigan, New York, and Oregon.

77. Alabama (as to public employment, housing, and public accommodations); Arkansas (as to public accommodations); Mississippi (as to public employment and employment by state-funded employers); and Wyoming (as to public and private employment). Note, however, that the Wyoming Fair Employment Commission Rules of Practice incorporate the federal definition of disability.

78. Florida, Hawaii, Iowa, Kentucky, Maryland, Missouri, Montana, Nebraska, New Jersey, North Carolina, Vermont, Virginia, Washington, and Wisconsin.

79. Florida, Iowa, Kentucky, Nebraska, and New Jersey.

80. Hawaii, Maryland, Missouri, Montana, North Carolina, Vermont, Virginia, Washington, and Wisconsin.

81. N.C. Gen. Stat. § 130A-148(i) (1997).

82. Ibid.

83. Florida, Iowa, Kentucky, Nebraska, and New Jersey.

84. Hawaii, Maryland, Missouri, Montana, Vermont, Virginia, Washington, and Wisconsin.

85. North Carolina.

86. *Missouri Rose City Oil Co. v. Missouri Comm'n on Human Rights*, 832 S.W.2d 314, 316–17 (Mo. Ct. App. 1992) (construing the statutory definition of disability to require the existence of a *condition* that might be perceived as a handicap).

87. Tex. Health & Safety § 85.082 (2001); Ky. Rev. Stat. Ann. § 214.181 (6)(d) (1998).

88. Arkansas, California, Florida, Hawaii, Kansas, Kentucky, Maine, Maryland, New Mexico, Ohio, Rhode Island, and Texas. See Table 6-1, col. B.

89. California, Florida, Kentucky, Maine, New Mexico, and Texas.

90. Arkansas and Maryland.

91. Ohio.

92. Illinois, North Carolina, and West Virginia.

93. *Benjamin R. v. Orkin Exterminating Co.*, 390 S.E.2d 814 (W.Va. 1990); *Burgess v. Your House of Raleigh, Inc.*, 388 S.E.2d 134 (N.C. 1990) (decided before the adoption of North Carolina's Communicable Disease Act, N.C. Gen. Stat. § 130A-148(i), which prohibits discrimination in continuing employment).

94. *Raintree Health Care Center v. Illinois Human Rights Comm'n*, 672 N.E.2d 1136, 1141 (Ill. 1996).

95. *Doe v. Jamaica Hosp.*, 608 N.Y.S.2d 518 (N.Y. App. Div. 1994) (mem.); *Syracuse Community Health Ctr. v. Wendi A.M.*, 604 N.Y.S.2d 406 (N.Y. App. Div. 1993), *aff'd*, 659 N.E.2d 760 (N.Y. 1995); *Petri v. Bank of N.Y. Co.*, 582 N.Y.S.2d 608 (N.Y. Sup. Ct. 1992); *H. S. v. Bd. of Regents of Southeast Missouri State Univ.*, 967 S.W.2d 665 (1998) (stating that there was no dispute that an HIV-positive employee was covered by the Missouri Human Rights Act).

96. *Beaulieu v. Clausen*, 491 N.W.2d 662 (Minn. Ct. App. 1992).

97. Ibid. at 666.

98. CDC, *H/ASR* 13 (June 2001): 7 (table 1).

99. Alabama, Georgia, Mississippi, North Carolina, Puerto Rico, and the U.S. Virgin Islands.

Chapter 7

This chapter is based on Lawrence O. Gostin and William J. Curran, "The Case against Compulsory Casefinding in Controlling AIDS: Testing, Screening, and Reporting," *American Journal of Law and Medicine* 12 (1987):1–47; Paul Cleary, Michael Barry, Kenneth Mayer, Allan M. Brandt, Gostin, and Harvey V. Fineberg, "Compulsory Premarital Screening for the Human Immunodeficiency Virus: Technical and Public Health Considerations," *JAMA* 258 (1987): 1757–62; and Gostin and Curran, "AIDS Screening, Confidentiality, and the Duty to Warn," *AJPH* 77 (1987): 361–65.

1. CDC, "Revised Guidelines for HIV Counseling, Testing, and Referral," *MMWR* 50 (November 9, 2001): 1–51; CDC, "HIV Testing—United States, 1996," *MMWR* 48 (January 29, 1999): 52–55.

2. Jesus Castilla, Paz Sobrino, Luis De La Fuente, Isabel Noguer, Luis Guerra, and Francisco Parras, "Late Diagnosis of HIV Infection in the Era of Highly Active Antiretroviral Therapy: Consequences for AIDS Incidence," *AIDS* 16 (September 27, 2002): 1945–51; Ronald O. Valdiserri, David R. Holtgrave and Gary R. West, "Promoting Early HIV Diagnosis and Entry into Care," *AIDS* 13 (December 3, 1999): 2317–30.

3. Mary L. Kamb, Martin Fishbein, John M. Douglas Jr., et al., "Efficacy of Risk-Reduction Counseling to Prevent Human Immunodeficiency Virus and Sexually Transmitted Diseases: A Randomized Controlled Trial," *JAMA* 280 (October 7, 1998):

1161–67; National Institute of Mental Health (NIMH) Multisite HIV Prevention Trial Group, "The NIMH Multisite HIV Prevention Trial: Reducing HIV Sexual Risk Behavior," *Science* 280 (June 19, 1998): 1889–94; Neil S. Wenger, Lawrence S. Linn, Maxwell Epstein, and Martin F. Shapiro, "Reduction of High-Risk Sexual Behavior among Heterosexuals Undergoing HIV Antibody Testing: A Randomized Clinical Trial," *AJPH* 81 (December 1991): 1580–85; Rochelle N. Shain, Jeanna M. Piper, Edward R. Newton, et al., "A Randomized Controlled Trial of a Behavioral Intervention to Prevent Sexually Transmitted Disease among Minority Women," *NEJM* 340 (January 14, 1999): 93–100; David R. Gibson, Jane Lovelle-Drache, James L. Sorensen, et al., "Effectiveness of Brief Counseling in Reducing HIV Risk Behavior in Injecting Drug Users: Final Results of Randomized Trials of Counseling with and without HIV Testing," *AIDS and Behavior* 3 (1999): 3–12; The Compendium of HIV Prevention Interventions with Evidence of Effectiveness, ‹www.cdc.gov/hiv/pubs/hivcompendium.pdf›.

4. Thomas C. Quinn, Maria J. Wawer, Nelson Sewankambo, et al., "Viral Load and Heterosexual Transmission of Human Immunodeficiency Virus Type 1," *NEJM* 342 (March 30, 2000): 921–29.

5. Charles C. J. Carpenter, Margaret A. Fischl, Scott M. Hammer, et al., "Antiretroviral Therapy for HIV Infection in 1998: Updated Recommendations of the International AIDS Society—USA Panel," *JAMA* 280 (July 1, 1998): 78–86; CDC, "Report of the NIH Panel to Define Principles of Therapy of HIV Infection and Guidelines for the Use of Antiretroviral Agents in HIV-infected Adults and Adolescents," *MMWR* 47 (April 24, 1998): 1–41.

6. Ralf Jürgens and Michael Palles, "HIV Testing and Confidentiality: A Discussion Paper" (Canadian HIV/AIDS Legal Network and Canadian AIDS Society, Montreal, 1997).

7. CDC, "Advancing HIV Prevention: New Strategies for a Changing Epidemic—United States, 2003," *MMWR* 52 (April 18, 2003): 329–32.

8. Scott E. Kellerman, J. Stan Lehman, Amy Lansky, Mark R. Stevens, Frederick M. Hecht, Andrew B. Bindman, and Pascale M. Wortley, "HIV Testing within At-Risk Populations in the United States and the Reasons for Seeking or Avoiding HIV Testing," *JAIDS* 31 (October 1, 2002): 202–10; CDC, "HIV Incidence among Young Men Who Have Sex with Men—Seven U.S. Cities, 1994–2000," *MMWR* 50 (June 1, 2001): 440–44.

9. Sten H. Vermund and Craig M. Wilson, "Barriers to HIV Testing—Where Next?" *Lancet* 360 (October 19, 2002): 1186–87.

10. CDC, "Advancing HIV Prevention: New Strategies for a Changing Epidemic," *MMWR* 52 (April 18, 2003): 328–32.

11. Julie Louise Gerberding, Harold W. Jaffe, "Dear Colleague Letter," April 21, 2003.

12. Ronald Bayer et al., "HIV Antibody Screening: An Ethical Framework for Evaluating Proposed Programs," *JAMA* 256 (October 3, 1986): 1768.

13. William C. Black and Gilbert Welch, "Screening for Disease," *American Journal of Radiology* 168 (1997): 3–11.

14. Michael A. Stoto, Donna A. Almario, and Marie C. McCormick, eds., *Reducing the Odds: Preventing Perinatal Transmission of HIV in the United States* (Washington, D.C.: National Academy Press, 1999), 22.

15. UNAIDS, "Guidelines for Using HIV Testing Technologies in Surveillance: Se-

lection, Evaluation, and Implementation" (UNAIDS and WHO, Geneva, July 2001), ‹http://www.unaids.org/publications/documents/epidemiology/surveillance/JC602-HIVSurvGuidel-E.pdf›.

16. William J. Kassler, "Advances in HIV Testing Technology and Their Potential Impact on Prevention," *AIDS Education and Prevention* 9, supp. B (June 1997): 27–40.

17. CDC, "Update: HIV Counseling and Testing Using Rapid Tests—United States, 1995," *MMWR* 47 (March 27, 1998): 211–15.

18. CDC, "Approval of a New Rapid Test for HIV Antibody," *MMWR* 51 (November 22, 2002): 1051–52.

19. Bernard M. Branson, "Home Sample Collection Tests for HIV Infection," *JAMA* 280 (November 18, 1998): 1699–701. Home sample collection kits, which are FDA-approved, are not the same as home-use test kits, which are not approved. In the former, the individual collects a personal sample at home and sends it to a laboratory for analysis; in the latter, the individual can analyze the sample at home.

20. Federal Trade Commission, *Consumer Alert, Home-Use Tests for HIV Can Be Inaccurate, FTC Warns* (Washington, D.C.: Federal Trade Commission, 1999), ‹www.ftc.gov/bcp/conline/pubs/alerts/hivalrt.htm›.

21. CDC, "Update: HIV Counseling and Testing Using Rapid Tests."

22. Bernard J. Turnock and Chester J. Kelly, "Mandatory Premarital Testing for Human Immunodeficiency Virus: The Illinois Experience," *JAMA* 261 (June 16, 1989): 3415–18; Paul D. Cleary et al., "Compulsory Premarital Screening for the Human Immunodeficiency Virus: Technical and Public Health Considerations," *JAMA* 258 (October 2, 1987): 1757.

23. Ronald Bayer, *Private Acts, Social Consequences: AIDS and the Politics of Public Health* (New York: Free Press, 1989).

24. Ruth R. Faden, Nancy E. Kass, and Madison Powers, "Warrants for Screening Programs: Public Health, Legal, and Ethical Frameworks," in *AIDS, Women, and the Next Generation: Towards a Morally Acceptable Public Policy for HIV Testing of Pregnant Women and Newborns*, edited by Ruth Faden, Gail Geller, and Madison Powers (New York: Oxford University Press, 1991), 3–26.

25. Colo. Rev. Stat. § 18-7-205.5 (2001).

26. N.Y. Public Health Law § 2500-f (1999).

27. N.C. Gen. Stat. § 15A-615 (1997).

28. Va. Code § 32.1–59 (1997).

29. Staff of Volume 8, "State Statutes Dealing with HIV and AIDS: A Comprehensive State-by-State Summary (1999 Edition)," *Law and Sexuality: A Review of Lesbian, Gay, Bisexual, and Transgender Legal Issues* 8 (1998): 1–65, ‹http://www.law.tulane.edu/tuexp/journals/l&s/law_sex.htm›.

30. CDC, "HIV Testing among Pregnant Women—United States and Canada, 1998–2001," *MMWR* 51 (November 15, 2002): 1013–16.

31. IOM, "Reducing the Odds: Preventing Perinatal Transmission of HIV in the United States" (Washington, D.C.: National Academy Press, 1999).

32. CDC, "Advancing HIV Prevention: New Strategies for a Changing Epidemic," *MMWR* 52 (April 18, 2003): 329–32; CDC, "Letter regarding Preventing Perinatal HIV Transmission: A Review of Prenatal Testing Approaches," April 22, 2003.

33. Ruth R. Faden, Tom L. Beauchamp, and Nancy M. P. King, *A History and Theory of Informed Consent* (New York: Oxford University Press, 1986), 25.

34. *Canterbury v. Spence*, 464 F.2d 772 (D.C. Cir. 1972).

35. In fact, a recent study revealed that fewer than one-third of physicians complied with legal requirements for STD screening, resulting in screening levels that did not meet practice guidelines for women and were practically nonexistent for men. Janet S. St. Lawrence, Daniel E. Montano, Danuta Kasprzyk, William R. Phillips, Keira Armstrong, and Jami S. Leichliter, "STD Screening, Testing, Case Reporting, and Clinical and Partner Notification Practices: A National Survey of US Physicians," *AJPH* 92 (2002): 1784–88.

36. *Hill v. Evans*, U.S. Dist. LEXIS 19878 (M.D. Ala. 1993).

37. *Schmerber v. California*, 384 U.S. 757, 767–68 (1966).

38. *Skinner v. Railway Labor Executives' Ass'n*, 489 U.S. 602 (1989); *Nat'l Treasury Employees Union v. Von Raab*, 489 U.S. 656 (1989).

39. In *Ferguson v. City of Charleston*, 532 U.S. 67 (2001), the Supreme Court held that a public hospital's policy of subjecting pregnant women to nonconsensual drug tests without a warrant, and turning positive test results over to police, violated the Fourth Amendment's proscription against unreasonable searches.

40. *Board of Ed. of Independent School Dist. No. 92 of Pottawatomie County v. Earls*, 122 S. Ct. 2559 (2002).

41. *Skinner*, 489 U.S. (1989) at 625.

42. *Veronia School Dist. 47J v. Acton*, 515 U.S. 646 (1995).

43. *Anonymous Fireman v. City of Willoughby*, 779 F. Supp. 402 (N.D. Ohio 1991).

44. *Plowman v. United States Dep't of Army*, 698 F. Supp. 627 (E.D. Va. 1988).

45. *Local 1812, Am. Fed'n of Gov't Employees v. United States Dep't of State*, 662 F. Supp. 50 (D.D.C. 1987).

46. *Haitian Ctrs. Council v. Sale*, 823 F. Supp 1028 (E.D.N.Y. 1993).

47. *Juveniles A,B,C,D,E*, 847 P.2d 455 (Wash. 1993).

48. *Harris v. Thigpen*, 941 F.2d 1495 (11th Cir. 1991).

49. Donna I. Dennis, "HIV Screening and Discrimination: The Federal Example," in *AIDS Law Today: A New Guide for the Public*, edited by Scott Burris, Harlon L. Dalton, and Judith Leonie Miller (New Haven: Yale University Press, 1993), 187.

50. *Glover v. Eastern Nebraska Community Office of Retardation*, 686 F. Supp. 243 (D. Neb. 1988), *aff'd*, 867 F.2d 461 (9th Cir. 1989); Steven Eisenstat, "An Analysis of the Rationality of Mandatory Testing for the HIV Antibody: Balancing Public Health Interest with the Individual's Privacy Interest," *University of Pittsburgh Law Review* 52 (1991): 327.

51. ADA, 42 U.S.C. § 12101–201 (1992).

52. 42 U.S.C. § 12112(d).

53. Lawrence O. Gostin, "The Resurgent Tuberculosis Epidemic in the Era of AIDS: Reflections on Public Health, Law, and Society," *University of Maryland Law Review* 81 (Winter 1995): 81; *City of Newark v. J. S.*, 652 A.2d 265, 273 (N.J. Super. Ct. Law Div. 1993).

54. 42 U.S.C. § 12181(7)(F).

55. *Bragdon v. Abbott*, 524 U.S. 624 (1998).

56. *State in Interest of J. G.*, 701 A.2d 1260 (N.J. 1997).

57. Scott Burris, "Public Health, 'AIDS Exceptionalism' and the Law," *John Marshall Law Review* 27 (Winter 1994): 251.

58. CDC, "Advancing HIV Prevention: New Strategies for a Changing Epidemic—United States, 2003," *MMWR* 52 (April 18, 2003): 329–32.

59. Stoto, Almario, and McCormick, *Reducing the Odds*, 22.

60. John Maxwell, Glover Wilson, and Gunnar Jungner, *Principles and Practice of Screening for Disease* (Geneva: WHO, 1968).

61. Henry J. Kaiser Family Foundation, *State Health Facts Online* (Washington, D.C.: Kaiser Family Foundation, 2002), ‹http://www.statehealthfacts.kff.org/cgi-bin/healthfacts.cgi?›; Amanda Watson, Stephanie Wasserman, and Julie Scales, *Issue Brief: HIV Reporting in the States* (Washington, D.C.: Health Policy Tracking Service, National Conference of State Legislatures, February 4, 2002).

Chapter 8

This chapter is based on Lawrence O. Gostin, John W. Ward, and A. Cornelius Baker, "National HIV Case Reporting for the United States: A Defining Moment in the History of the Epidemic," *NEJM* 337 (October 16, 1997): 1162–67, and Gostin and James G. Hodge Jr., "The 'Names Debate': The Case for National HIV Reporting in the United States," *Albany Law Review* 61 (1998): 679–743.

1. CDC, *H/ASR* 13 (Atlanta: CDC, December 2001): 1–44, ‹http://www.cdc.gov/hiv/stats/hasr1302.pdf›.

2. CDC, "Updated Guidelines for Evaluating Public Health Surveillance Systems: Recommendations from the Guidelines Working Group," *MMWR* 50 (July 27, 2001): 1–36; Allyn K. Nakashima and Patricia L. Fleming, "HIV/AIDS Surveillance in the United States, 1981–2001," *JAIDS* 32 (February 1, 2003): 68–85.

3. John M. Karon, Patricia L. Fleming, Richard W. Steketee, and Kevin M. DeCock, "HIV in the United States at the Turn of the Century: An Epidemic in Transition," *AJPH* 91 (July 2001): 1060–68.

4. CDC, "Guidelines for National Human Immunodeficiency Virus Case Surveillance, Including Monitoring for Human Immunodeficiency Virus Infection and Acquired Immunodeficiency Syndrome," *MMWR* 48 (December 10, 1999): 1–28.

5. IOM, *Confronting AIDS: Directions for Public Health, Health Care, and Research* (Washington, D.C.: National Academy Press, 1986).

6. Donald P. Francis, James W. Curran, and Max Essex, "Epidemic Acquired Immune Deficiency Syndrome: Epidemiologic Evidence for a Transmissible Agent," *Journal of the National Cancer Institute* 71 (July 1983): 1–4; Henry Masur et al., "An Outbreak of Community-Acquired *Pneumocystis Carinii* Pneumonia: Initial Manifestation of Cellular Immune Dysfunction," *NEJM* 305 (December 10, 1981): 1431–38.

7. Francoise Barre-Sinoussi et al., "Isolation of a T-Lymphotropic Retrovirus from a Patient at Risk for Acquired Immune Deficiency Syndrome (AIDS)," *Science* 220 (May 20, 1983): 868–71; Robert C. Gallo et al., "Frequent Detection and Isolation of Cytopathic Retroviruses (HTLV-III) from Patients with AIDS and at Risk for AIDS," *Science* 224 (May 4, 1984): 500–503.

8. CDC, "Provisional Public Health Service Interagency Recommendations for Screening Donated Blood and Plasma for Antibody to the Virus Causing Acquired Immunodeficiency Syndrome," *MMWR* 34 (February 22, 1985): 1–5.

9. Ronald Bayer, *Private Acts, Social Consequences: AIDS and the Politics of Public Health* (New York: Free Press, 1989).

10. Alan S. Perelson, Avidan U. Neumann, Martin Markowitz, John M. Leonard, and David D. Ho, "HIV-1 Dynamics in Vivo: Virion Clearance Rate, Infected Cell Life-Span, and Viral Generation Time," *Science* 271 (March 15, 1996): 1582–86.

11. Clinical Practices for the Treatment of HIV Infection, *Guidelines for the Use of Antiretroviral Agents in HIV-infected Adults and Adolescents*, (Washington, D.C.: Clinical Practices for the Treatment of HIV Infection, February 4, 2002): 1–96, ⟨http://www.aidsinfo.nih.gov/guidelines/adult/AAMay23.pdf⟩.

12. National Institute of Allergy and Infectious Diseases, *Fact Sheet* (Bethesda, Md.: NIH, January 2002); CDC, "Recommendations for Preventing Transmission of Human Immunodeficiency Virus and Hepatitis B Virus to Patients during Exposure-prone Invasive Procedures," *MMWR* 40 (July 12, 1991): 1–9.

13. Perinatal HIV Guidelines Working Group, *Public Health Service Task Force Recommendations for Use of Antiretroviral Drugs in Pregnant HIV-1 Infected Women for Maternal Health and Interventions to Reduce Perinatal HIV-1 Transmission in the United States* (Washington, D.C.: Perinatal HIV Guidelines Working Group, February 4, 2002): 1–47 ⟨http://www.aidsinfo.nih.gov/guidelines/perinatal/perinatal.pdf⟩.

14. CDC, "Advancing HIV Prevention: New Strategies for a Changing Epidemic— United States, 2003," *MMWR* 52 (April 18, 2003): 329–32.

15. Patricia L. Fleming, Pascale M. Wortley, John M. Karon, Kevin M. DeCock, and Robert S. Janssen, "Tracking the HIV Epidemic: Current Issues, Future Challenges," *AJPH* 90 (July 2000): 1037–41.

16. Phillip S. Rosenburg, "HIV in the Late 1990s: What We Don't Know May Hurt Us," *AJPH* 91 (July 2001): 1016–17.

17. CDC, "HIV and AIDS—United States, 1981–2000," *MMWR* 50 (June 1, 2001): 430–34.

18. Amanda Watson, Stephanie Wasserman, and Julie Scales, *Issue Brief: HIV Reporting in the States* (Washington, D.C.: Health Policy Tracking Service, National Conference of State Legislatures, February 4, 2002).

19. Janet S. St. Lawrence, Daniel E. Montano, Danuta Kasprzyk, William R. Phillips, Keira Armstrong, and Jami S. Leichliter, "STD Screening, Testing, Case Reporting, and Clinical and Partner Notification Practices: A National Survey of US Physicians," *AJPH* 92 (2002): 1784–88.

20. CDC, *H/ASR: U.S. HIV and AIDS Cases Reported through December 2001* (Atlanta: CDC, December 2001).

21. CDC, "HIV Infection Reporting—United States," *MMWR* 38 (July 21, 1989): 496–99.

22. HIV Criminal Law and Policy Project, "HIV Reporting" (2002), ⟨http://www.hivcriminallaw.org/laws/reporting.cfm⟩.

23. James W. Buehler et al., "The Supplement to HIV/AIDS Surveillance Project:

An Approach for Monitoring HIV Risk Behaviors," *Public Health Reports* 111, supp. 1 (1996): 133–37.

24. James G. Kahn, "The Cost-Effectiveness of HIV Prevention Targeting: How Much More Bang for the Buck?" *AJPH* 86 (December 1996): 1709–12.

25. Mary L. Kamb et al., "Efficacy of Risk Reduction Counseling to Prevent Human Immunodeficiency Virus and Sexually Transmitted Diseases: A Randomized Controlled Trial: Project RESPECT Study Group," *JAMA* 280 (October 7, 1998): 1161–67.

26. Pascale M. Wortley et al., "Using HIV/AIDS Surveillance to Monitor Public Health Efforts to Reduce Perinatal Transmission of HIV," *JAIDS* 11 (February 1, 1996): 205–6.

27. CDC, "Unrecognized HIV Infection, Risk Behavior, and Perceptions of Risk among Young Black Men Who Have Sex with Men—Six U.S. Cities, 1994–1998," *MMWR* 51 (August 23, 2002): 733–36.

28. Todd Summers, Freya Spielberg, Chris Collins, and Thomas Coates, "Voluntary Counseling, Testing, and Referral: New Technologies, Research, and Findings Create Dynamic Opportunities," *JAIDS* 25, supp. 2 (December 15, 2000): S128–S135; Mary L. Kamb et al., "Efficacy of Risk-Reduction Counseling to Prevent Human Immunodeficiency Virus and Sexually Transmitted Diseases," *JAMA* 280 (October 7, 1998): 1161–67.

29. Clinical Practices for the Treatment of HIV Infection, *Guidelines for the Use of Antiretroviral Agents in HIV-infected Adults and Adolescents* (Washington, D.C.: Clinical Practices for the Treatment of HIV Infection, February 4, 2002):1–96, ⟨http://www.aidsinfo. nih.gov/guidelines/adult/AAMay23.pdf⟩.

30. CDC, "Update: Trends in AIDS Incidence—United States, 1996," *MMWR* 46 (September 19, 1997): 861–67.

31. D. D. Brewer and J. J. Potter, "Name-Based Surveillance for HIV-infected Persons," *Annals of Internal Medicine* 132 (June 6, 2000): 922–23; Ronald Bayer and Kathleen Toomey, "HIV Prevention and the Two Faces of Partner Notification," *AJPH* 82 (August 1992): 1158–64.

32. P.L. 106–345, 114 Stat. 1319 (2000).

33. 42 U.S.C.A. § 300ff-11 (2001).

34. ACLU, *HIV Surveillance and Name Reporting*; Anna Forbes, "Naming Names—Mandatory Name-Based HIV Reporting: Impact and Alternatives," *AIDS Policy and Law* 11 (May 1996): 1–4.

35. Frederick M. Hecht et al., "Does HIV Reporting by Name Deter Testing?" *AIDS* 14 (August 18, 2000): 1801–8; AIDS Action Foundation, *Should HIV Test Results Be Reportable?: A Discussion of the Key Policy Questions* (Washington, D.C.: AIDS Action Foundation, 1993).

36. CDC, *HIV and AIDS: Are You at Risk* (Atlanta: CDC, 2000), ⟨http://www.cdc. gov/hiv/pubs/brochure/atrisk.htm⟩; CDC, *HIV Counseling, Testing, and Referral Standards and Guidelines* (Atlanta: CDC, 1994).

37. Hecht et al., "Does HIV Reporting by Name Deter Testing?"

38. Amy Lansky, J. Stan Lehman, Jill Gatwood, Frederick M. Hecht, and Patricia L. Fleming, "Changes in HIV Testing after Implementation of Name-Based HIV Case Surveillance in New Mexico," *AJPH* 92 (November 1, 2002): 1757.

39. William J. Woods et al., "Name-Based Reporting of HIV-Positive Test Results as a Deterrent to Testing," *AJPH* 89 (July 1999): 1097–100.

40. CDC, "Anonymous or Confidential HIV Counseling and Voluntary Testing in Federally Funded Testing Sites—United States, 1995–1997," *MMWR* 48 (June 25, 1999): 509–13; Andrew B. Bindman et al., "Multistate Evaluation of Anonymous HIV Testing and Access to Medical Care," *JAMA* 280 (October 28, 1998): 1416–20.

41. Frederick M. Hecht et al., "Named Reporting of HIV: Attitudes and Knowledge of Those at Risk," *Journal of General Internal Medicine* 12 (1997): 108.

42. ACLU, *Comments on CDC Draft "Guidelines for National HIV Case Surveillance, Including Monitoring for HIV Infection and Acquired Immunodeficiency Syndrome (AIDS)," 63 Fed. Reg. 237, 68289 (December 10, 1998)* (New York: ACLU, January 11, 1999), ⟨http://www.aclu.org/congress/l011299a.html⟩.

43. Andrew B. Bindman et al., "Multistate Evaluation of Anonymous HIV Testing and Access to Medical Care: Multistate Evaluation of Surveillance of HIV (MESH) Study Group" *JAMA* 280 (October 28, 1998): 1416–20.

44. CDC, "Anonymous or Confidential HIV Counseling and Voluntary Testing."

45. These states are Alabama, Idaho, Iowa, Mississippi, Nevada, North Carolina, North Dakota, South Carolina, Tennessee, and Wyoming. Amanda Watson, Stephanie Wasserman, and Julie Scales, *Issue Brief: HIV Reporting in the States* (Washington, D.C.: Health Policy Tracking Service, National Conference of State Legislatures, February 4, 2002).

46. HIV Testing Action Coalition, *Statement of the National HIV Testing Action Coalition on the Necessity for Maintaining Anonymous HIV Testing Sites in All States* (Washington, D.C.: HIV Testing Action Coalition, 1997).

47. John G. Taylor, "HIV Home-Testing Kits Leave Counseling Gaps," *Fresno Bee*, February 20, 1997.

48. Daniel Fox, "From TB to AIDS: Value Conflicts in Reporting Disease," *Hastings Center Report* (December 1986): S11–14.

49. Richard C. Paddock, "Thieves Steal Computer Containing Confidential List of 60 AIDS Victims," *Los Angeles Times*, July 9, 1987.

50. "Log, Said to List AIDS Test-Takers, Is Lost," *NYT*, April 23, 1989.

51. Sue Landry, "AIDS List Is Out: State Investigating Breach," *St. Petersburg Times*, September 20, 1996.

52. *Tarrant City Hospital District v. Huges*, 734 S.W.2d 675 (Tex. App. 1987).

53. Pub. Act 87–763, § 693.40(3)(A) (1991).

54. *Whalen v. Roe*, 429 U.S. 589 (1977).

55. Joy Pritts et al., *The State of Health Privacy: An Uneven Terrain: A Comprehensive Survey of State Health Privacy Statutes* (Washington, D.C.: Health Privacy Project, 1999); Lawrence O. Gostin, Zita Lazzarini, Verla S. Neslund, and Michael T. Osterholm, "The Public Health Information Infrastructure: A National Review of the Law on Health Information Privacy," *JAMA* 275 (June 26, 1996): 1921–27.

56. 42 U.S.C. § 242m(d) (2001).

57. Lynda Richardson, "AIDS Group Urges New York to Start Reporting of HIV," *NYT*, January 13, 1998.

58. "Is There a Viable Alternative To Name-Based HIV Reporting?," *AIDS Policy and Law* 12 (October 31, 1997): 1, 8–9.

59. John W. Ward et al., "Annotation: What Will Be the Role of HIV Infection Reporting?," *AJPH* 84 (December 1994): 1888–89.

60. CDC, "Evaluation of HIV Case Surveillance through the Use of Non-Name Unique Identifiers—Maryland and Texas, 1994–1996," *MMWR* 46 (January 9, 1998): 1254–71.

61. "Is There a Viable Alternative to Name-Based Reporting?"

62. CDC, "Evaluation of HIV Case Surveillance through the Use of Non-Name Unique Identifiers—Maryland and Texas, 1994–1996."

63. Texas Department of Health, Bureau of HIV and STD Prevention, *Unique Identifier Reporting for HIV Infection Surveillance* (Austin: Texas Department of Health, November 1997), and *Questions and Answers: HIV Reporting by Name* (Austin: Texas Department of Health, 1999): 1–14, ⟨http://www.tdh.state.tx.us/hivstd/hivrept/pdf/hivname2.pdf⟩.

64. Liza Solomon et al., "Evaluation of a Statewide Non-Name-Based HIV Surveillance System," *JAIDS* 22 (November 1, 1999): 272–80.

65. San Francisco AIDS Foundation, *Executive Summary of the HIV Surveillance and Reporting Policy Statement of the San Francisco AIDS Foundation* (San Francisco: San Francisco AIDS Foundation, 1997); ACLU, *HIV Surveillance and Name Reporting* (New York: ACLU, October 1997).

66. HIV Criminal Law and Policy Project, "HIV Reporting" (2002).

67. Sonia Bhatnager, "HIV Reporting and Partner Notification in New York State," *Fordham University Law Journal* 26 (May 1999): 1482–83.

Chapter 9

This chapter is based on Lawrence O. Gostin and James G. Hodge Jr., "Piercing the Veil of Secrecy in HIV/AIDS and Other Sexually Transmitted Diseases: Theories of Privacy and Disclosure in Partner Notification," *Duke Journal of Gender Law and Policy* 5 (Spring 1998): 9–88; Gostin and William J. Curran, "AIDS Screening, Confidentiality, and the Duty to Warn," *AJPH* 77 (March 1987): 361–65; and Hodge and Gostin, "Handling Cases of Wilful Exposure through HIV Partner Counseling and Referral Services," *Rutgers Women's Law Reporter* 22 (Summer–Fall 2001): 45–62.

1. Susan P. Connor, "The Pox in Eighteenth-Century France," in *The Secret Malady: Venereal Disease in Eighteenth-Century Britain and France*, edited by Linda E. Merians (Lexington: University Press of Kentucky, 1996): 15, 17.

2. Theodor Rosebury, *Microbes and Morals: The Strange Story of Venereal Disease* (New York: Viking Press, 1971), 6.

3. Linda E. Merians, *The Secret Malady: Venereal Disease in Eighteenth-Century Britain and France* (Lexington: University of Kentucky Press, 1996), 1.

4. IOM, *The Hidden Epidemic: Confronting Sexually Transmitted Diseases*, edited by Thomas R. Eng and William T. Butler (Washington, D.C.: National Academy Press, 1997), 151–52.

5. WHO, *Control of Sexually Transmitted Diseases* (Geneva: WHO, 1985), 47–51.

6. Frances M. Cowan et al., "The Role and Effectiveness of Partner Notification in STD Control: A Review," *Genitourinary Medicine* 72 (August 1996): 247–52.

7. "Reglementation" refers to the government-regulated medical inspection of prostitutes. For more on this, see Gostin and Hodge, "Piercing the Veil of Secrecy."

8. Michael J. Adler, "The Terrible Peril: A Historical Perspective on the Venereal Diseases," *British Medical Journal* 281 (July 19, 1980): 206.

9. Thomas Parran, "The Eradication of Syphilis as a Practical Public Health Objective," *JAMA* 92 (1931): 73.

10. Allan M. Brandt, *No Magic Bullet: A Social History of Venereal Disease in the United States since 1880*, expanded ed. (New York: Oxford University Press, 1987), 150–51.

11. ASTHO et al., *Guide to Public Health Practice: HIV Partner Notification Strategies* (Washington, D.C.: Public Health Foundation, 1988), 1; Lawrence K. Altman, "Case of HIV Transmission Is First to Be Linked to Kiss," *NYT*, July 11, 1997.

12. Susan Sontag, *Illness as Metaphor and AIDS and Its Metaphors* (New York: Doubleday, 1990), 153.

13. Chandler Burr, "The AIDS Exception: Privacy vs. Public Health," *Atlantic Monthly*, June 1997, 57–67.

14. Ronald Bayer, "Public Health Policy and the AIDS Epidemic: An End to HIV Exceptionalism?," *NEJM* 324 (May 23, 1991): 1500–1504.

15. Lynda Richardson, "Progress on AIDS Brings Movement for Less Secrecy," *NYT*, August 21, 1997; *contra* Gabriel Rotello, "AIDS Is Still an Exceptional Disease," *NYT*, August 22, 1997.

16. Peter G. Pappas, "Syphilis 100 Years Ago: Parallels with the AIDS Pandemic," *International Journal of Dermatology* 32 (October 1993): 708–9.

17. Emily Erbelding, "HIV and Sexually Transmitted Diseases," *CRIA Update* 7 (Spring 1998), ⟨http://www.thebody.com/cria/spring98/diseases.html⟩.

18. Ronald Bayer and Kathleen E. Toomey, "HIV Prevention and the Two Faces of Partner Notification," *AJPH* 82 (August 1992): 1158–64.

19. Ronald Bayer, *Private Acts, Social Consequences: AIDS and the Politics of Public Health* (New York: Free Press, 1989), 124.

20. Editorial, "The AIDS Establishment's Conspiracy of Silence," *Washington Post*, October 1, 1994.

21. At least thirty-two states have enacted HIV/AIDS-specific partner notification laws: Arizona, California, Connecticut, Florida, Georgia, Hawaii, Idaho, Illinois, Indiana, Iowa, Kansas, Louisiana, Maryland, Michigan, Minnesota, Missouri, Montana, Nebraska, New Hampshire, New Mexico, New York, North Dakota, Ohio, Pennsylvania, Rhode Island, South Carolina, Texas, Utah, Virginia, West Virginia, Wisconsin, and Wyoming. Delaware, the District of Columbia, and New Jersey require mandatory court orders; the remaining states mandate partner notification under general communicable disease efforts. Stephanie Wasserman and Amanda Watson, *Partner Notification Programs* (Washington, D.C.: Health Policy Tracking Service, Issue Brief, March 15, 2000), ⟨http://stateserv.hpts.org/HPTS2001/issue⟩.

22. ASTHO et al., *Guide to Public Health Practice*; WHO, *Global Programme on AIDS and*

Programme of STD, Consensus Statement from Consultation on Partner Notification for Preventing HIV Transmission (Geneva: WHO, 1989): 2–3.

23. 42 U.S.C. § 300ff-46 (1990).

24. 42 U.S.C. § 201 *et seq.* (1996).

25. CDC, "Announcement 00005A: HIV/AIDS Surveillance and HIV Incidence and Prevalence Cooperative Agreements Finding, Characterizing, and Referring Persons with Recent Infection," ‹http://www.cdc.gov/od/pgo/funding/00005AGd.htm›; David R. Holtgrave, "Human Immunodeficiency Virus Counseling, Testing, Referral, and Partner Notification Services," *Archives of Internal Medicine* 153 (May 24, 1993): 1225–30.

26. CDC, "HIV Partner Notification Support Services," *Operational Guidance Outline* (Atlanta: CDC, 1997): 1–8.

27. Gary R. West and Kathleen A. Stark, "Partner Notification for HIV Prevention: A Critical Reexamination," *AIDS Education and Prevention* 9 (June 1997): 68–78.

28. CDC, "Advancing HIV Prevention: New Strategies for a Changing Epidemic—United States, 2003," *MMWR* 52 (April 18, 2003): 329–32.

29. William Sundbeck, "It Takes Two to Tango: Rethinking Negligence Liability for the Sexual Transmission of AIDS," *Health Matrix* 5 (Summer 1995): 397–441; Daniel M. Oyler, "Interspousal Tort Liability for Infliction of a Sexually Transmitted Disease," *Journal of Family Law* 29 (1990–91): 519; Richard Carl Schoenstein, "Standards of Conduct, Multiple Defendants, and Full Recovery of Damages in Tort Liability for the Transmission of Human Immunodeficiency Virus," *Hofstra Law Review* 18 (Summer 1989): 32–87.

30. *Estate of Behringer v. Medical Center at Princeton*, 592 A.2d 1251, 1281 n. 19 (N.J. Super. 1991); *State v. Yonts*, 84 S.W.3d 516 (Mo. Ct. App. 2002).

31. *Mussivand v. David*, 544 N.E.2d 265, 273 (Ohio 1989).

32. Gregory G. Sarno, Annotation, "Tort Liability for Infliction of Infectious or Venereal Disease," *American Law Reports 4th* 40 (1985 and supp. 1996): 1089.

33. Eric L. Schulman, "Sleeping with the Enemy: Combating the Sexual Spread of HIV-AIDS through a Heightened Legal Duty," *John Marshall Law Review* 29 (Summer 1996): 957–93.

34. See, e.g., *C. A. U. v. R. L.*, 438 N.W.2d 441 (Minn. Ct. App. 1989); *Doe v. Johnson*, 817 F. Supp. 1382 (W.D. Mich. 1993); and *Neal v. Neal*, 873 P.2d 881 (Idaho Ct. App. 1993).

35. *Tarasoff v. Regents of University of California*, 551 P.2d 334 (Cal. 1976); *Thompson v. County of Alameda*, 614 P.2d 728 (Cal. 1980).

36. *Tarasoff*, 551 P.2d at 340.

37. *Alberts v. Devine*, 479 N.E.2d 113 (Mass. 1985), *cert. denied*, 474 U.S. 1013 (1985); *Reisner v. Regents of Univ. of Cal.*, 37 Cal. Rptr. 2d 518 (Ct. App. 1995); *Garcia v. Santa Rosa Health Care Corp.*, 925 S.W.2d 372, 377 (Tex. App. 1996); *Sealed Case*, 67 F.3d 965 (D.C. Cir. 1995); Peter F. Lake, "Revisiting Tarasoff," *Albany Law Review* 58 (1994): 97–173.

38. Kenneth E. Labowitz, "Beyond Tarasoff: AIDS and the Obligation to Breach Confidentiality," *St. Louis University Public Law Review* 9 (1990): 495–517; Joseph D. Piorkowski Jr., "Between a Rock and a Hard Place: AIDS and the Conflicting Physicians'

Duties of Preventing Disease Transmission," *Georgetown Law Journal* 76 (October 1987): 169–202.

39. Christine E. Stenger, "Taking Tarasoff Where No One Has Gone Before: Looking at 'Duty to Warn' under the AIDS Crisis," *St. Louis University Public Law Review* 15 (1996): 471–504.

40. Janet S. St. Lawrence, Daniel E. Montano, Danuta Kasprzyk, William R. Phillips, Keira Armstrong, and Jami S. Leichliter, "STD Screening, Testing, Case Reporting, and Clinical and Partner Notification Practices: A National Survey of US Physicians," *AJPH* 92 (2002): 1784–88.

41. "Name Brands: The Effects of Intrusive HIV Legislation on High-Risk Demographic Groups," *Harvard Law Review* 113 (June 2000): 2098–115.

42. Ronald Bayer and Lawrence O. Gostin, "Legal and Ethical Issues in AIDS," in *Current Topics in AIDS* 2, edited by M. S. Gottlieb et al. (New York: John Wiley and Sons, 1989), 264–65; Hermes Fernandez, "Is AIDS Different?," *Albany Law Review* 61 (1998): 1053–77.

43. Karen Rothenberg et al. "The AIDS Project: Creating a Public Health Policy-Rights and Obligations of Health Care Workers," *Maryland Law Review* 48 (Fall 1989): 93–211; Julie E. Maher et al., "Partner Violence, Partner Notification, and Women's Decision to Have an HIV Test," *JAIDS* 25 (November 1, 2000): 276–82; Andrea C. Gielan, Linda Fogarty, Patricia O'Campo, and Kay Anderson, "Women Living with HIV: Disclosure, Violence, and Social Support," *Journal of Urban Health* 77 (September 2000): 480–91.

44. Morton E. Winston, "AIDS, Confidentiality, and the Right to Know," *Public Affairs* 2 (1988): 91–104.

45. James F. Childress, "Contact Tracing: A Liberal-Communitarian Perspective," *Responsive Community* (Winter 1990–91): 74.

46. Dennis H. Osmond, Andrew B. Bindman, Krean Uranizan, Stan J. Lehman, et al., "Name-Based Surveillance and Public Health Intervention for Persons with HIV Infection," *Annals of Internal Medicine* 131 (November 16, 1999): 775–79.

47. Andrew T. Pavia et al., "Partner Notification for Control of HIV: Results After 2 Years of a Statewide Program in Utah," *AJPH* 83 (October 1993): 1418–24; CDC, "Notification of Syringe-Sharing and Sexual Partners of HIV Infected Persons—Pennsylvania, 1993–1994," *MMWR* 44 (1995): 202–4; Beth A. Macke, Michael H. Hennessy, and Mary McFarlane, "Predictors of Time Spent on Partner Notification in Four U.S. Sites," *Sexually Transmitted Infections* 76 (October 2000): 371–74.

48. Caswell A. Evans and C. J. O'Connell, *Contact Tracing and Partner Notification: A Report of the Special Initiative on AIDS* (Washington, D.C.: American Public Health Association, 1988), 6.

49. Jon K. Andrus et al., "Partner Notification: Can It Control Epidemic Syphilis?," *Annals of Internal Medicine* 112 (April 1, 1990): 539–43.

50. Hawazin Faruki et al., "A Community Based Outbreak of Infection with Penicillin-Resistant *Neisseria gonorrhea* Not Producing Penicillinase (Chromosomally Mediate Resistance)," *NEJM* 313 (September 5, 1985): 607.

51. Barry P. Katz et al., "Efficiency and Cost-Effectiveness of Field Follow-up for

Patients with Chlamydia Trachomatis Infection in a Sexually Transmitted Diseases Clinic," *Sexually Transmitted Diseases* 15 (January–March 1988): 11–16.

52. Suzanne E. Landis, Victor J. Schoenbach, David J. Weber, et al., "Results of a Randomized Trial of Partner Notification in Cases of HIV Infection in North Carolina," *NEJM* 326 (January 9, 1992): 101–6; Matthew Carmody, "Mandatory HIV Partner Notification: Efficacy, Legality, and Notions of Traditional Public Health," *Texas Forum on Civil Liberties and Civil Rights* 4 (Summer–Fall 1999): 107–37.

53. Catherine Baker, Drew Johnson, and Harold Rasmussen, "HIV Partner Counseling and Referral," *FOCUS: A Guide to AIDS Research and Counseling* 14 (February 1999): 1–4.

54. Kathleen E. Toomey and Willard Cates Jr., "Partner Notification for the Prevention of HIV Infection," *AIDS* 3, supp. 1 (1989): S57–62.

55. Nathan Clumeck et al., "A Cluster of HIV Infection among Heterosexual People without Apparent Risk Factors," *NEJM* 321 (November 23, 1989): 1460–62.

56. Neil Graham, Scott L. Zeger, Lawrence P. Park, Sten H. Vermund, Roger Detels, et al., "The Effects on Survival of Early Treatment of Human Immunodeficiency Virus Infection," *NEJM* 326 (April 16, 1992): 1037–42.

57. Michael W. Adler, "Contact Tracing," *British Medical Journal* 284 (1982): 1211; Ralph H. Henderson, "Control of Sexually Transmitted Disease in the United States—A Federal Perspective," *British Journal of Venereal Disease* 53 (August 1977): 211; Richard S. Pattman and Elspeth M. Gould, "Partner Notification for HIV Infection in the United Kingdom: A Look Back on Seven Years' Experience in Newcastle upon Tyne," *Genitourinary Medicine* 69 April 1993): 94–97.

58. Nancy E. Spencer et al., "Partner Notification for Human Immunodeficiency Virus Infection in Colorado: Results across Index Case Groups and Costs," *International Journal of STD and AIDS* 4 (January–February 1993): 26, 31; Beth A. Macke and Julie E. Maher, "Partner Notification in the United States," *American Journal of Preventive Medicine* 17 (October 1999): 230–42.

59. Richard E. Hoffman et al., "Comparison of Partner Notification at Anonymous and Confidential HIV Test Sites in Colorado," *JAIDS* 8 (April 1, 1995): 406–10; Robin Sheridan, "Public Health versus Civil Liberties: Washington State Imposes HIV Surveillance and Strikes the Proper Balance," *Seattle University Law Review* 24 (Winter 2001): 941–68.

60. Andrus et al., "Partner Notification," 539–43; Suzanne E. Landis, Victor J. Schoenbach, David J. Weber, et al., "Results of a Randomized Trial of Partner Notification in Cases of HIV Infection in North Carolina," *NEJM* 326 (January 9, 1992): 101–6.

61. Andrew D. Oxman et al., "Partner Notification for Sexually Transmitted Diseases: An Overview of the Evidence," *Canadian Journal of Public Health* 85, supp. 1 (July–August 1994): S41–S47.

62. Gabriel Rotello, "AIDS Is Still an Exceptional Disease," *NYT*, August 22, 1997.

63. Samuel R. Friedman, Editorial, "Network Methodologies, Contact Tracing, Gonorrhea, and Human Immunodeficiency Virus," *Sexually Transmitted Diseases* 23 (November–December 1996): 523–25.

64. Richard Rothenberg and Jerry Narramore, "The Relevance of Social Network Concepts to Sexually Transmitted Disease Control," *Sexually Transmitted Diseases* 23 (January–February 1996): 24–29.

Chapter 10

This chapter is based on Lawrence O. Gostin, *Public Health Law: Power, Duty, Restraint* (New York: Milbank Memorial Fund and University of California Press, 2000); Gostin, "The Politics of AIDS: Compulsory State Powers, Public Health, and Civil Liberties," *Ohio State Law Review* 49 (1989): 1018–42; James G. Hodge Jr. and Gostin, "Handling Cases of Wilful Exposure through HIV Partner Counseling and Referral Services," *Rutgers Women's Law Reporter* 22 (Summer–Fall 2001): 45–62.

1. Eleanor Singer, Teresa Rogers, and Mary Corcoran, "The Polls: A Report: AIDS," *Public Opinion Quarterly* 51 (Winter 1987): 580–95.

2. *Time/CNN/Yankelovich Partners Poll* (Time, CNN, October 31, 1997), ‹http://www.ropercenter.uconn.edu›; *AIDS and the Safety of America's Blood Supply Survey by American Association of Blood Banks* (Gallup Organization, March 29–April 16, 1993), ‹http://www.ropercenter.uconn.edu›.

3. David L. Kirp, *Learning by Heart: AIDS and School Children in America's Communities* (New Brunswick, N.J.: Rutgers University Press, 1989); Lawrence O. Gostin and David W. Webber, "The AIDS Litigation Project: HIV/AIDS in the Courts in the 1990s, Part 2," *APPJ* 13 (Spring 1998): 3–19.

4. William F. Buckley Jr., "Identify All the Carriers," *NYT*, March 18, 1986 (recommending that persons with HIV infection be tattooed on their forearms and buttocks).

5. J. F. Grutsch and A. D. J. Robertson, "The Coming of AIDS: It Didn't Start with the Homosexuals and It Won't End with Them," *American Spectator*, March 1986, 12; "Florida Considering Locking Up Some Carriers of the AIDS Virus," *NYT*, January 27, 1988 (state proposing "special lock-up" wards"); Tamar Lewin, "Rights of Citizens and Society Raise Legal Muddle on AIDS," *NYT*, October 14, 1987 (Senator Jesse Helms and Pat Robertson suggest that "quarantine may be necessary"); Singer, Rogers, and Corcoran, "The Polls" (in five national opinion polls, 28–51 percent of respondents said that "people with AIDS should be put into quarantine in special places").

6. David J. Rothman, "The Single Disease Hospital: Why Tuberculosis Justifies a Departure That AIDS Does Not," *Journal of Law, Medicine, and Ethics* 21 (Fall–Winter 1993): 296–302.

7. Jennifer Brown, "A Troublesome Maternal-Fetal Conflict: Legal, Ethical, and Social Issues Surrounding Mandatory AZT Treatment of HIV Positive Pregnant Women," *Buffalo Public Interest Law Journal* 18 (2000): 67–94.

8. Robin Marantz Henig, "AIDS: A New Disease's Deadly Odyssey," *NYT Magazine*, February 6, 1983, 36: "Innocent bystanders caught in the path of a new disease, they can make no behavioral decisions to minimize their risk: hemophiliacs cannot stop taking bloodclotting medication; surgery patients cannot stop getting transfusions; women cannot control the drug habits of their mates; babies cannot choose their mothers."

9. Randy Schilts, *And the Band Played On: People, Politics, and the AIDS Epidemic* (New York: Penguin Books, 1988); David Altman, *AIDS in the Mind of America* (Garden City, N.Y.: Anchor Press/Doubleday, 1986).

10. Francis M. Pottenger, "Is Another Chapter in Public Phthisiophobia About to be Written?," *California State Journal of Medicine* 1 (1903): 81.

11. Diane V. Havlir et al., "Maintenance Antiretroviral Therapies in HIV-infected Subjects with Undetectable Plasma HIV RNA after Triple-Drug Therapy," *NEJM* 339 (October 29, 1998): 1261–68.

12. Brain Conway et al., "Development of Drug Resistance in Patients Receiving Combinations of Zidovudine, Didanosine, and Nevirapine," *AIDS* 15 (July 6, 2001): 1269–74; Douglas L. Mayer, "Prevalence and Incidence to Zidovudine and Other Antiretroviral Drugs," *American Journal of Medicine* 102 (May 19, 1997): 70–75; Martin S. Hirsch, "Antiretroviral Drug Resistance Testing in Adults with HIV Infection: Implications for Clinical Management," *JAMA* 279 (June 24, 1998): 1984–91.

13. Andrew Carr, "Improvements of the Study, Analysis, and Reporting of Adverse Events Associated with Antiretroviral Therapy," *Lancet* 360 (July 6, 2002): 81–85.

14. E. Fuller Torrey and Mary T. Zdanowicz, "We've Tried Mandatory Treatment—and It Works," *City Journal* 9 (Summer 1999): 82–85; Gina Kolata, "Discovery That AIDS Can Be Prevented in Babies Raises Debate on Mandatory Testing," *NYT*, November 3, 1994.

15. *Washington v. Harper*, 494 U.S. 210, 227 (1990) (upholding forced administration of antipsychotic medication if inmate is dangerous to himself or others and treatment is in the inmate's medical interest); *McCormick v. Stalder*, 105 F.3d 1059, 1061 (5th Cir. 1997) (finding that the state's compelling interest in reducing spread of TB justifies involuntary treatment); *United States v. Bechara*, 935 F. Supp. 892, 894 (S.D. Tex. 1996) (upholding involuntary sedation of deportee to ensure public safety).

16. *Reynolds v. McNichols*, 488 F.2d 1378 (10th Cir. 1973) (upholding mandatory physical examination, treatment, and detention of person suspected of having venereal disease); *People ex rel. Baker v. Strautz*, 54 N.E. 2d 441 (Ill. 1944) (same); *Rock v. Carney*, 185 N.W. 798 (Mich. 1921) (upholding physical examination, but only on reasonable grounds).

17. *In re City of New York v. Doe*, 614 N.Y.S.2d 8 (N.Y. App. Div. 1994) (upholding continued detention for TB treatment based on the fact that public health could not be protected by less restrictive means); *In re City of New York v. Antoinette R.*, 630 N.Y.S.2d 1008 (1995) (finding that clear and convincing evidence existed to detain women for treatment of TB based on past noncompliance).

18. Lawrence O. Gostin, "The Resurgent Tuberculosis Epidemic in the Era of AIDS: Reflections on Public Health, Law, and Society," *Maryland Law Review* 54 (1995): 1–131.

19. Joseph Barbera et al., "Large-Scale Quarantine following Biological Terrorism in the United States: Scientific Examination, Logistic and Legal Limits, and Possible Consequences," *JAMA* 286 (December 5, 2001): 2711–17.

20. P. Pagano, "Quarantine Considered for AIDS Victims," *California Law* 4 (March 1984): 17; John A. Gleason, "Quarantine: An Unreasonable Solution to the AIDS Dilemma," *University of Cincinnati Law Review* 55 (1986): 217–35.

21. Abram S. Benenson, ed., *Control of Communicable Diseases Manual,* 16th ed. (American Public Health Association, 1995), 541–43.

22. CDC, *HIV/AIDS Update* (Atlanta: CDC, December 2000): 1, ‹www.cdc.gov/nchstp/od/news/At-a-Glance.pdf›.

23. Paul Slovic, John Monahan, and Donald MacGregor, "Violence Risk Assessment and Risk Communication: The Effects of Using Actual Cases, Providing Instruction, and Employing Probability versus Frequency Formats," *Law and Human Behavior* 24 (June 2000): 271–96.

24. Deborah Merritt, "Communicable Disease Control and Constitutional Law: Controlling AIDS," *New York University Law Review* 61 (November 1986): 759; Wendy Parmet, "AIDS and Quarantine: The Revival of an Archaic Doctrine," *Hofstra Law Review* 14 (Fall 1985): 53–90.

25. *O'Connor v. Donaldson,* 422 U.S. 563, 580 (1975) (Berger, C.J., concurring); *Addington v. Texas,* 441 U.S. 418, 425–27 (1979); *Vitek v. Jones,* 445 U.S. 480, 491–92 (1980); *Project Release v. Prevost,* 722 F.2d 960, 971 (2d Cir. 1983).

26. *William Arthur Greene v. Hugh S. Edwards, M.D.,* 263 S.E.2d 661, 663 (1980).

27. Jennifer Frey, "Nushawn's Girls," *Washington Post,* June 1, 1999; Lynda Richardson, "Man Faces Felony Charge in HIV Case," *NYT,* August 20, 1998.

28. "HIV-Positive Woman Gets Revenge through Lengthy String of Affairs," *Washington Times,* August 1, 1998.

29. Kristina Sauerwein, "Man's Deadly Legacy Triggers Frantic Race," *St. Louis Post-Dispatch,* April 11, 1997.

30. Barnaby C. Wittels and Stephen Robert LaCheen, "The Persecution of Ed Savitz," *Philadelphia Inquirer,* June 1, 1993.

31. Lynda Richardson, "Wave of Laws Aimed at People with HIV," *NYT,* September 25, 1998; "Criminal Exposure to HIV: Evolving Laws and Court Cases," *AIDS Policy and Law* (Bonus Report) 13 (July 24, 1998): 1.

32. See, e.g., Denise M. Bonilla, "Prostitute with HIV Sentenced to 10 Years," *Los Angeles Times,* April 2, 2003; John-John Williams IV, "Two S. Dakotans Sentenced for Spreading HIV," *Argus Leader,* March 26, 2003; "Failure to Disclose Serostatus Increasingly Leads to Lawsuits," *AIDS Policy and Law,* February 14, 2003.

33. Jeffrey D. Fisher et al., "Dynamics of Sexual Risk Behavior in HIV-infected Men Who Have Sex with Men," *AIDS and Behavior* 2 (1998): 101–13; Linda M. Niccolai, D. Dorst, Leann Myers, and Patricia J. Kissinger, "Disclosure of HIV Status to Sexual Partners: Predictors and Temporal Patterns," *Sexually Transmitted Diseases* 26 (May 1999): 281–85; Christine J. De Rosa and Gary Marks, "Preventive Counseling of HIV-Positive Men and Self-Disclosure of Serostatus to Sex Partners: New Opportunities for Prevention," *Health Psychology* 17 (May 1998): 224–31.

34. "Continued Sexual Risk Behavior among HIV-Seropositive, Drug-Using Men," *MMWR* 45 (February 23, 1996): 151–59; Carol F. Kwiatkowski and Robert E. Booth, "HIV-Seropositive Drug Users and Unprotected Sex," *AIDS and Behavior* 2 (1998): 151.

35. Michael D. Stein et al., "Sexual Ethics: Disclosure of HIV-Positive Status to Partners," *Archives of Internal Medicine* 158 (February 9, 1998): 253.

36. Thomas A. Coburn, "Introduction of the HIV Prevention Act of 1996," *Cong. Rec.* (August 1, 1996): E1446–E1447.

37 *Report of the Presidential Commission on the Human Immunodeficiency Virus Epidemic* (Washington, D.C.: GPO, June 24, 1988), 130–31.

38. Lawrence O. Gostin, "The Politics of AIDS: Compulsory State Powers, Public Health, and Civil Liberties," *Ohio State Law Review* 49 (Fall 1989): 1017–58.

39. *Grayned v. City of Rockford*, 408 U.S. 104, 108–9 (1972).

40. A separate line of cases have been prosecuted under the military code of justice. These cases fall under two types of actions: (1) violation of "safe-sex" orders (*United States v. Barrows*, 48 M.J. 783 [A.C.C.A. 1998]; *United States v. Womack*, 29 M.J. 88 [1989]; *but see United States v. Perez*, 33 M.J. 392 (1991) [overturning conviction for violation of safe-sex order when the government did not prove that an HIV-infected man with a vasectomy could spread the disease]), and (2) criminal assault through knowing exposure or transmission of the disease (*United States v. Schoolfield*, 48 M.J. 132 [C.M.A. 1994] [upholding aggravated assault conviction for unprotected and undisclosed sex with five partners]; *United States v. Bygrave*, 40 M.J. 839 [1994] [upholding assault conviction for unprotected consensual sex]; *United States v. Joseph*, 33 M.J. 960 [N-M.C.M.R. 1991] [affirming aggravated assault conviction for one sexual encounter using a condom but not warning partner]). The Supreme Court held that removing a soldier from the military rolls after a conviction for violation of safe-sex order does not violate constitutional proscriptions of ex post facto laws or double jeopardy. *Clinton v. Goldsmith*, 119 S. Ct. 1538 (1999).

41. *Blacks Law Dictionary* 370 (6th ed. 1991); J. C. Smith and Brian Hogan, *Criminal Law*, 3d ed. (1973): 17–23.

42. Robert Boorstin, "Criminal and Civil Litigation on Spread of AIDS Appears," *NYT*, June 19, 1987.

43. Model Penal Code § 2.02 (1998) (a person is not guilty of an offense unless he acted purposely, knowingly, recklessly, or negligently).

44. Prosecutors can also charge persons with reckless endangerment, but usually this is a lesser included offense rather than a stand-alone charge. Perhaps the reason is that reckless endangerment is considered an insufficiently serious charge. Donald H. J. Hermann, "Criminalizing Conduct Related to HIV Transmission," *St. Louis University Public Law Review* 9 (1990): 351–78.

45. Kathleen M. Sullivan and Martha A. Field, "AIDS and the Coercive Power of the State," *Harvard Civil Rights–Civil Liberties Law Review* 23 (Winter 1988): 139–97.

46. *Smallwood v. State*, 680 A.2d 512 (Md. 1996).

47. *State v. Hinkhouse*, 912 P.2d 921, *modified*, 915 P.2d 489 (Oreg. Ct. App. 1996).

48. *State v. Bird*, 692 N.E.2d 1013 (1998).

49. Model Penal Code § 5.01(1)(a) (1998).

50. *State v. Smith*, 621 A.2d 493 (N.J. Super. Ct.), *cert. denied*, 634 A.2d 523 (N.J. 1993) (inmate biting guard during an altercation).

51. *Weeks v. State*, 834 S.W.2d 559 (Tex. Ct. App. 1992), *petition for habeas corpus denied sub nom. Weeks v. Scott*, 55 F.3d 1059 (5th Cir. 1995) (inmate spitting at guard); *Bird*, 692 N.E.2d 1013.

52. *State v. Haines*, 545 N.E.2d 834 (Ind. Ct. App. 1989) (throwing bloody wig at police officers after attempting suicide).

53. Jason Strait, "Man Guilty of Giving Son HIV Virus," *Associated Press* (December

6, 1998); Michele Munz, "Father Is Found Guilty of Giving His Son HIV-Tainted Injection, Jury Recommends Life in Prison on Assault Conviction," *St. Louis Post-Dispatch*, December 6, 1998.

54. Bruce Schultz, "Dr. Schmidt Found Guilty—Jury Says Physician Tried to Kill Lover with HIV Injection," *Baton Rouge Advocate*, October 24, 1998; *State v. Schmidt*, No. 99–1412 (La. App. July 26, 2000); *State v. Caine*, 652 So.2d 611 (La. App. 1995) (upholding second-degree murder charge against a burglar who stabbed a victim with a needle and shouted "I'll give you AIDS").

55. *Haines*, 545 N.E.2d 834.

56. Model Penal Code § 211.1(1)(a) (1998).

57. *Scroggins v. State*, 401 S.E.2d 13 (Ga. Ct. App. 1990), *Brock v. State*, 555 So. 2d 285 (Ala. Crim. App. 1989), and *Commonwealth v. Brown*, 605 A.2d 429 (Pa. Super. Ct. 1992).

58. *Bird*, 692 N.E.2d 1013.

59. *Newman v. State of Indiana*, 677 N.E.2d 590 (Ind. Ct. App. 1997) (battery conviction for shaking nasal mucous, tears, and saliva onto arresting officers).

60. Model Penal Code §211.1(2) (1998).

61. *United States v. Sturgis*, 48 F.3d 784 (4th Cir. 1995) (the mouth and teeth are deadly weapons, finding that HIV can be transmitted from a bite wound); *United States v. Moore*, 846 F.2d 1163 (8th Cir. 1988) (the mouth and teeth are deadly weapons, finding that HIV transmission is unlikely, but other infections are more likely).

62. Patricia Davis, "Man Accused of Knowingly Passing HIV," *Washington Post*, June 19, 2002.

63. Model Penal Code § 2.02(2)(b)(ii) (1998).

64. Minn. Stat. Ann. § 145.36 (1998) (prohibiting willful exposure of anyone affected with a contagious or infectious disease in any public place); Utah Code Ann. § 26-6-5 (1953) (prohibiting willful or knowing introduction of any communicable or infectious disease into any community).

65. Lawrence O. Gostin, "Controlling the Resurgent Tuberculosis Epidemic: A Fifty State Survey of Tuberculosis Statutes and Proposals for Reform," *JAMA* 269 (January 13, 1993): 255–61.

66. Allan M. Brandt, "AIDS in Historical Perspective: Four Lessons from the History of Sexually Transmitted Diseases," *AJPH* 78 (April 1988): 367–71; Stephen V. Kenney, "Criminalizing HIV Transmission: Lessons from History and a Model for the Future," *Journal of Contemporary Health Law and Policy* 8 (Spring 1992): 245–73.

67. William Curran, Lawrence O. Gostin, and Mary Clark, *Acquired Immunodeficiency Syndrome: Legal and Regulatory Policy Analysis* (1986, republished by U.S. Department of Commerce 1988): i–ii, 204–7.

68. *New York Society of Surgeons v. Axelrod*, 572 N.E.2d 605 (1991); *Plaza v. Estate of Wisser*, 626 N.Y.S.2d 446, 452 (App. Div. 1995).

69. Fla. Stat. Ann. § 384.24 (1997) and Idaho Code § 39–601 (1948) (explicitly defining "venereal disease" to include HIV).

70. National Council of State Legislatures, *Criminalization of HIV Transmission and Exposure: Health Policy Tracking Service*, March 15, 2001, ⟨http://www.stateserv.hpts.org⟩; David L. McColgin and Elizabeth T. Hey, "Criminal Law," in *AIDS and the Law*, 3d ed., edited by David W. Webber (New York: John Wiley and Sons, 1997, with 2000 Supp.),

259, 287, n. 134; Mark H. Jackson, "The Criminalization of HIV," in *AIDS Agenda: Emerging Issues in Civil Rights*, edited by Nan D. Hunter and William B. Rubenstein (New York: New Press, 1992), 239; J. Kelly Strader, "Criminalization as a Policy Response to a Public Health Crisis," *John Marshall Law Review* 27 (Winter 1994): 435–47.

71. 18 U.S.C. § 1118 (1994) (persons who know that they are HIV-infected may not "donate or sell blood, semen, tissues, organs or other bodily fluids for use by another, except as determined necessary for medical research or testing").

72. CARE, 42 U.S.C. § 300ff-47 (1994) (state certifying that it can prosecute knowing, and with intent to expose others to HIV, donation of blood, semen or breast milk, sexual activity, or sharing needles). CARE recommends that states use a "specific intent" standard and does not require an HIV-specific statute.

73. In addition to the most common form of HIV-specific criminal statutes (which generally apply to persons living with HIV/AIDS), some state statutes apply only when a law enforcement official is assaulted or otherwise exposed to HIV, provide enhanced penalties for the commission of a sexual offense while infected with HIV, or specifically target HIV-infected prostitutes.

74. For example, Missouri House Bill 1756 (2002) criminalizes intentional transmission of HIV and explicitly states that the "use of condoms is not a defense to a violation of this section."

75. Donald C. Ainslie, "Question Bioethics: AIDS, Sexual Ethics, and the Duty to Warn," *Hastings Center Report* 29 (September–October 1999): 26–35; Ronald Bayer, "AIDS Prevention—Sexual Ethics and Responsibility," *NEJM* 334 (June 6, 1996): 1540–42.

76. *State v. Thomas*, 983 P.2d 245 (1999).

77. Zita Lazzarini, Sarah Bray, and Scott Burris, "Evaluating the Impact of Criminal Laws on HIV Sexual Risk Behavior," *Journal of Law, Medicine, and Ethics* 30 (Summer 2002): 239–53.

78. South Dakota ST § 34-22-12.1.

79. *Missouri v. Mahan*, 971 S.W.2d 307, 313–14 (Mo. 1998) (upholding criminalization of "grave and unjustifiable risk" as applied to unprotected sexual intercourse); *People v. Russell*, 630 N.E.2d 794, 796 (Ill.), *cert. denied*, 115 S. Ct. 97 (1994); *People v. Dempsey*, 610 N.E.2d 208, 222–24 (Ill. App. Ct. 1993); *Louisiana v. Gambrella*, 633 So. 2d 595 (La. App. 1993) (upholding HIV-specific criminal statute).

80. *People v. Russell*, 630 N.E.2d 794 (S. Ct. Ill.), *cert. denied*, 115 S. Ct. 97 (1994); *Michigan v. Jensen*, 586 N.W.2d 748 (1998) (statute requiring infected persons to give notice of HIV status prior to sexual intercourse is not overbroad).

81. *People v. Jensen*, 586 N.W.2d 748, 752–54 (Ct. App. Mich. 1998).

82. *State v. Stark*, 832 P.2d 109, 116 (Wash. Ct. App. 1992) ("any reasonably intelligent person would understand . . . that the term ['expose'] refers to engaging in . . . unprotected sexual intercourse").

83. Lazzarini, Bray, and Burris, "Evaluating the Impact of Criminal Laws."

84. Richard Elliott and Miriam Maluwa, *Criminal Law, Public Health, and HIV Transmission* (Geneva: UNAIDS, June 2002).

85. Gene P. Shultz, "AIDS: Public Health and the Criminal Law," *St. Louis University Public Law Review* 7 (1988): 65–113; Michael L. Closen, Mary Anne Bobinski, Donald

H. J. Hermann, et al., "Criminalization of an Epidemic: HIV/AIDS and Criminal Exposure Laws," *Arkansas Law Review* 46 (1994): 921–83; Harlon Dalton, "Law and Responsibility Lecture Series: Shaping Responsible Behavior—Lessons from the AIDS Front," *Washington and Lee Law Review* 56 (Summer 1999): 931–52.

86. Harlon L. Dalton, "Criminal Law," in *AIDS Law Today: A New Guide for the Public*, edited by Scott Burris, Harlon L. Dalton, and Judith Leonie Miller (New Haven: Yale University Press, 1993), 242.

Chapter 11

This chapter is based on the Report of the Working Group on HIV Testing, Counseling, and Prophylaxis after Sexual Assault. The members of the Working Group were Dianne D. Alexander; Allan Brandt, Ph.D.; Renee Brant, M.D.; Robert Carr; David Chambers, J.D.; Paul D. Cleary, Ph.D.; Deborah Cotton, M.D., M.P.H.; Lawrence O. Gostin (chair), J.D.; Zita Lazzarini, J.D., M.P.H.; Kenneth H. Mayer, M.D.; Ruth Purtilo, Ph.D., P.T.; San Juanita Rangel; Veronica Reed Ryback, A.C.S.W., L.I.C.S.W.; Nancy Scannell; Daniel Silverman, M.D.; Helene Tomlinson; and Susan M. Wolf, J.D. The data and reasoning are updated to reflect new information on HIV and sexual assault. The Working Group report was summarized in Gostin, Lazzarini, Alexander, Brandt, Mayer, and Silverman, "HIV Testing, Counseling, and Prophylaxis after Sexual Assault," *JAMA* 271 (November 23–30, 1994): 1436–44.

1. Allan M. Brandt, *No Magic Bullet: A Social History of Venereal Disease in the United States since 1880*, rev. ed. (New York: Oxford University Press, 1987); Elizabeth Fee and Daniel M. Fox, eds., *AIDS: The Burden of History* (Berkeley: University of California Press, 1988).

2. Susan Brownmiller, *Against Our Will: Men, Women, and Rape* (New York: Simon and Schuster, 1975).

3. Allan M. Brandt, "Historical Perspective," in *AIDS Law Today: A Guide for the Public*, edited by Scott Burris, Harlon L. Dalton, and Judith Leonie Miller (New Haven: Yale University Press, 1993), 46–53.

4. Angela M. Downs and Isabelle De Vincenzi, "Probability of Heterosexual Transmission of HIV: Relationship to the Number of Unprotected Sexual Contacts," *JAIDS* 11 (April 1, 1996): 388–95; Carole Jenny et al., "Sexually Transmitted Diseases in Victims of Rape," *NEJM* 322 (March 1990): 713–16.

5. CDC, "Public Health Service Guidelines for the Management of Health-Care Worker Exposures to HIV and Recommendations for Postexposure Prophylaxis," *MMWR* 47 (May 15, 1998): 1–28.

6. William C. Holmes and Gail B. Slap, "Sexual Abuse of Boys: Definition, Prevalence, Correlates, Sequelae, and Management," *JAMA* 280 (December 2, 1998): 1855–62.

7. Callie Marie Rennison, *Criminal Victimization, 2001: Changes 2000–2001, with Trends 1993–2001* (Washington, D.C.: U.S. Department of Justice, Office of Justice Programs, Bureau of Justice Statistics, National Crime Victimization Survey, NCJ 194610, September 2002), 8–10.

8. Howard N. Snyder, *Sexual Assault of Young Children as Reported to Law Enforcement: Victim, Incident, and Offender Characteristics* (Washington, D.C.: U.S. Department of Justice, Office of Justice Programs, Bureau of Justice Statistics, NCJ 182990, July 2000); Jennifer Clarke, Michael D. Stein, Mindy Sobota, Margaret Marisi, and Lucy Hanna, "Physical Aggression by Persons with a History of Childhood Abuse," *Archives of Internal Medicine* 159 (September 13, 1999): 1920–24.

9. Rennison, *Criminal Victimization*.

10. Ellen R. Wiebe, Susan E. Comay, Margaret McGregor, and Sylvia Ducceschi, "Offering HIV Prophylaxis to People Who Have Been Sexually Assaulted: 16 Months' Experience in a Sexual Assault Service," *Canadian Medical Association Journal* 162 (March 7, 2000): 641–45.

11. Donald B. Louria et al., "HIV Heterosexual Transmission: A Hypothesis about an Additional Potential Determinant," *International Journal of Infectious Diseases* 4 (2000): 110–16; Phyllis J. Kanki et al., "Slower Heterosexual Spread of HIV-2 Than HIV-1," *Lancet* 343 (April 16, 1994): 943–46; Diarmuid O'Donovan et al., "Maternal Plasma Viral RNA Levels Determine Marked Differences in Mother-to-Child Transmission Rates of HIV-1 and HIV-2 in the Gambia," *AIDS* 14 (March 10, 2000): 441–48.

12. U.S. Department of Justice, "HIV in Prisons, 2000," *Bureau of Justice Statistics Bulletin* 1 (October 2002): 1–12; Laura M. Maruschak, *HIV in Prisons and Jails, 1999*, Bureau of Justice Statistics Bulletin, NCJ 187456 (Washington, D.C.: U.S. Department of Justice, Office of Justice Programs, Bureau of Justice Statistics, October 30, 2001), 1–11; Anne Spaulding et al., "Human Immunodeficiency Virus in Correctional Facilities: A Review," *Clinical Infectious Diseases* 35 (August 1, 2002): 305–12.

13. Nancy S. Padian, Stephen C. Shiboski, Sarah O. Glass, and Eric Vittinghoff, "Heterosexual Transmission of Human Immunodeficiency Virus (HIV) in Northern California: Results from a Ten-Year Study," *American Journal of Epidemiology* 146 (August 15, 1997): 350–57.

14. King K. Holmes, David W. Johnson, and Henry J. Trostle, "An Estimate of the Risk of Men Acquiring Gonorrhea by Sexual Contact with Infected Females," *American Journal of Epidemiology* 91 (February 1970): 170–74, and Richard R. Hooper et al., "Cohort Study of Venereal Disease, I: The Risk of Gonorrhea Transmission from Infected Women to Men," *American Journal of Epidemiology* 108 (August 1978): 136–44.

15. CDC, *STD Fact Sheet*, Publication CDC-79-8195 (Atlanta: CDC, 1979).

16. Franklin N. Judson, "Epidemiology of Sexually Transmitted Hepatitis B Infections in Heterosexuals: A Review," *Sexually Transmitted Diseases* 8, supp. (October–December 1981): 336–43.

17. CDC, "Management of Possible Sexual, Injecting-Drug-Use, or Other Nonoccupational Exposure to HIV, Including Considerations for Antiretroviral Therapy: Public Health Service Statement," *MMWR* 47 (September 25, 1998): 1–14; Timothy D. Mastro and Isabelle de Vincenzi, "Probabilities of Sexual HIV-1 Transmission," *AIDS* 10, supp. A (1996): S75–S82; Padian, Shiboski, Glass, and Vittinghoff, "Heterosexual Transmission of Human Immunodeficiency Virus (HIV) in Northern California."

18. CDC, "Management of Possible Sexual, Injecting-Drug-Use, or Other Nonoccupational Exposure to HIV."

19. Myron S. Cohen, Diane C. Shugars, and Susan A. Fiscus, "Limits on Oral Trans-

mission of HIV-1," *Lancet* 356 (July 22, 2000): 272; Joan Stephenson, "HIV Risk from Oral Sex Higher Than Many Realize," *JAMA* 283 (March 8, 2000): 1279.

20. Nancy S. Padian et al., "Clinical and Immunological Correlates of the Heterosexual Transmission of HIV," *Program and Abstracts of the Twenty-eighth Interscience Conference on Antimicrobial Agents and Chemotherapy* (Washington, D.C.: American Society of Microbiology, 1988).

21. Lucy Dorrell et al., "Absence of Specific Mucosal Antibody Responses in HIV-Exposed Uninfected Sex Workers from the Gambia," *AIDS* 14 (June 16, 2000): 1117–22.

22. Max Essex, Luis E. Soto-Ramirez, Boris Renjifo, Wei-Kung Wang, and Ton-Hou Lee, "Genetic Variation within Human Immunodeficiency Viruses Generates Rapid Changes in Tropism, Virulence, and Transmission," *Leukemia* 11, supp. (April 1997): 93–94.

23. Thomas C. Quinn et al., "Viral Load and Heterosexual Transmission of Human Immunodeficiency Virus Type 1: Rakai Project Study Group," *NEJM* 342 (March 30, 2000): 921–29; Peter Greenhead et al., "Parameters of Human Immunodeficiency Virus Infection of Human Cervical Tissue and Inhibition by Vaginal Virucides," *Journal of Virology* 74 (June 2000): 5577–86.

24. Diane V. Havlir et al., "Maintenance Antiretroviral Therapies in HIV-infected Subjects with Undetectable Plasma HIV RNA after Triple-Drug Therapy," *NEJM* 339 (October 29, 1998): 1261–68.

25. Ronald H. Gray et al., "Probability of HIV-1 Transmission per Coital Act in Monogamous, Heterosexual, HIV-1-Discordant Couples in Rakai, Uganda," *Lancet* 357 (April 2001): 1149–53; Thomas C. Wright Jr. et al., "Human Immunodeficiency Virus 1 Expression in the Female Genital Tract in Association with Cervical Inflammation and Ulceration," *American Journal of Obstetrics and Gynecology* 184 (February 2001): 279–85.

26. Guido Vanham et al., "The HIV-2 Genotype and the HIV-1 Syncytium-Inducing Phenotype Are Associated with a Lower Virus Replication in Dendritic Cells," *Journal of Medical Virology* 60 (March 2000): 300–312.

27. John H. Greist and James W. Jefferson, "Anxiety Disorders," in *Review of General Psychiatry*, 5th ed. (New York: Lange Medical Books/McGraw Hill, 2000); Melissa A. Jenkins, Philip J. Langlais, Dean Delis, and Ronald Cohen, "Learning and Memory in Rape Victims with Post-Traumatic Stress Disorder," *American Journal of Psychiatry* 155 (February 1998): 278–79.

28. Ann W. Burgess and Lytle L. Holmstrom, "Rape Trauma Syndrome," *American Journal of Psychiatry* 131 (September 1974): 981–86.

29. American Psychiatric Association, *Diagnostic and Statistical Manual of Mental Disorders*, 3d ed., rev. (Washington, D.C.: American Psychiatric Association, 1987); Jenny A. Petrak and Elizabeth A. Campbell, "Post-Traumatic Stress Disorder in Female Survivors of Rape Attending a Genitourinary Medicine Clinic: A Pilot Study," *International Journal of STD and AIDS* 10 (August 1999): 531–35.

30. James Pilcher, "Rape Victims Worry about AIDS," *Associated Press* (February 26, 2000), ⟨http://www.aegis.com/news/ap/2000/ap000215.html⟩.

31. Daniel C. Silverman, "Sharing the Crisis of Rape: Counseling the Mates and Families of Victims," *American Journal of Orthopsychiatry* 48 (January 1978): 166–73; Lytle L. Holmstrom and Ann W. Burgess, "Rape: The Husband's and Boyfriend's Ini-

tial Reactions," *Family Coordinator* 28 (1979): 321–30; Priscilla N. White and Judith C Rollins, "Rape: A Family Crisis," *Family Relations* 30 (1981): 103–9.

32. National Organization for Victim Assistance, ‹http://try-nova.org›.

33. Dean G. Kilpatrick, Christine N. Edmunds, and Anne K. Seymour, *Rape in America: A Report to the Nation* (Arlington, Va.: National Victim Center, 1992).

34. In counseling children and adolescents after sexual assault, service providers must balance the importance of delivering information with the constraints posed by the psychological and developmental needs, and the special legal position, of minors. A full discussion is outside the scope of this chapter.

35. Unpublished data, Boston Beth Israel Hospital, Rape Crisis Intervention Program, 1993.

36. Wiebe, Comay, McGregor, and Ducceschi, "Offering HIV Prophylaxis to People Who Have Been Sexually Assaulted."

37. Committee on Adolescence, "Care of the Adolescent Sexual Assault Victim," *Pediatrics* 107 (June 2001): 1476–79; Felicia H. Stewart and James Trussell, "Prevention of Pregnancy Resulting from Rape: A Neglected Preventive Health Measure," *American Journal of Preventive Medicine* 19 (November 2000): 228–29.

38. Ai Ee Ling et al., "Failure of Routine HIV-1 Tests in a Case Involving Transmission with Preseroconversion Blood Components during the Infectious Window Period," *JAMA* 284 (July 12, 2000): 210–14.

39. Lyle R. Petersen et al., "Duration of Time from Onset of Human Immunodeficiency Virus Type 1 Infectiousness to Development of Detectable Antibody: The HIV Seroconversion Study Group," *Transfusion* 34 (April 1994): 283–89.

40. CDC, "Persistent Lack of Detectable HIV-1 Antibody in a Person with HIV Infection—Utah, 1995," *MMWR* 45 (March 8, 1996): 181–85.

41. Willi Kurt Roth, Marijke Weber, and Erhard Seifried, "Feasibility and Efficacy of Routine PCR Screening of Blood Donations for Hepatitis C Virus, Hepatitis B Virus, and HIV-1 in a Blood-Bank Setting," *Lancet* 353 (January 30, 1999): 359–63.

42. *Pennsylvania v. Ritchie*, 480 U.S. 39 (1987).

43. *State v. McLellan*, 767 A.2d 953 (N.H. 2001) (finding sexual assault defendant has the right to an in-camara review of victim's confidential records because defendant showed reasonable probability that the records contained information relevant to the defense); *Commonwealth v. Fuller*, 667 N.E.2d 847 (Mass. 1996) (finding that defendant must meet an even higher burden to obtain the victim's otherwise confidential records).

44. *Commonwealth v. Fuller*, 667 N.E.2d 847 (Mass. 1996).

45. *Commonwealth v. Bishop*, 617 N.E. 2d 990 (Mass. 1993).

46. *Commonwealth v. Oliveira*, 728 N.E.2d 320 (Mass. 2000); *Commonwealth v. Tripolone*, 681 N.E.2d 1216 (Mass. 1997); Rachel M. Capoccia, "Piercing the Veil of Tears: The Admission of Rape Crisis Counselor Records in Acquaintance Rape Trials," *Southern California Law Review* 68 (July 1995): 1335–90.

47. Julie L. Gerberding and David K. Henderson, "Management of Occupational Exposures to Blood-borne Pathogens: Hepatitis B Virus, Hepatitis C Virus, and Human Immunodeficiency Virus," *Clinical Infectious Diseases* 14 (1992): 1179–85.

48. David K. Henderson, "HIV Postexposure Prophylaxis in the Twenty-first Century," *Emerging Infectious Diseases* 7 (March–April 2001): 254–58; Susan A. Wang et al.,

"Experience of Health Care Workers Taking Postexposure Prophylaxis after Occupational HIV Exposures: Finding of the HIV Postexposure Prophylaxis Registry," *Infection Control and Hospital Epidemiology* 21 (December 2000): 780–85.

49. Laurent Mandelbrot et al., "Lamivudine-Zidovudine Combination for Prevention of Maternal-Infant Transmission of HIV-1," *JAMA* 285 (April 25, 2001): 2083–93.

50. Joshua D. Bamberger, Craig R. Waldo, Julie Louise Gerberding, and Mitchell H. Katz, "Post-Exposure Prophylaxis for Human Immunodeficiency Virus (HIV) Infection following Sexual Assault," *American Journal of Medicine* 106 (March 1999): 323–26.

51. Steven D. Pinkerton, David R. Holtgrave, and Frederick R. Bloom, "Cost-Effectiveness of Post-Exposure Prophylaxis following Sexual Exposure to HIV," 12 *AIDS* (June 18, 1998): 1067–78.

52. Julie Louise Gerberding, "Occupational Exposure to HIV in Health Care Settings," *NEJM* 348 (February 27, 2003): 826–33.

53. CDC, "Updated U.S. Public Health Service Guidelines for the Management of Occupational Exposures to HBV, HCV, and HIV and Recommendations for Postexposure Prophylaxis," *MMWR* 50 (RR-11) (June 29, 2001): 1–52 (recommending a four-week regimen of two drugs for most HIV exposures and an additional third drug for exposures that pose an increased risk of transmission).

54. Global AIDS and Tuberculosis Relief Act of 2000, P.L. 106–264, Title 22 U.S.C. § 6822 (2000).

55. Federal Bureau of Investigation, *Crime in the United States—2000* (Washington, D.C.: Federal Bureau of Investigation, 2001), ⟨http://www.fbi.gov/ucr/cius_00/contents.pdf⟩.

56. Jodi M. Brown, Patrick A. Langan, and David J. Levin, "Felony Sentences in State Courts, 1996," in *Bureau of Justice Statistics Bulletin* (Washington, D.C.: U.S. Department of Justice Office of Justice Programs, May 1999).

57. CARE, P.L. 101–381, Title 42 U.S.C. § 300ff-48 (1991).

58. Ann Dietrich, *Testing of Violent Sex Offenders* (Washington, D.C.: Health Policy Tracking Service, Issue Brief, February 27, 2001), ⟨http://stateserv.hpts.org/⟩.

59. 42 U.S.C. § 3756(f) (1995).

60. Dietrich, *Testing of Violent Sex Offenders.*

61. Steven G. Deeks, "Durable HIV Treatment Benefit Despite Low-Level Viremia: Reassessing Definitions of Success or Failure," *JAMA* 286 (July 11, 2001): 224–26; Edward L. Murphy et al., "Highly Active Antiretroviral Therapy Decreases Mortality and Morbidity in Patients with Advanced HIV Disease," *Annals of Internal Medicine* 135 (July 3, 2001): 17–26.

62. Woraphot Tantisiriwat and William G. Powderly, "Prophylaxis of Opportunistic Infections," *Infectious Disease Clinics of North America* 14 (December 2000): 929–44.

63. Steve Estreich and Greta E. Forster, "Sexually Transmitted Diseases and Rape," *NEJM* 323 (October 18, 1990): 1141–42.

64. Lisa Speissegger, Stephanie Wilson, and Amanda Watson, *Criminal Transmission and Exposure* (Washington, D.C.: Health Policy Tracking Service, Issue Brief, July 1, 2002), ⟨http://stateserv.hpts.org/⟩.

65. "The right of the people to be secure in their persons, houses, papers, and effects, against unreasonable searches and seizures, shall not be violated, and no War-

rants shall issue, but upon probable cause, supported by Oath or affirmation, and particularly describing the place to be searched, and the persons or things to be seized." U.S. Const., amend. IV.

66. *Schmerber v. California*, 384 U.S. 757 (1966).

67. Ibid.

68. *Mincey v. Arizona*, 437 U.S. 385 (1978).

69. *U.S. v. Ward*, 131 F.3d 335 (3d Cir. 1997).

70. Mark H. Jackson, "The Criminalization of HIV," in *AIDS Agenda: Emerging Issues in Civil Rights*, edited by Nan D. Hunter and William B. Rubenstein (New York: New Press, 1992), 239–70.

71. *National Treasury Employees Union v. Von Raab*, 489 U.S. 656 (1989); *Skinner v. Railway Labor Executives' Association*, 489 U.S. 602 (1989).

72. *Griffin v. Wisconsin*, 483 U.S. 868, 873 (1987), quoting *New Jersey v. T. L. O.*, 469 U.S. 325, 351 (1985).

73. *Vernonia School Dist. 47J v. Acton*, 515 U.S. 646 (1995); *Chandler v. Miller*, 520 U.S. 305 (1997).

74. *Ferguson v. City of Charleston*, 532 U.S. 67, 82–84 (2001).

75. *U.S. v. Ward*, 131 F.3d 335 (3d Cir. 1997); *Matter of Juveniles A, B, C, D, E*, 847 P.2d 455 (Wash. 1993).

76. *Barlow v. Ground*, 943 F.2d 1132 (9th Cir. 1991); *Glover v. Eastern Neb. Com. Office of Retardation*, 867 F.2d 461, 463 (8th Cir. 1989); CDC, "Management of Possible Sexual, Injecting-Drug-Use, or Other Nonoccupational Exposure to HIV, Including Considerations for Antiretroviral Therapy," *MMWR* 47 (September 25, 1998): 1–14.

77. *State in Interest of J. G.*, 701 A.2d 1260 (N.J. 1997); Steven Eisenstat, "An Analysis of the Rationality of Mandatory Testing for the HIV Antibody: Balancing the Governmental Public Health Interests with the Individual's Privacy Interest," *University of Pittsburgh Law Review* 52 (Winter 1991): 327–82.

78. *Schmerber v. California*, 384 U.S. 757 (1966); *Skinner v. Railway Labor Executives' Association*, 489 U.S. 656 (1989).

Chapter 12

This chapter is based on Lawrence O. Gostin, "A Proposed National Policy on Health Care Workers Living with HIV/AIDS and Other Blood-borne Pathogens," *JAMA* 284 (October 18, 2000): 1965–70. See also Gostin, "The HIV-infected Health Care Professional: Public Policy, Discrimination, and Patient Safety," *Archives of Internal Medicine* 151 (April 1991): 663–65, and Gostin, "HIV-infected Physicians and the Practice of Seriously Invasive Procedures," *Hastings Center Report* 19 (January–February 1989): 32–39. The author is grateful to Julie L. Gerberding and Robert Janssen of the Centers for Disease Control and Prevention for their assistance and insights. The opinions in this chapter do not necessarily represent the views of the U.S. Department of Health and Human Services.

1. Carol Ciesielski et al., "The 1990 Florida Dental Investigation: The Press and the Science," *Annals of Internal Medicine* 121 (December 1, 1994): 886–88; CDC, "Update:

Investigations of Persons Treated by HIV-infected Health-Care Workers," *MMWR* 42 (May 7, 1993): 329–31.

2. Gostin, "The HIV-infected Health Care Professional."

3. In fact, HCWs run a greater risk of acquiring HIV infection in the health care setting than patients. CDC, "Surveillance of Health Care Workers with HIV/AIDS" (Atlanta, 2002), ‹http://www.cdc.gov/hiv/pubs/facts/hcwsurv.htm›. As of 2001, HCWs made up 5.1 percent of the AIDS cases reported to the CDC; fifty-seven HCWs were known to have acquired HIV through occupational exposure.

4. CDC, "Recommendations for Preventing Transmission of Human Immunodeficiency Virus and Hepatitis B Virus to Patients during Exposure-prone Invasive Procedures," *MMWR* 40 (July 12, 1991): 1–9.

5. American College of Surgeons, "Statement on the Surgeon and HIV Infection," *Bulletin of the American College of Surgeons* 83 (February 1998): 27–29.

6. P.L. 102–141, Title VI, § 663, 42 U.S.C. § 300ee-2 (2001).

7. William L. Roper to State Health Departments, June 16, 1992, on file with the CDC.

8. Patti Miller Tereskerz, Richard D. Pearson, and Janine Jagger, "Infected Physicians and Invasive Procedures: National Policy and Legal Reality," *Milbank Quarterly* 77 (1999): 511–29; Phillip L. McIntosh, "When the Surgeon Has HIV: What to Tell Patients about the Risk of Exposure and the Risk of Transmission," *University of Kansas Law Review* 44 (February 1996): 315–64.

9. Committee on Pediatric AIDS and Committee on Infectious Diseases, "Issues Related to Human Immunodeficiency Virus Transmission in Schools, Child Care, Medical Settings, the Home, and Community," *Pediatrics* 104 (August 1999): 318–24; AIDS/TB Committee of the Society for Healthcare Epidemiology of America, "Management of Healthcare Workers Infected with Hepatitis B Virus, Hepatitis C Virus, Human Immunodeficiency Virus, or Other Bloodborne Pathogens," *Infection Control and Hospital Epidemiology* 18 (May 1997): 349–63; American College of Surgeons, "Statement on the Surgeon and HIV Infection."

10. Alicia Noble, Troyen A. Brennan, and Andrew L. Hyams, "*Snyder v. American Association of Blood Banks*: A Re-examination of Liability for Medical Practice Guideline Promulgators," *Journal of Evaluation in Clinical Practice* 4 (February 4, 1998): 49–62.

11. Todd Summers, "Public Policy for Health Care Workers Infected with Human Immunodeficiency Virus," *JAMA* 285 (February 21, 2001): 882.

12. Linda T. Kohn, Janet M. Corrigan, and Molla S. Donaldson, eds., *To Err Is Human: Building a Safer Health System* (Washington, D.C.: National Academy Press, 1999).

13. Edward N. Robinson Jr. and Ruth de Bliek, "The College Student, the Dentist, and the North Carolina Senator: Risk Analysis and Risk Management of HIV Transmission from Health Care Worker to Patient," *Medical Decision Making* 16 (January–March 1996): 86–91.

14. Julie Louise Gerberding, "Occupational Exposure to HIV in Health Care Settings," *NEJM* 348 (February 27, 2003): 826–33.

15. Florence Lot et al., "Probable Transmission from an Orthopedic Surgeon to a Patient in France," *Annals of Internal Medicine* 130 (January 5, 1999): 1–6; Alain Blanchard et al., "Molecular Evidence for Nosocomial Transmission of Human Immuno-

deficiency Virus from a Surgeon to One of His Patients," *Journal of Virology* 72 (1998): 4537–40.

16. Christophe P. Goujon et al., "Phylogenetic Analyses Indicate an Atypical Nurse-to-Patient Transmission of Human Immunodeficiency Virus Type 1," *Journal of Virology* 74 (2000): 2525–32.

17. Laurie M. Robert et al., "Investigations of Patients of Health Care Workers Infected with HIV," *Annals of Internal Medicine* 122 (May 1, 1995): 653–57; Audrey S. Rodgers et al., "Investigation of Potential HIV Transmission to Patient of an HIV-infected Surgeon," *JAMA* 269 (April 14, 1993): 1795–1801.

18. CDC, *Fact Sheet: HIV and Its Transmission* (Atlanta: CDC, January 31, 2001), ⟨http://www.cdc.gov/hiv/pubs/facts/transmission.htm⟩.

19. Michael Donnely et al., "Are HIV Lookbacks Worthwhile? Outcome of an Exercise to Notify Patients Treated by an HIV Infected Health Care Worker," *Communicable Disease and Public Health* 2 (June 1999): 126–29.

20. Michael S. Saag et al., "HIV Viral Load Markers in Clinical Practice," *Nature Medicine* 2 (June 1996): 625–29.

21. Panel for Clinical Practices for the Treatment of HIV, *Guidelines for the Use of Antiretroviral Agents in HIV-infected Adults and Adolescents*, April 23, 2001, ⟨http://www.hivatis.org/guidelines/adult/Apr23_01/text/index.html⟩.

22. Thomas C. Quinn et al., "Viral Load and Heterosexual Transmission of Human Immunodeficiency Virus Type 1," *NEJM* 342 (March 30, 2000): 921–29; Matthew G. Law et al., "Modeling the Effect of Combination Antiretroviral Treatments on HIV Incidence," *AIDS* 15 (July 6, 2001): 1287–94.

23. R. Stefan Ross, Sergei Viazov, and Michael Roggendorf, "Risk of Hepatitis C Transmission from Infected Medical Staff to Patients: Model-based Calculations for Surgical Settings," *Archives of Internal Medicine* 160 (August 14–28, 2000): 2312–16.

24. Rafael Harpaz et al., "Transmission of Hepatitis B Virus to Multiple Patients from a Surgeon without Evidence of Inadequate Infection Control," *NEJM* 334 (February 29, 1996): 549–54.

25. Siew L. Ngui, Ruth P. F. Watkins, Julia Heptonstall, and Chong G. Teo, "Selective Transmission of Hepatitis B Virus after Percutaneous Exposure," *Journal of Infectious Diseases* 181 (March 2000): 838–43; R. Stefan Ross, Sergei Vlazov, and Michael Roggendorf, "Provider-to-Patient Transmission of Hepatitis B Virus," *Lancet* 353 (January 23, 1999): 324–25; The Incident Investigation Team and Others, "Transmission of Hepatitis B to Patients from Four Infected Surgeons without Hepatitis B e Antigen," *NEJM* 336 (January 16, 1997): 178–84.

26. Hepatitis B Outbreak Investigation Team, "An Outbreak of Hepatitis B Associated with Reusable Subdermal Electroencephalogram Electrodes," *Canadian Medical Association Journal* 162 (April 18, 2000): 1127–31.

27. Yvan J. F. Hutin et al., "An Outbreak of Hospital-Acquired Hepatitis B Virus Infection among Patients Receiving Chronic Hemodialysis," *Infection Control and Hospital Epidemiology* 20 (November 1999): 731–35.

28. CDC, "Recommendations for Prevention and Control of Hepatitis C Virus (HCV) Infection and HCV-Related Chronic Disease," *MMWR* 47 (October 16, 1998): 1–39.

29. Juan I. Esteban et al., "Transmission of Hepatitis C by a Cardiac Surgeon," *NEJM* 334 (February 29, 1996): 555–60.

30. R. Stefan Ross et al., "Transmission of Hepatitis C Virus from a Patient to an Anesthesiology Assistant to Five Patients," *NEJM* 343 (December 21, 2000): 1851–54.

31. Xavier Bosch, "Hepatitis C Outbreak Astounds Spain," *Lancet* 351 (May 9, 1998): 1415.

32. R. Stefan Ross et al., "Risk of Hepatitis C Virus Transmission from an Infected Gynecologist to Patients," *Archives of Internal Medicine* 102 (April 2002): 805–10; Georgia J. Duckworth et al., "Transmission of Hepatitis C Virus from a Surgeon to a Patient," *Communicable Disease and Public Health* 2 (September 1999): 188–92; Anonymous, "Hepatitis C Virus Transmission from Health Care Worker to Patient," *Communicable Disease Report Weekly* 5 (June 30, 1995): 121.

33. Ross, Viazov, and Roggendorf, "Risk of Hepatitis C Transmission from Infected Medical Staff to Patients."

34. American College of Surgeons, "Statement on the Surgeon and Hepatitis," *Bulletin of the American College of Surgeons* 84 (April 1999): 21–24.

35. CDC, "Guidelines for Prevention of Transmission of Human Immunodeficiency Virus and Hepatitis B Virus to Health-Care and Public-Safety Workers," *MMWR* 38 (1989): 1–36.

36. 29 C.F.R. § 1910.1030 (2001).

37. American Academy of Orthopaedic Surgeons, *Advisory Statement: Preventing the Transmission of Bloodborne Pathogens* (August 8, 2001), ⟨http://www.aaos.org/wordhtml/papers/advistmt/prevent.htm⟩; Alicia Mangram et al., "Guideline for Prevention of Surgical Site Infection, 1999," *Infection Control and Hospital Epidemiology* 20 (1999): 247–78.

38. CDC, "Updated U.S. Public Health Service Guidelines for the Management of Occupational Exposures to HBV, HCV, and HIV and Recommendations for Postexposure Prophylaxis," *MMWR* 50 (June 29, 2001): 1–52.

39. Julie Gerberding, "Provider-to-Patient HIV Transmission: How to Keep It Exceedingly Rare," *Annals of Internal Medicine* 130 (January 5, 1999): 64–65: "Unfortunately, for most patient infections . . . recontact is either not recognized or not reported in time to initiate prophylactic treatment."

40. Correspondence from Janet Heinrich, Director of Health Care-Public Health Issues, GAO, to Representative Pete Stark, entitled "Occupational Safety: Selected Cost and Benefit Implications of Needlestick Prevention Devices for Hospitals, November 17, 2000," ⟨http://www.cdc.gov/niosh/pdfs/GOA-01-60R.pdf⟩; National Institute for Occupational Safety and Health, "Preventing Needlestick Injuries in Health Care Settings" (Washington, D.C., November 1999), ⟨http://www.cdc.gov/niosh/2000-108.html⟩.

41. P.L. 106–430 (2000).

42. Bernard Lo and Robert Steinbrook, "Health Care Workers Infected with the Human Immunodeficiency Virus," *JAMA* 267 (February 26, 1992): 1100–1105.

43. Lawrence O. Gostin, Chai Feldblum, and David W. Webber, "Disability Discrimination in America: HIV/AIDS and Other Health Conditions," *JAMA* 281 (February 24, 1999): 745–52.

44. 42 U.S.C. § 12113(b) (2001).

45. 42 U.S.C. § 12112(b)(5)(A) (2001).

46. *Parks v. Female Health Care Assoc., Ltd.*, No. 96 C 7133, 1997 WL 285870 (N.D. Ill. May 23, 1997).

47. Joe Zopolsky, "HIV-infected Healthcare Workers and Practice Modification," *North Dakota Law Review* 78 (2002): 77–98 (summarizing state and federal case law for applying the ADA to HCWs infected with HIV).

48. *School Bd. of Nassau County v. Arline*, 480 U.S. 273, 287 (1987).

49. 29 C.F.R. §1630 pt. 1630, App. (2001).

50. Ryan J. Rohlfsen, "HIV-infected Surgical Personnel under the ADA: Do They Pose a Threat or Are Reasonable Accommodations Possible," *Journal of Contemporary Health Law and Policy* 16 (1999): 127–44.

51. *Scoles v. Mercy Health Corp.*, 887 F. Supp. 765 (E.D. Pa. 1994); Adam G. Forrest, "Is There a Significant Risk or High Probability of HIV Transmission from an Infected Health Care Worker to Others?: The Sixth Circuit's Answer Lies in *Mauro v. Borgess Medical Center*," *Creighton Law Review* 32 (June 1999): 1763–1803.

52. Jeffrey A. Van Detta, "Typhoid Mary Meets the ADA: A Case Study of the Direct Threat Standard under the Americans with Disabilities Act," *Harvard Journal of Law and Public Policy* 22 (Summer 1999): 853–949.

53. *Bradley v. Univ. of Texas M. D. Anderson Cancer Ctr.*, 3 F.3d 922, 924 (5th Cir. 1993).

54. *Onishea v. Hopper*, 171 F.3d 1289 (11th Cir. 1999) (en banc), *cert. denied sub. nom*, *Davis v. Hopper*, 528 U.S. 1114 (2000).

55. Robert S. Rhodes, Gordon L. Telford, Walter J. Hierholzer Jr., and Mark Barnes, "Bloodborne Pathogen Transmission from Health-care Workers to Patients: Legal Issues and Provider Prospective," *Surgical Clinics of North America* 75 (December 1995): 1205–17.

56. *Estate of Mauro v. Borgess Med. Ctr.*, 137 F.3d 398, 404 (6th Cir. 1998); *Doe v. Univ. of Maryland Med. Sys. Corp.*, 50 F.3d 1261, 1266 (4th Cir. 1995). *But see Tolman v. Doe*, 988 F. Supp. 582 (E.D. Va. 1997) (determining that an HIV-infected cardiologist followed the CDC's guidelines; thus the cardiologist had a valid defamation claim against his partner in practice who implied to patients that the cardiologist was unfit for practice).

57. *Estate of Mauro*, 137 F.3d 398.

58. *Parks v. Female Health Care Assoc.*, 1997 WL 285870 (N.D. Ill., 1997).

59. For the few exceptions, see *Doe by Lavery v. Attorney General*, 44 F.3d 715, *opinion superseded by* 62 F.3d 1424 (9th Cir. 1995), *judgment vacated by* 518 U.S. 101, and *Doe v. Westchester County Med. Ctr. State Div. of Human Rights*, No. 91-504-2, N.Y.L.J. (December 26, 1990): 30.

60. *Doe v. Univ. of Maryland Med. Sys. Corp.*, 50 F.3d 1261, 1264.

61. *Leckelt v. Bd. of Comm'rs*, 909 F.2d 820 (5th Cir. 1990).

62. *Waddell v. Valley Forge Dental Associates, Inc.*, 276 F.3d 1275 (11th Cir. 2001).

63. *Doe v. Washington Univ.*, 780 F. Supp. 628 (E.D. Mo. 1991).

64. David W. Webber, ed., *AIDS and the Law* (New York: John Wiley and Sons, 1997, with 2000 Supp.).

65. *Estate of Mauro*, 137 F.3d 398; *Leckelt v. Bd. of Comm'rs*, 909 F.2d 820.

66. *Doe v. Univ. of Maryland Med. Sys. Corp.*, 50 F.3d 1261; *Doe v. Washington Univ.*, 780 F. Supp. 628.

67. Norman Fost, "Patient Access to Information on Clinicians Infected with Blood-borne Pathogens," *JAMA* 284 (October 18, 2000): 1975–76.

68. Jennifer Tuboku-Metzger, Linda Chiarello, Ronda L. Sinkowitz-Cochran, An-nelise Casano, and Denise Cardo, "Public Attitudes and Opinions toward Physicians and Dentists Infected with Bloodborne Viruses: Results of a National Survey," CDC, 2003.

69. Byron B. Rediger, "Living in a World with HIV: Balancing Privacy, Privilege, and the Right to Know between Patients and Health Care Professionals," *Hamline Journal of Public Law and Policy* 21 (Spring 2000): 443–87; Patti Miller Tereskerz, Richard D, Pearson, and Janine Jagger, "Infected Physicians and Invasive Procedures: National Policy and Legal Reality," *Milbank Quarterly* 77 (1999): 511–29

70. Norman Daniels, "HIV-infected Professionals, Patient Rights, and the 'Switch-ing' Dilemma," *JAMA* 267 (March 11, 1992): 1368–71; American College of Surgeons, "Statement on the Surgeon and HIV Infection" (maintaining that the CDC's policy to-ward HCWs with HIV is "intrusive in the extreme").

71. Lawrence Gostin, "CDC Guidelines on HIV or HBV-Positive Health Care Pro-fessionals Performing Exposure-prone Invasive Procedures," *Law, Medicine, and Health Care* 19 (Spring–Summer 1991): 140–43.

72. "Proceedings of the Consensus Conference on Infected Health Care Workers: Risk for Transmission of Bloodborne Pathogens," *Canada Communicable Disease Report* 24S4, supp. (July 15, 1998), ⟨http://www.hc-sc.gc.ca/hpb/lcdc/publicat/ccdr/98vol24/24s4/⟩.

73. *Estate of Behringer v. Princeton Med. Ctr.*, 592 A.2d 1251 (N.J. Super. Ct. Law Div. 1991).

74. *In re Milton S. Hershey Med. Ctr.*, 634 A.2d 159 (Pa. 1993).

75. *Faya v. Almaraz*, 620 A.2d 327 (Md. 1993).

76. *Williamson v. Waldman*, 696 A.2d 14 (N.J. 1997) (granting emotional distress dam-ages to cleaning employee who feared contracting AIDS after she was pricked by a dis-carded lancet while cleaning a medical office); *Madrid v. Lincoln County Med. Ctr.*, 923 P.2d 1154 (N.M. 1996) (granting emotional distress damages without evidence of actual exposure to worker who feared exposure to HIV when body fluid samples she was trans-porting to a lab leaked).

77. Eric S. Fisher, "Aidsphobia: A National Survey of Emotional Distress Claims for the Fear of Contracting AIDS," *Tort and Insurance Law Journal* 33 (Fall 1997): 169–226.

78. *Majca v. Beekil*, 701 N.E.2d 1084 (Ill. 1998); *K. A. C. v. Benson*, 527 N.W.2d 553 (Minn. 1995); *Brzoska v. Olsen*, 688 A.2d 1355 (Del. 1995); *Kerins v. Hartley*, 33 Cal. Rptr. 2d 172 (Cal. Ct. App. 1994).

79. *Leckelt v. Bd. of Comm'rs*, 909 F.2d 820 (5th Cir. 1990).

80. *Watson v. City of Miami Beach*, 177 F.3d 932 (11th Cir. 1999); *EEOC v. Prevo's Fam-ily Market, Inc.*, 135 F.3d 1089 (6th Cir. 1998).

81. *Doe v. High-Tech Inst.*, 972 P.2d 1060 (Colo. Ct. App. 1998).

82. Benjamin Schatz, "Supporting and Advocating for HIV-Positive Health Care Workers," *Bulletin of the New York Academy of Medicine* 72 (1995): 263–72.

83. Gay and Lesbian Medical Association to CDC, June 26, 1996.

84. American College of Surgeons, "Statement on the Surgeon and HIV Infection."

85. Julie Gerberding, "The Infected Health Care Provider," *NEJM* 334 (February 29, 1996): 594–95.

86. Julia S. Garner, "Hospital Infections Practices Advisory Committee: Guideline for Isolation Precautions in Hospitals," *Infection Control and Hospital Epidemiology* 17 (January 1996): 53–80; Susan E. Beekman et al., "Temporal Association between Implementation of Universal Precautions and a Sustained Progressive Decrease in Percutaneous Exposures to Blood," *Clinical Infectious Diseases* 18 (April 1994): 562–69.

Chapter 13

This chapter is based on Lawrence O. Gostin, *Public Health Law: Power, Duty, Restraint* (Berkeley: Milbank Memorial Fund and University of California Press, 2000).

1. Athena P. Kouris, Marc Bulterys, Steven R. Nesheim, and Francis K. Lee, "Understanding the Timing of HIV Transmission from Mother to Infant," *JAMA* 285 (February 14, 2001): 709–12. Approximately one-third of the transmission in nonbreastfeeding, untreated women occurs during gestation and the remaining two-thirds occurs during delivery.

2. Edward M. Connor, Rhoda S. Sperling, Richard Gelber, et al., "Reduction of Maternal-Infant Transmission of Human Immunodeficiency Virus Type 1 with Zidovudine Treatment," *NEJM* 331 (November 3, 1994): 1173–80; Catherine Peckham and Diana Gibb, "Mother-to-Child Transmission of the Human Immunodeficiency Virus," *NEJM* 333 (August 3, 1995): 298–302; Marc Bulterys and Mary Glenn Fowler, "HIV/AIDS in Infants, Children, and Adolescents," *Pediatric Clinics of North America* 47 (February 2000): 241–60.

3. Perinatal HIV Guidelines Working Group, *Public Health Service Task Force Recommendations for the Use of Antiretroviral Drugs in Pregnant HIV-1-Infected Women for Maternal Health and Interventions to Reduce Perinatal HIV-1 Transmission in the United States* (Rockville, Md.: HIV/AIDS Treatment Information Service, August 20, 2002): 1–50, ⟨http://www.aidsinfo.nih.gov/guidelines/perinatal/perinatal.pdf⟩.

4. Mary Lou Lindegren, Robert H. Byers, Pauline Thomas, et al., "Trends in Perinatal Transmission of HIV/AIDS in the United States," *JAMA* 282 (August 11, 1999): 531–38.

5. John P. A. Ioannidis, Elaine J. Abrams, Arthur Ammann, et al., "Perinatal Transmission of Human Immunodeficiency Virus Type 1 by Pregnant Women with RNA Virus Loads ⟨1000," *Journal of Infectious Diseases* 183 (February 15, 2001): 539–45; Laurent Mandelbrot, Aline Landreau-Mascaro, Claire Rekacewicz, et al., "Lamivudine-Zidovudine Combination for the Prevention of Maternal-Infant Transmission of HIV-1," *JAMA* 285 (April 25, 2001): 2083–93; Nathan Shaffer, "Combination Prophylaxis for Prevention of Maternal-Infant HIV Transmission: Beyond 076," *JAMA* 285 (April 25, 2001): 2129–31; M. F. Rogers and Nathan Shaffer, "Reducing the Risk of Maternal-Infant Transmission of HIV by Attacking the Virus," *NEJM* 341 (August 5, 1999): 441–42; Lynne M. Mofenson, John S. Lambert, Richard E. Stiehm, et al., "Risk Factors for Perinatal Transmission of Human Immunodeficiency Virus Type 1 in Women Treated with Zidovudine," *NEJM* 341 (August 5, 1999): 385–93.

6. CDC, *HIV Strategic Plan through 2005* (Atlanta: CDC, 2001); Mary Glenn Fowler, R. J. Simonds, and Anuvat Roongpisuthipong, "Update on Perinatal HIV Transmission," *Pediatric Clinics of North America* 47 (February 2000): 21–38.

7. CDC, *Status of Perinatal HIV Prevention: U.S. Declines Continue* (Atlanta: CDC, 2002), ⟨http://www.cdc.gov/hiv/pubs/facts/perinatl.htm⟩.

8. Zita Lazzarini and Lorilyn Rosales, "Legal Issues concerning Public Health Efforts to Reduce Perinatal HIV Transmission," *Yale Journal of Health Policy, Law, and Ethics*, forthcoming.

9. CDC, "Characteristics of Persons Living with AIDS," *Surveillance Supplemental Report* 7 (February 21, 2001): 1–16, ⟨http://www.cdc.gov/hiv/stats/hasrsupp71.htm⟩.

10. CDC, *HIV/AIDS among US Women: Minority and Young Women at Continuing Risk* (Atlanta: CDC, 2002), ⟨http://www.cdc.gov/hiv/pubs/facts/women.htm⟩.

11. John M. Karon, Philip S. Rosenberg, Geraldine McQuillan, et al., "Prevalence of HIV Infection in the United States, 1984 to 1992," *JAMA* 276 (July 10, 1996): 126–31.

12. CDC, "Advancing HIV Prevention: New Strategies for a Changing Epidemic— United States, 2003," *MMWR* 52 (April 18, 2003): 329-32; CDC, "HIV Testing among Pregnant Women—United States and Canada, 1998–2001," *MMWR* 51 (November 15, 2002): 1013–16.

13. Patricia Reaney, "Number of U.S. Newborns with HIV Plummets," *Toronto (Canada) Globe and Mail*, July 9, 2002.

14. CDC, "HIV Testing among Pregnant Women" (in 2000 preliminary data indicated that 766 [93 percent] of 824 HIV-infected women in 25 states knew their HIV status before delivery); CDC, "Prenatal Discussion of HIV Testing and Maternal HIV Testing—14 States, 1996–1997," *MMWR* 48 (May 21, 1999): 401–4; Rachel A. Royce, Emmanuel B. Walter, M. Isabel Fernandez, et al., "Barriers to Universal Prenatal HIV Testing in 4 US Locations in 1997," *AJPH* 91 (May 2001): 727–33; Esther Joo, Anne Carmack, Elizabeth Garcia-Bunuel, et al., "Implementation of Guidelines for HIV Counseling and Voluntary HIV Testing of Pregnant Women," *AJPH* 90 (February 2000): 273–76.

15. Royce, Walter, Fernandez, et al., "Barriers to Universal Prenatal HIV Testing."

16. Mayris P. Webber, Penelope Demas, Evelyn Enriquez, et al., "Pilot Study of Expedited HIV-1 Testing of Women in Labor at an Inner-City Hospital in New York City," *American Journal of Perinatology* 18 (2001): 49–57; Joo, Carmack, Garcia-Bunuel, et al., "Implementation of Guidelines for HIV Counseling and Voluntary HIV Testing."

17. USPHS, "Recommendations of the U.S. Public Health Service Task Force on the Use of Zidovudine to Reduce Perinatal Transmission of Human Immunodeficiency Virus," *MMWR* 43 (August 5, 1994): 1–20, USPHS, "Public Health Service Task Force's Recommendations for the Use of Antiviral Drugs in Pregnant Women Infected with HIV-1 for Maternal Health and for Reducing Perinatal HIV-1 Transmission in the United States," *MMWR* 47 (January 30, 1998): 1–30 (updating the 1994 guidelines), and CDC, *Guidelines for the Use of Antiretroviral Agents in Pediatric HIV Infection* (Atlanta: CDC, 2001):1–68, ⟨http://www.aidsinfo.nih.gov/guidelines/pediatric/pediatric/pdf⟩. In 2003 the CDC issued updated guidelines for HIV testing, including screening pregnant women.

18. USPHS, "United States Public Health Service Recommendations for Human Immunodeficiency Virus Counseling and Voluntary Testing for Pregnant Women," *MMWR* 44 (July 1, 1995): 1–15.

19. Lynne M. Mofenson, "U.S. Public Health Service Task Force Recommendations for Use of Antiretroviral Drugs in Pregnant HIV-1 Infected Women for Maternal Health and Interventions to Reduce Perinatal HIV-1 Transmission in the United States," *MMWR* 51 (November 22, 2002): 1–38.

20. CARE Amendments of 1996, P.L. 104–146, 42 U.S.C. 300ff-34 (1994).

21. Secretary of Health Determines Required Newborn HIV Testing Not Routine Practice, 65 Fed. Reg. 3367–3374 (Washington, D.C.: HHS, January 20, 2000).

22. Ibid.

23. Amanda Watson, *Reducing Perinatal Transmission* (Washington, D.C.: Health Policy Tracking Service, 2000), ⟨http://stateserv.hpts.org⟩.

24. Mayris P. Webber, Penelope Demas, Evelyn Enriquez, et al., "Pilot Study of Expedited HIV-1 Testing of Women in Labor at an Inner-City Hospital in New York City," *American Journal of Perinatology* 18 (2001): 49–57.

25. Miriam Davis, "Workshop I Summary," in *Reducing the Odds: Preventing Perinatal Transmission of HIV in the United States*, edited by Michael A. Stoto, Donna A. Almario, and Marie C. McCormick (Washington, D.C.: National Academy Press, 1999), 190–202.

26. Evan R. Myers, Joseph W. Thompson, and Kit Simpson, "Cost-Effectiveness of Mandatory Compared with Voluntary Screening for Human Immunodeficiency Virus in Pregnancy," *Obstetrics and Gynecology* 91 (February 1998): 174–81; William A. Grobman and Patricia M. Garcia, "The Cost-Effectiveness of Voluntary Intrapartum Rapid Human Immunodeficiency Virus Testing for Women without Adequate Prenatal Care," *American Journal of Obstetrics and Gynecology* 181, pt. 1 (November 1999): 1062–71; Maarten J. Postma, Eduard J. Beck, S. Mandalia, et al., "Universal HIV Screening of Pregnant Women in England: Cost-Effectiveness Analysis," *British Medical Journal* 318 (June 19, 1999): 1656–59; Manuel E. Rivera-Alsina, Christine C. Rivera, Nanette Rollene, et al., "Voluntary Screening Program for HIV in Pregnancy: Cost-Effectiveness," *Journal of Reproductive Medicine* 46 (March 2001): 243–48.

27. Gina V. Hanna and Harold E. Fox, "HIV in Pregnancy—More Patients, Choices," *OBG Management* (July 2001): 58–75; Lynne Mofenson and James McIntyre, "Advances and Research Directions in the Prevention of Mother-to-Child HIV-1 Transmission," *Lancet* 355 (June 24, 2000): 2237–44; Alex H. Krist, "Obstetric Care in Patients with HIV Disease," *American Family Physician* 63 (January 2001): 107–16.

28. American Academy of Pediatrics and the American College of Obstetricians and Gynecologists, "Joint Statement of the American Academy of Pediatrics and the American College of Obstetricians and Gynecologists on Human Immunodeficiency Virus Screening," *Pediatrics* 104 (July 1999): 128.

29. Mofenson, "U.S. Public Health Service Task Force Recommendations for Use of Antiretroviral Drugs in Pregnant HIV-1 Infected Women.

30. CDC, "Prenatal Discussion of HIV Testing and Maternal HIV Testing"; National Alliance of State and Territorial AIDS Directors, *An Overview of Recent State Policies, Programs, Data Collection, and Evaluation Activities Related to Reducing Perinatal HIV*

Transmission: 1998 Summary Report (Washington, D.C.: NASTAD Issue Brief, July 1998), ‹http://www.stateserv.hpts.org›, (listing laws passed by individual states).

31. CDC, "Revised Guidelines for HIV Counseling, Testing, and Referral and Revised Recommendations for HIV Screening of Pregnant Women," *MMWR* 50 (November 9, 2001): 59–86.

32. Ibid.

33. CDC, "Advancing HIV Prevention: New Strategies for a Changing Epidemic—United States, 2003," *MMWR* 52 (April 18, 2003): 329–32.

34. Martha A. Field, "Testing for AIDS: Uses and Abuses," *American Journal of Law and Medicine* 16 (1990): 34–35.

35. CDC, "Update—HIV Counseling and Testing Using Rapid Tests," *MMWR* 47 (March 27, 1998): 211–15.

36. CDC, "HIV Testing among Pregnant Women."

37. Watson, *Reducing Perinatal Transmission*.

38. Zita Lazzarini and Lorilyn Rosales, "Legal Issues concerning Public Health Efforts to Reduce Perinatal HIV Transmission," *Yale Journal of Health Policy, Law, and Ethics*, forthcoming; Watson, *Reducing Perinatal Transmission*. Arkansas, California, Connecticut, Delaware, Florida, Indiana, Iowa, Maryland, Michigan, New Jersey, Tennessee, Texas, Virginia, and Washington State have enacted laws regarding HIV counseling of pregnant women. Counseling is required in California, Connecticut, Delaware, Indiana, Iowa, Maryland, New Jersey, Virginia, and Washington State.

39. Watson, *Reducing Perinatal Transmission*. Arkansas, Connecticut, Michigan, New York, Tennessee, and Texas have opt-out procedures.

40. Md. HEALTH-GENERAL Code Ann. § 18–338.2 (2000).

41. Nathan Schaffer, "Combination Prophylaxis for Prevention of Maternal Infant HIV Transmission: Beyond 076," *JAMA* 285 (April 25, 2001): 2129–31.

42. Howard Minkoff, "Prevention of Mother-to-Child Transmission of HIV," *Clinical Obstetrics and Gynecology* 44 (June 2001): 210–25.

43. Nancy E. Kass, Holly A. Taylor, and Jean Anderson, "Treatment of Human Immunodeficiency Virus during Pregnancy: The Shift from an Exclusive Focus on Fetal Protection to a More Balanced Approach," *American Journal of Obstetrics and Gynecology* 182 (April 2000): 856–59; Mardge H. Cohen, "Women and HIV: Creating an Ambiance of Caring," *Journal of the American Medical Women's Association* 56 (Winter 2001): 9–10.

44. Karen H. Rothenberg and Stephen J. Paskey, "The Risk of Domestic Violence and Women with HIV Infection: Implications for Partner Notification, Public Policy, and the Law," *AJPH* 85 (November 1995): 1569–76; Sally Zierler, William E. Cunningham, R. Anderson, et al., "Violence Victimization after HIV Infection in a U.S. Probability Sample of Adult Patients in Primary Care," *AJPH* 90 (February 2000): 208–15.

45. Ronald Bayer, "Rethinking the Testing of Babies and Pregnant Women for HIV Infection," *Journal of Clinical Ethics* 7 (Spring 1996): 85–86.

Chapter 14

This chapter is based on the results of the syringe law project, supported by the Centers for Disease Control and Prevention, the Association of State and Territorial Health

Officials, the Association of Schools of Public Health, and the Henry J. Kaiser Family Foundation. The legal issues presented were developed from a consultation in May 1996 at the Carter Presidential Center under the auspices of the CDC and leading medical, public health, substance abuse, and criminal justice organizations. The data and analysis have been updated as of December 2002.

The chapter draws on Lawrence O. Gostin, "The Legal Environment Impeding Access to Sterile Syringes and Needles: The Conflict between Law Enforcement and Public Health," *JAIDS* 18, supp. 1 (July 1998): S60–S70; Gostin and Zita Lazzarini, "Prevention of HIV/AIDS among Injection Drug Users: The Theory and Science of Public Health and Criminal Justice Approaches to Disease Prevention," *Emory Law Journal* 46 (Spring 1997): 587–696; Gostin, Lazzarini, T. Stephen Jones, and Kathleen Flaherty, "Prevention of HIV/AIDS and Other Blood-borne Diseases among Injecting Drug Users: A National Survey on the Regulation of Syringes and Needles," *JAMA* 277 (January 1, 1997): 53–62; Gostin, "The Needle-borne HIV Epidemic: Causes and Public Health Responses," *Behavioral Sciences and the Law* 9 (1991): 287–304; Gostin, "The Inter-connected Epidemics of Drug Dependency and AIDS," *Harvard Civil Rights–Civil Liberties Law Review* 26 (Winter 1991): 113–84; and Gostin, "An Alternative Public Health Vision for a National Drug Strategy: 'Treatment Works,'" *Houston Law Review* 28 (January 1991): 285–308.

1. For the purpose of this chapter, the word "syringe" includes both syringes and needles, as well as other drug-injection equipment capable of transmitting blood-borne infection, such as "cookers" used to heat and prepare the drug for injection.

2. Scottish physician Alexander Wood introduced the hypodermic syringe in 1853. Norman Howard-Jones, "The Origins of Hypodermic Medication," *Scientific American* 224 (January 1971): 96–102.

3. Heather Sidwell and Amanda Watson, updated by Julie Scales, *Needle Exchange and Access to Sterile Syringes* (Washington, D.C.: Health Policy Tracking Service, April 2001), ⟨http://stateserv.hpts.org⟩.

4. Dean R. Gerstein and Henrick J. Harwood, eds., *Treating Drug Problems* (Washington, D.C.: National Academy Press, 1990–92), 58–104.

5. Alex Wodak, "Harm Reduction: Australia as a Case Study," *Bulletin of the New York Academy of Medicine* 72 (Winter 1995): 339–47; John Strang, "Harm Reduction for Drug Users: Exploring the Dimensions of Harm, Their Measurement, and Strategies for Reductions," *APPJ* 7 (January 1, 1992): 145–52; Scott Burris, Peter Lurie, and Mitzi Ng, "Harm Reduction in the Health Care System: The Legality of Prescribing and Dispensing Syringes to Drug Users," *Health Matrix* 11 (Winter 2001): 5–64.

6. Charles E. Cherubin and Joseph D. Sapira, "The Medical Complications of Drug Addiction and the Medical Assessment of the IV Drug Users: Twenty-Five Years Later," *Annals of Internal Medicine* 119 (November 15, 1993): 1017–28.

7. Jonathan A. Cohn, "HIV-1 Infection in Injection Drug Users," *Infectious Disease Clinics of North America* 16 (September 2002): 745–70.

8. CDC, *H/ASR* 13 (Atlanta: CDC, December 2001): 14 (table 5), ⟨http://www.cdc.gov/hiv/stats/hasr1302.pdf⟩.

9. Jacques Normand, David Vlahov, and Lincoln E. Moses, eds., *Preventing HIV*

Transmission: The Role of Sterile Needles and Bleach (Washington, D.C.: National Academy Press, 1995).

10. Robert A. Hahn, Ida M. Onorato, T. Stephen Jones, and John Dougherty, "Prevalence of HIV Infection among Intravenous Drug Users in the United States," *JAMA* 261 (May 12, 1989): 2677–84; Rebecca D. Prevots, David M. Allen, J. Stan Lehman, Timothy A. Green, Lyle R. Peterson, and Marta Gwinn, "Trends in HIV Seroprevalence among Injection Drug Users Entering Drug Treatment Centers, United States, 1988–1993," *American Journal of Epidemiology* 143 (April 1, 1996): 733–42.

11. Donald C. Des Jarlais et al., "HIV-1 Infection among Intravenous Drug Users in Manhattan, from 1977 through 1987," *JAMA* 261 (February 17, 1989): 1008–12.

12. CDC, *H/ASR* 13 (Atlanta: CDC, December 2001): 18–20 (tables 9–11), ⟨http://www.cdc.gov/hiv/stats/hasr1302.pdf⟩.

13. Dawn Day, *Health Emergency 2003: The Spread of Drug-Related AIDS and Hepatitis C among African Americans and Latinos* (Princeton, N.J.: Dogwood Center, 2003).

14. Harvey W. Feldman and Patrick Biernacki, "The Ethnography of Needle Sharing among Intravenous Drug Users and Implications for Public Policies and Intervention Strategies," in *National Institute on Drug Abuse: Needle Sharing among Intravenous Drug Abusers: National and International Perspectives, NIDA Monograph No. 80*, edited by Robert J. Battjes and Roy W. Pickens (Rockville, Md.: National Institute on Drug Abuse, 1988), 28–39; Phillippe Bourgois, "The Moral Economics of Homeless Heroin Addicts: Confronting Ethnography, HIV Risk, and Everyday Violence in San Francisco Shooting Encampments," *Substance Abuse and Misuse* 33 (September 1998): 2323–51.

15. CDC, *H/ASR* 13 (Atlanta: CDC, December 2001): 14 (table 5); Henry J. Kaiser Family Foundation, *Key Facts: Women and HIV/AIDS* (Menlo Park, Calif.: Kaiser Family Foundation, May 2001).

16. CDC, *H/ASR*, 24 (table 15).

17. ABA, "American Bar Association Report and Resolution on Needle Exchange Programs," August 1997.

18. Denise Paone, Stephanie Caloir, Quihu Shi, and Don C. Des Jarlais, "Sex, Drugs, and Syringe Exchange in New York City: Women's Experiences," *Journal of American Women's Association* 50 (May–August 1995): 109–14.

19. Normand, Vlahov, and Moses, *Preventing HIV Transmission*.

20. CDC, *H/ASR*, 14 (table 5).

21. T. Stephen Jones and David Vlahov, "Use of Sterile Syringes and Aseptic Drug Preparation Are Important Components of HIV Prevention among Injection Drug Users," *JAIDS* 18, supp. 1 (July 1998): S1–S5; Don C. Des Jarlais, Holly Hagan, Samuel R. Friedman, et al., "Maintaining Low HIV Seroprevalence in Populations of Injecting Drug Users," *JAMA* 274 (October 18, 1995): 1226–31; Don C. Des Jarlais et al., "HIV Incidence among Injecting Drug Users in New York City Syringe-Exchange Programmes," 348 *Lancet* (October 12, 1996): 987–91; W. Wayne Weibel et al., "Risk Behavior and HIV Seroincidence among Out-of-Treatment Injection Drug Users: A Four Year Prospective Study," *JAIDS* 12 (July 1996): 282–89.

22. John K. Watters et al., "Syringe and Needle Exchange as HIV/AIDS Prevention for Injection Drug Users," *JAMA* 271 (January 12, 1994): 115–20, and Edward H. Kaplan and Robert Heimer, "HIV Prevalence among Intravenous Drug Users:

Model-Based Estimates from New Haven's Legal Needle Exchange," *JAIDS* 5 (1992): 163–69.

23. Christina Hartgers et al., "The Impact of the Needle and Syringe-Exchange Programme in Amsterdam in Injecting Risk Behavior," *AIDS* 3 (September 1989): 571–76, and Bengt Ljunberg et al., "HIV Prevention among Injecting Drug Users: Three Years' Experience from a Syringe Exchange Program in Sweden," *JAIDS* 4 (1991): 890–95.

24. Alex Wodak, "A Report of the National Advisory Committee on Acquired Immunodeficiency Syndrome's Workshop on Human Immunodeficiency Virus Infection and Intravenous Drug Abuse," *Medical Journal of Australia* 149 (October 3, 1988): 373–76.

25. New York City Department of Health, *The Pilot Needle Exchange Study in New York City—A Bridge to Treatment: A Report on the First Ten Months' Operation* (New York: New York City Department of Health, December 1989).

26. Peter Lurie, Arthur L. Reingold, et al., *The Public Health Impact of Needle Exchange Programs in the United States and Abroad: Summary, Conclusions, and Recommendations* (Atlanta: CDC, 1993).

27. Donna E. Shalala, *Report to the Committee on Appropriations for the Departments of Labor, Health and Human Services, and Education and Related Agencies: Needle Exchange Programs in America: Review of Published Studies and Ongoing Research* (Washington, D.C.: HHS, February 18, 1997); NIH, *NIH Consensus Development Statement: Interventions to Prevent HIV Risk Behaviors* (Bethesda, Md.: NIH, February 11–13, 1997), ⟨http://consensus.nih.gov/cons/104/104_statement.htm⟩.

28. Joseph Guydish et al., "Evaluating Needle Exchange: Are There Negative Effects?," *AIDS* 7 (June 1993): 871–76.

29. Don C. Des Jarlais and Samuel R. Friedman, "The Psychology of Preventing AIDS among Intravenous Drug Users," *American Psychologist* 43 (November 1988): 865–69.

30. Stephen K. Koester, "Copping, Running, and Paraphernalia Laws: Contextual Variables and Needle Risk Behavior among Injection Drug Users in Denver," *Human Organization* 53 (Fall 1994): 287–95; Josiah D. Rich et al., "High Street Prices of Syringes Correlate with Strict Syringe Possession Laws," *American Journal of Drug and Alcohol Abuse* 26 (August 2000): 481–87.

31. Scott Burris, Joseph Welsh, Mitzi Ng, Mei Li, and Alyssa Ditzler, "State Syringe and Drug Possession Laws Potentially Influencing Safe Syringe Disposal by Injection Drug Users," *JAPA* 42 (November–December 2002): S94–S98.

32. *Doe v. Bridgeport Police Department*, 198 F.R.D. 325 (D. Conn. 2001).

33. *Roe v. City of New York*, 2002 U.S. Dist. LEXIS 22307 at 2 (S.D.N.Y. Nov. 19, 2002).

34. Ibid.; *L. B. v. Town of Chester*, 2002 U.S. Dist. LEXIS 22305 (S.D.N.Y. Nov. 19, 2002).

35. Patricia Case, Theresa Meehan, and T. Stephen Jones, "Arrests and Incarceration of Injection Drug Users for Syringe Possession in Massachusetts: Implications for HIV Prevention," *JAIDS* 18, supp. 1 (July 1998): S71–S75.

36. Gregory R. Veal, "The Model Drug Paraphernalia Act: Can We Outlaw Head Shops—and Should We?," *Georgia Law Review* 16 (1981): 137–69.

37. U.S. House of Representatives, *Drug Paraphernalia: Hearing before the House Select Committee on Narcotics Abuse and Control*, 96th Cong., 1st sess., 1979 (Washington, D.C.: GPO, 1979), 6 (Statement of Sue Rusche).

38. D.C. Code 1967 § 22–3601 (prohibiting the possession of "any instrument, tool, or other implement . . . that is usually employed or may be employed in the commission of a crime").

39. *Geiger v. City of Eagan*, 618 F.2d 26 (8th Cir. 1980).

40. *Village of Hoffman Estates v. Flipside, Hoffman Estates, Inc.*, 455 U.S. 489, *reh'g denied*, 456 U.S. 950 (1982).

41. Neb. Rev. Stat. § 28–441 (Reissue 1995).

42. Neb. Rev. Stat. § 28–439 (Reissue 1995).

43. *Commonwealth v. Lacey*, 344 Pa. Super. 576, 496 A.2d 1256 (1985).

44. Scott Burris, Steffanie A. Strathdee, and Jon S. Vernick, *Syringe Access Law in the United States: A State of the Art Assessment of Law and Policy* (Washington, D.C., and Baltimore: Center for Law and the Public's Health at Georgetown University Law Center and Johns Hopkins University, 2002), ⟨http://www.publichealthlaw.net/Research/PDF/syringe.pdf⟩; Burris, Vernick, Alyssa Ditzler, and Strathdee, "The Legality of Selling or Giving Syringes to Injection Drug Users," *JAPA* 42 (November–December 2002): S13–S18.

45. Ind. Code § 35-48-4-8.5 (2000).

46. 21 U.S.C.A. § 857 (1986), Historical and Statutory Notes.

47. 21 U.S.C. § 857 (1986), reenacted as 21 U.S.C. § 863 (1990).

48. Although the absence of the public health voice in paraphernalia control efforts has not been explained, a thorough discussion of the AIDS epidemic and early syringe exchange efforts in New York City sheds some insight. See Warwick Anderson, "The New York Needle Trial: The Politics of Public Health in the Age of AIDS," *AJPH* 81 (November 1991): 1506–17.

49. *United States v. Murphy*, 977 F.2d 503 (10th Cir. 1992); *United States v. 57,261 Items of Drug Paraphernalia*, 869 F.2d 955 (6th Cir.), *cert. denied*, 493 U.S. 933 (1989).

50. 21 U.S.C. § 857 (1986), reenacted as 21 U.S.C. § 863 (1990).

51. *Posters 'N' Things, Ltd. v. United States*, 511 U.S. 513 (1994).

52. Daniel Abrahamson, "Federal Law and Syringe Prescription and Dispensing," *Health Matrix* 11 (Winter 2001): 65–71.

53. 21 U.S.C. § 863(e)(5), (7) (1994).

54. Chris Pascal, "Intravenous Drug Abuse and AIDS Transmission: Federal and State Laws Regulating Needle Availability," in *National Institute on Drug Abuse, Needle Sharing among Intravenous Drug Abusers: National and International Perspectives, NIDA Monograph No. 80*, edited by Robert J. Battjes and Roy W. Pickens (Rockville, Md.: National Institute on Drug Abuse, 1988), 119–35.

55. David F. Musto, *The American Disease: Origins of Narcotic Control* (New York: Oxford University Press, 1987), 1–2.

56. Ibid., 5: "By 1900, America had developed a comparatively large addict population, perhaps 250,000, along with a fear of addiction and addicting drugs."

57. Musto, *The American Disease*, 5.

58. 1914 N.Y. Laws ch. 363.

59. Association of the Bar of the City of New York, Committee on Medicine and Law, "Legalization of Non-Prescription Sale of Hypodermic Needles: A Response to the AIDS Crisis," *Record of the Association of the Bar of the City of New York* 41 (November 1986): 809, 811.

60. M. Daniel Fernando, *AIDS and Intravenous Drug Use: The Influence of Morality, Politics, Social Science, and Race in the Making of a Tragedy* (Westport, Conn.: Praeger Publishers, 1993), 44, 55.

61. Samuel R. Friedman, Theresa Perlis, and Don C. Des Jarlais, "Laws Prohibiting Over-the-Counter Syringe Sales to Injection Drug Users: Relations to Population Density, HIV Prevalence, and HIV Incidence," *AJPH* 91 (May 2001): 791–93.

62. Sidwell and Watson, updated by Scales, *Needle Exchange and Access to Sterile Syringes.*

63. *People v. Bellfield,* 230 N.Y.S.2d 79, 80 (1961), *Dayton v. State,* 250 A.2d 503, 506 (Del. 1969); *People v. Salerno,* 185 N.Y.S.2d 169, 173 (1959).

64. *People v. Saul,* 176 N.Y.S.2d 405–7 (1958); *People v. Strong,* 365 N.Y.S.2d 310, 311 (App. Div. 1975).

65. *Minnesota ex rel. Whipple v. Martinson,* 256 U.S. 41 (1921).

66. *Commonwealth v. Jefferson,* 387 N.E.2d 579, 581 (Mass. 1979).

67. *People v. Goldberg,* 369 N.Y.S.2d 989, 991 (1975): "It is clear that a doctor who issues a prescription or dispenses controlled substances for non-medical purposes is not acting 'in the course of his professional practice only.'"

68. Canadian HIV/AIDS Legal Network, *The Provision of HIV Related Services to People Who Inject Drugs: A Discussion of Ethical Issues* (Canada: Canadian HIV/AIDS Legal Network, 2002).

69. Zita Lazzarini, "An Analysis of Ethical Issues in Prescribing and Dispensing Syringes to Injection Drug Users," *Health Matrix* 11 (Winter 2001): 85–128; Josiah D. Rich et al., "Prescribing Syringes to Prevent HIV: A Survey of Infectious Disease and Addiction Medicine Physicians in Rhode Island," *Substance Use and Misuse* 36 (April 2001): 535–50; Scott Burris, Peter Lurie, Daniel Abrahamson, and Josiah D. Rich, "Physician Prescribing of Sterile Injection Equipment to Prevent HIV Infection: Time for Action," *Annals of Internal Medicine* 133 (August 1, 2000): 218–26.

70. Maxwell J. Mehlman, "Liability for Prescribing Intravenous Injection Equipment to IV Drug Users," *Health Matrix* 11 (Winter 2001): 73–84.

71. Phillip Coffin, "Syringe Availability as HIV Prevention: A Review of Modalities," *Journal of Urban Health* 77 (September 2000): 306–30.

72. Benjamin Junge et al., "Pharmacy Access to Sterile Syringes for Injection Drug Users: Attitudes of Participants in a Syringe Exchange Program," *JAPA* 39 (January–February 1999): 17–22.

73. Phillip O. Coffin et al., "More Pharmacists in High-Risk Neighborhoods of New York City Support Selling Syringes to Injection Drug Users," *JAPA* 42 (November–December 2002): S62–S67; Don C. Des Jarlais, Courtney McKnight, and Patricia Friedmann, "Legal Syringe Purchases by Injection Drug Users, Brooklyn and Queens, New York City, 2000–2001," *JAPA* 42 (November–December 2002): S73–S76.

74. Alice A. Gleghorn, Gilbert Gee, and David Vlahov, "Pharmacists' Attitudes about Pharmacy Sale of Needles/Syringes and Needle Exchange Programs in a City without Needle/Syringe Prescription Laws," *JAIDS* 18, supp. 1 (July 1998): S89–S93.

75. R. Ettelson, "Sell Needles and Syringes to IV Drug Abusers?," *Pharmacy Times* 57 (1991): 107–14.

76. Wilson M. Compton et al., "Legal Needle Buying in St. Louis," *AJPH* 82 (April 1992): 595–96; J. P. Croatto et al., "The Role of the Pharmacist in Preventing a 'Second Wave' of the HIV Epidemic among IV Drug Users," *Australian Journal of Pharmacy* 68 (1987): 602–4; Alan Glantz, Clare Byrne, and Paul Jackson, "Role of Community Pharmacies in Prevention of AIDS among Injecting Drug Misusers: Findings of a Survey in England and Wales," *British Medical Journal* 299 (October 28, 1989): 1076–79.

77. William A. Zellmer, "Pharmacist Involvement in Needle Exchange Programs," *American Pharmacy* NS34 (September 1994): 48–51.

78. Jeff Stryker, "IV Drug Use and AIDS: Public Policies and Dirty Needles," *Journal of Health Policy, Politics, and Law* 14 (1989): 719–40.

79. Stephen K. Koester, "Copping, Running, and Paraphernalia Laws: Contextual Variables and Needle Risk Behavior among Injection Drug Users in Denver," *Human Organization* 53 (1994): 287–95.

80. Mytri P. Singh et al., "Update: Syringe Exchange Programs—United States, 1998," *MMWR* 50 (May 18, 2001): 384–88.

81. Denise Paone et al., "Syringe Exchange Programs—United States, 1994–1995," *MMWR* 44 (October 25, 1995): 684–85, 691 (55 percent of SEPs were "legal" because they operated in a state with no syringe prescription law or under an exemption to the law; 32 percent were "illegal-but-tolerated" because the program operated in a state with a prescription law but had received a formal vote of support from a local elected body; and 13 percent were "illegal/underground" because the program operated in a state with a prescription law and had no formal support); Scott Burris, Davis Finucane, Heather Gallagher, and Joseph Grace, "The Legal Strategies Used in Operating Syringe Exchange Programs in the United States," *AJPH* 86 (August 1996): 1161–66 (25 percent of SEPs operated under claims of lawfulness, 52 percent had received formal authorization, and 17 percent operated without a legal foundation and were subject to prosecution).

82. Burris, Strathdee, and Vernick, *Syringe Access Law*.

83. N.Y. Public Health Law § 3381; N.Y. Comp. Codes R. & Regs., Title 10, § 80.135.

84. *Spokane County Health District v. Brockett*, 839 P.2d 324 (Wash. 1992).

85. As of September 2001, the Board of Health of Allegheny County, Pa., encompassing Pittsburgh, had voted to authorize a legal SEP but had not implemented the decision.

86. Burris, Strathdee, and Vernick, *Syringe Access Law*.

87. Title V, Section 505 of the Consolidated Appropriations—FY 2001, P.L. 106–554, § 505, 114 Stat. 2763 (Dec. 21, 2000).

88. U.S. General Accounting Office, *Needle Exchange Programs: Research Suggests Promise as an AIDS Prevention Strategy* (Washington, D.C.: GPO, 1993).

89. Normand, Vlahov, and Moses, *Preventing HIV Transmission*.

90. NIH, *NIH Consensus Development Statement*.

91. Shalala, *Report to the Committee on Appropriations . . . : Needle Exchange Programs*; Presidential Advisory Council on HIV/AIDS, *Presidential Advisory Council on HIV/AIDS*

Resolution on Needle Exchange Programs (Washington, D.C.; Presidential Advisory Council on HIV/AIDS, March 17, 1998).

92. *Allen v. City of Tacoma*, No. 89-2-09067-3 (Wash. Super. Ct., Pierce County, May 9, 1990).

93. Washington Rev. Code, par. 70.24.400 (Supp. 1990).

94. *Spokane County Health District v. Brockett*, 839 P.2d 324.

95. J. Keller, "Needle Exchange: HIV Prevention Takes on the Law," *Exchange* 17 (1992): 1–7.

96. National Center for HIV, STD, and TB Prevention, *HIV Prevention Bulletin: Medical Advice for Persons Who Inject Illicit Drugs* (Atlanta: CDC, May 9, 1997), ‹http://www.cdc.gov/idu/pubs/hiv_prev.htm›.

97. American Medical Association, House of Delegates Resolution 231 (I-94), Policy H-95.958 Syringe and Needle Exchange Programs; Normand, Vlahov, and Moses, *Preventing HIV Transmission*.

98. Scott Burris, ed., *Deregulation of Hypodermic Needles and Syringes as a Public Health Measure: A Report on Emerging Policy and Law in the United States* (Washington, D.C.: AIDS Coordinating Committee of the ABA, 2000).

99. Donald C. Des Jarlais et al., "Continuity and Change within an HIV Epidemic: Injecting Drug Users in New York City, 1984 through 1992," *JAMA* 271 (January 12, 1994): 121–27; John K. Watters, Michelle J. Estilo, George L. Clark, and Jennifer Lorvick, "Syringe and Needle-Exchange as HIV/AIDS Prevention for Injection Drug Users," *JAMA* 271 (January 12, 1994): 115–20.

100. Jennifer A. Taussig, Beth Weinstein, Scott Burris, and T. Stephen Jones, "Syringe Laws and Pharmacy Regulations Are Structural Constraints on HIV Prevention in the United States," *AIDS* 14, supp. 1 (2000): S47–S51; Samuel L. Groseclose et al., "Impact of Increased Access to Needles and Syringes on Practices of Injecting-Drug Users and Police Officers—Connecticut, 1992–1993," *JAIDS* 10 (September 1, 1995): 82–89.

101. Normand, Vlahov, and Moses, *Preventing HIV Transmission*.

102. David R. Holtgrave et al., "Cost and Cost-Effectiveness of Increasing Access to Sterile Syringes and Needles as an HIV Prevention Intervention in the United States," *JAIDS* 18, supp. 1 (July 1998): S133–S138.

Chapter 15

This chapter is adapted from Larry O. Gostin, Paul D. Cleary, Kenneth H. Mayer, Allan M. Brandt, and Eva H. Chittenden, "Screening Immigrants and International Travelers for the Human Immunodeficiency Virus," *NEJM* 322 (June 14, 1990): 1743–46.

1. U.S. Congress, Staff of House Committee on the Judiciary, *Grounds for Exclusion of Aliens under the Immigration and Nationality Act: Historical Background and Analysis*, 100th Cong., 2d sess., 1988 (Washington, D.C.: GPO, 1988); Carol L. Wolchok, "AIDS at the Frontier: United States Immigration Policy," *Journal of Legal Medicine* 10 (March 1989): 127–42; David F. Musto, "Quarantine and the Problem of AIDS," *Milbank Quarterly* 64,

supp. 1 (1986): 97–117; Brian D. Gushulak and Douglas W. MacPherson, "Population Mobility and Infectious Diseases: The Diminishing Impact of Classical Infectious Diseases and New Approaches for the Twenty-first Century," *Clinical Infectious Diseases* 31 (September 2000): 776–80.

2. Howard Markel and Alexandra Minna Stern, "The Foreignness of Germs: The Persistent Association of Immigrants and Disease in American Society," *Milbank Quarterly* 80 (2002): 757–88; Howard Markel, *When Germs Travel: American Stories of Imported Disease* (New York: Pantheon Books, 2003).

3. Bureau of Consular Affairs, "Human Immunodeficiency Virus (HIV) Testing Requirements for Entry into Foreign Countries" (February 2002), ⟨http://travel.state.gov/HIVtestingreqs.html⟩.

4. William J. Curran and Lawrence O. Gostin, *A World Wide Survey of AIDS Legislation* (Geneva: WHO, 1990).

5. Alana Klein, *HIV and Immigration: Final Report* (Canadian HIV/AIDS Legal Network, 2001), ⟨http://www.aidslaw.ca⟩.

6. Suzanne B. Goldberg, "Immigration Issues and Travel Restrictions," in *Encyclopedia of AIDS: A Social, Political, Cultural, and Scientific Record of the HIV Epidemic*, edited by Raymond A. Smith (Chicago: Fitzroy Dearborn, 1998).

7. "Official Wants TB, HIV Tests for All U.K. Immigrants," *AIDS Policy and Law* 18 (January 20, 2003).

8. National Commission on AIDS, *Resolution on U.S. Visa and Immigration Policy* (Washington, D.C.: National Commission on AIDS, December 1989); ABA, *Policy on AIDS* (Chicago: ABA, August 1989); Lesbian and Gay Immigration Rights Task Force, "Congress Ignores Gay and Lesbian Immigrants in Passing New Immigration Legislation," December 18, 2000, ⟨http://www.lgirtf.org/ignores.html⟩; Yves Sorokobi, "The African Services Committee Helps Immigrants Fight AIDS," June 1999, ⟨http://www.wnyc.org/new/news/arts/sorokobi061699.html⟩.

9. Resolution of the Delegates Calling on All Governments to Permit Entry to HIV-infected Travelers, June 9, 1989, Montreal, Fifth International Conference on AIDS, June 4–9, 1989; Statement by the League of Red Cross and Red Crescent Societies Regarding Participation in the Sixth International Conference on AIDS, November 21, 1989, Sixth International Conference on AIDS, San Francisco, June 20–24, 1990; Amnesty International, *Crimes of Hate, Conspiracy of Silence, Torture, and Ill-treatment Based on Sexual Identity* (ACT 40/016/2001, June 22, 2001): 49–52.

10. Immigration and Nationality Act § 212(a)(1)(A)(i) (1998).

11. Supplemental Appropriations Act of 1987, S. 518, P.L. 100–71, H.R. 1827 (July 11, 1987).

12. 51 Fed. Reg. 32, 540–44 (1987); 52 Fed. Reg. 21, 607 (effective Dec. 1, 1987).

13. National Commission on AIDS, *AIDS and Immigration: An Overview of United States Policy* (Washington, D.C.: National Commission on AIDS, 1989).

14. INS, Press Release, *In re Hans Paul Verhoef* (Washington, D.C.: INS, April 7, 1989).

15. DOS, *Cable no. 136115* (Washington, D.C.: DOS, April 27, 1990).

16. INS, *Medical Examination of Aliens Seeking Adjustment of Status, Form I-693* (Washington, D.C.: INS, September 1, 1987), ⟨http://www.ins.usdoj.gov/graphics/formsfee/forms/files/I-693.pdf⟩.

17. As a result of the Homeland Security Act of 2002, the functions of the INS were transferred to the Department of Homeland Security as of March 1, 2003. Department of Homeland Security, "Authority of the Secretary of Homeland Security: Delegations of Authority: Immigration Laws," 68 Fed. Reg. 10922-24, March 6, 2003.

18. INS, *HIV Infection: Inadmissibility and Waiver Policies* (Washington, D.C.: INS, July 10, 1998), ⟨http://www.ins.usdoj.gov/graphics/publicaffairs/factsheets/hivfs.htm (last modified Nov. 8, 2001)⟩.

19. "IJ Grants Asylum to HIV Positive Man, General Council Issues HIV Instructions," *Interpreter Release* 73 (July 8, 1996): 901–2.

20. Goldberg, "Immigration Issues and Travel Restrictions."

21. UNAIDS, Second Ad Hoc Thematic Meeting, New Delhi, December 9–11 1998, "Migration and HIV/AIDS," UNAIDS/PCB(7)/98.5, October 28, 1998.

22. Gregory K. Folkers and Anthony S. Fauci, "The AIDS Research Model: Implications for Other Infectious Diseases of Global Health Importance," *JAMA* 286 (July 25, 2001): 458–61; William H. Foege, "Global Public Health: Targeting Inequities," *JAMA* 279 (June 24, 1998): 1931–32.

23. Lawrence O. Gostin, Scott Burris, and Zita Lazzarini, "The Law and the Public's Health: A Study of Infectious Disease Law in the United States," *Columbia Law Review* 99 (January 1999): 59–128.

24. CDC, *HIV/AIDS Update* (Atlanta: CDC, December 2000), 1 ⟨www.cdc.gov/nchstp/od/news/At-a-Glance.pdf⟩.

25. BCIS, "Applications for Immigration Benefits," April 2003, ⟨http://www.immigration.gov/graphics/shared/aboutus/statistics/msrfeb03/BENEFIT.htm⟩.

26. BCIS, *Asylum* (April 2003), ⟨http://www.immigration.gov/graphics/shared/aboutus/statistics/msrfeb03/ASYLUM.htm⟩.

27. INS, *2001 Statistical Yearbook of the Immigration and Naturalization Service* (Washington, D.C.: Forthcoming), ⟨http://www.immigration.gov/graphics/aboutins/statistics/TEMP01yrbk/temp2001.pdf⟩.

28. Eleftherios Mylonakis et al., "Report of a False-Positive HIV Test Result and the Potential Use of Additional Tests in Establishing HIV Serostatus," *Archives of Internal Medicine* 160 (August 2000): 2386–88.

29. Ai Ee Ling et al., "Failure of Routine HIV-1 Tests in a Case Involving Transmission with Preseroconversion Blood Components during the Infectious Window Period," *JAMA* 284 (July 12, 2000): 210–14.

30. Beatrice Divine et al., *Revised Guidelines for HIV Counseling, Testing, and Referral—Draft* (Atlanta: CDC, October 17, 2000).

31. Robert S. Janssen et al., "The Serostatus Approach to Fighting the HIV Epidemic: Prevention Strategies for Infected Individuals," *AJPH* 91 (July 2001): 1019–24.

32. National Immigration Project of the National Lawyer's Guild ⟨http://www.nlg.org/nip⟩.

33. Diane V. Havlir et al., "Maintenance Antiretroviral Therapies in HIV-infected Subjects with Undetectable Plasma HIV RNA after Triple-Drug Therapy," *NEJM* 339 (October 29, 1998): 1261–68.

34. San Francisco AIDS Foundation, ⟨http://www.sfaf.org/policy/immigration⟩.

35. CDC, "1999 USPHS/IDSA Guidelines for the Prevention of Opportunistic In-

fections in Persons Infected with Human Immunodeficiency Virus: U.S. Public Health Service (USPHS) and Infectious Diseases Society of America (IDSA)," *MMWR* 48 (August 20, 1999): 1–59; Panel on Clinical Practices for Treatment of HIV Infection, *Guidelines for the Use of Antiretroviral Agents in HIV-infected Adults and Adolescents* (Washington, D.C.: HHS, August 13, 2001).

36. INS, *HIV Infection: Inadmissibility and Waiver Policies* (Washington, D.C.: INS, last updated November 8, 2001), ⟨http://www.ins.usdoj.gov/graphics/publicaffairs/factsheets/hivfs.htm⟩.

37. Kathleen A. Maloy et al., *Effect of the 1996 Welfare and Immigration Reform Laws on Immigrants' Ability and Willingness to Access Medicaid and Health Care Services*, Synthesis Report from Center for Health Services Research and Policy, School of Public Health and Health Services (Washington, D.C.: George Washington University Medical Center, May 2000).

38. *Haitian Centers Council v. Sale*, 823 F. Supp. 1029 (E.D.N.Y. 1993).

39. *Congressional Record*, February 17, 1993, 2865.

40. World Health Assembly, *International Health Regulations, 1969*, 3d annotated ed. (Geneva: WHO, 1983), art. 81.

41. WHO, "International Health Regulations (1969)," *Weekly Epidemiological Record* 60 (October 4, 1985): 311.

42. Immigration and Nationality Act of 1990, par. 210 (b)(6), 245 A(c)(5), 8 C.F.R 245 a, 2(t) (1990).

43. Lawrence Geiter, ed., *Ending Neglect: The Elimination of Tuberculosis in the United States* (Washington, D.C.: National Academy Press, 2000).

Chapter 16

1. Bernhard Schwartlander, Geoff Garnett, Neff Walker, and Roy Anderson, "AIDS in a New Millennium," *Science* 289 (July 7, 2000): 64–67.

2. UNAIDS and WHO, *AIDS Epidemic Update* (Geneva: UNAIDS and WHO, December 2002), ⟨http://www.unaids.org/worldaidsday/2002/press/Epiupdate.html⟩.

3. UNICEF, UNAIDS, and WHO, *Young People and HIV/AIDS: Opportunity in Crisis* (Paris: UNICEF, UNAIDS, and WHO, 2002); Todd Summers, Jennifer Kates, and Gillian Murphy, *The Tip of the Iceberg: The Global Impact of HIV/AIDS on Youth* (Menlo Park, Calif.: Henry J. Kaiser Family Foundation, 2002).

4. UNAIDS and World Bank, *HIV and Human Development: The Devastating Impact of AIDS* (Geneva: UNAIDS, 1999).

5. CDC, "The Global HIV and AIDS Epidemic, 2001," *MMWR* 50 (June 1, 2001): 434–39.

6. UNAIDS and WHO, *AIDS Epidemic Update* (December 2002).

7. Liz McGregor, "Botswana Battles against Extinction," *The Guardian*, July 8, 2002.

8. Karen A. Stanecki, *The AIDS Pandemic in the 21st Century* (Washington, D.C.: U.S. Census Bureau, 2002).

9. UNAIDS and WHO, *AIDS Epidemic Update* (Geneva: UNAIDS and WHO, December 2001), ⟨http://www.unaids.org/epidemic_update/report_dec01/index.html⟩.

10. Elisabeth Rosenthal, "Despite Law, China's H.I.V. Patients Suffer Bias," *NYT*, January 14, 2003.

11. Bernhard Schwartlander, Geoff Garnett, Neff Walker, and Roy Anderson, "AIDS in a New Millennium," *Science* 289 (July 7, 2000): 64–67; Elisabeth Rosenthal, "With Ignorance as the Fuel, AIDS Speeds across China," *NYT*, December 30, 2001.

12. Kofi A. Annan, "In Africa, AIDS Has a Woman's Face," *NYT*, December 29, 2002.

13. Patricia Reaney, "Women Make up 50 Percent of AIDS Sufferers," *Washington Post*, November 26, 2002; UNAIDS and WHO, *AIDS Epidemic Update* (December 2002).

14. Joan Stephenson, "Growing, Evolving HIV/AIDS Pandemic Is Producing Social and Economic Fallout," *JAMA* 289 (January 1, 2003): 31–33.

15. Anne Buve, Kizito Bishikwabo-Nsarhaza, and Gladys Mutangadura, "The Spread and Effect of HIV-1 Infection in Sub-Saharan Africa," *Lancet* 359 (June 8, 2002): 2011–17.

16. Thomas C. Quinn, "Global Burden of the HIV Pandemic," *Lancet* 348 (July 13, 1996): 99–106.

17. The orphan crisis has grown considerably, changing the landscape of the family, particularly in Sub-Saharan Africa. More than 13 million children under age fifteen have lost one or both parents to AIDS; by 2010, this number is expected to grow to 25 million. Governments and international agencies have remained somewhat complacent in the face of this crisis, perhaps due to the traditional African social system that has absorbed many of the most vulnerable children. UNAIDS, UNICEF, and USAID, *Children on the Brink, 2002: A Joint Report on Orphan Estimates and Program Strategies* (Washington, D.C.: UNAIDS, UNICEF, and USAID, July 2002); Geoff Foster, "Supporting Community Efforts to Assist Orphans in Africa," *NEJM* 346 (June 13, 2002): 1907–10.

18. UNAIDS, UNICEF, and USAID, *Children on the Brink, 2002*.

19. UNAIDS and World Bank, *HIV and Human Development: The Devastating Impact of AIDS* (Geneva: UNAIDS, 1999).

20. Kevin M. DeCock and Robert S. Janssen, "An Unequal Epidemic in an Unequal World," *JAMA* 288 (July 10, 2002): 236–38.

21. UNAIDS and WHO, *AIDS Epidemic Update* (December 2002).

22. Editorial, "Health Aid for Poor Countries," *NYT*, January 3, 2002.

23. Barton Gellman, "AIDS Is Declared Threat to Security," *Washington Post*, April 30, 2000; Stephenson, "Growing, Evolving HIV/AIDS Pandemic Is Producing Social and Economic Fallout."

24. Colin Powell, United Nations General Assembly Special Session on HIV/AIDS: Opening Session, New York: June 25, 2001, ⟨http://www.kaisernetwork.org/health_cast/uploaded_files/ACF427.pdf⟩.

25. UNAIDS and WHO, *AIDS Epidemic Update* (December 2002); UNAIDS and World Bank, *HIV and Human Development*.

26. WHO, "Commission on Macroeconomics and Health," Geneva, 2001.

27. World Bank, *Confronting AIDS: Public Priorities in a Global Epidemic* (New York: Oxford University Press, 1997); Martha Ainsworth, Lieve Fransen, and Mead Over,

eds., *Confronting AIDS: Evidence from the Developing World* (Brussels: European Commission, 1998).

28. DeCock and Janssen, "An Unequal Epidemic."

29. Thomas C. Quinn, "Global Burden of the HIV Pandemic," *Lancet* 348 (July 13, 1996): 99–106.

30. Carmen Perez-Casas et al., *HIV/AIDS Medicines Pricing Report: Setting Objectives—Is There a Political Will?* (Geneva: Médecins Sans Frontières, July 6, 2000), ‹http://www.accessmed-msf.org/resources/tools.shtm›.

31. World Bank, *Confronting AIDS*.

32. UNAIDS and WHO, *AIDS Epidemic Update* (December 2002).

33. World Bank, *Confronting AIDS*.

34. Paula Brewer, ed., *AIDS in India: Harvard AIDS Review* (Boston: Harvard AIDS Institute, Fall 1995).

35. Donald G. McNeil Jr., "AIDS and Death Hold No Sting for Fatalistic Men at African Bar," *NYT*, November 29, 2001; McNeil Jr., "Rare Condoms, Deadly Odds for Truck-Stop Prostitutes," *NYT*, November 29, 2001.

36. Elisabeth Rosenthal, "A Poor Ethnic Enclave in China Is Shadowed by Drugs and HIV," *NYT*, December 21, 2001; Rosenthal, "Spread of AIDS in Rural China Ignites Protests," *NYT*, December 11, 2001; Rosenthal, "AIDS Speeds across China."

37. "UNAIDS Executive Director Says AIDS Battle Must Be Fought on the Global Political Stage," *UNAIDS Press Release*, July 7, 2002, ‹http://www.unaids.org/whatsnew/press/eng/pressarc02/Barcelona_070702.html›.

38. Belinda Beresford, "Nkosi Johnson: Child Who Became the Campaigning Face of AIDS in South Africa," *The Guardian*, June 2, 2001, ‹http://www.guardian.co.uk/aids/story/0,7369,500309,00.html›.

39. Douglas Kirby, *No Easy Answers: Research Findings on Programs to Reduce Teen Pregnancy* (Washington, D.C.: National Campaign to Prevent Teen Pregnancy, 1997).

40. Scott Burris, Peter Lurie, and Mitzi Ng, "Harm Reduction in the Health Care System: The Legality of Prescribing and Dispensing Syringes to Drug Users," *Health Matrix* 11 (Winter 2001): 5–64.

41. William Jefferson Clinton, "AIDS Is Not a Death Sentence," *NYT*, December 1, 2002.

42. OHCHR and UNAIDS, *HIV/AIDS and Human Rights International Guidelines*, Third International Consultation on HIV/AIDS and Human Rights, Geneva, July 25–26, 2002, HR/PUB/2002/1 (New York: United Nations, 2002).

43. NIH, *New Model Suggests That AID Drugs May Not Abolish HIV Infection* (Bethesda, Md.: NIH, 1999), ‹http://www.nih.gov/news/pr/oct99/niaid-06a.htm›.

44. Annan, "In Africa, AIDS Has a Woman's Face."

45. Thomas C. Quinn, "Global Burden of the HIV Pandemic," *Lancet* 348 (July 13, 1996): 99–106.

46. UAC Secretariat, *Twenty Years of HIV in the World: Evolution of the Epidemic and Response in Uganda* (Kampala: UAC, June 2001), ‹http://www.aidsuganda.org/20%20years%20of%20HIV.pdf›.

47. Helen Epstein, "AIDS: The Lesson of Uganda," *New York Review of Books*, July 5, 2001.

48. UAC, National AIDS Documentation Centre, ⟨http://www.aidsuganda.org/hiv_aids.htm⟩.

49. UNAIDS, *Report on the Global HIV/AIDS Epidemic* (Geneva: UNAIDS, June 2000).

50. Stephen Morrison and Bates Gill, eds., *Averting a Full-Blown HIV/AIDS Epidemic in China* (Washington, D.C.: CSIS Press, 2003).

51. Editorial, "Thabo Mbeki and AIDS," *NYT*, November 4, 2001; "Mbeki's AIDS Experts Split over Link to HIV," *The Guardian*, April 5, 2001, ⟨http://www.guardian.co.uk/aids/story/0,7369,468704,00.html⟩.

52. Thabo Mbeki, quoted in "Mbeki: HIV Not Only Cause of AIDS," *Associated Press*, September 10, 2000, ⟨http://www.aegis.com/news/ap/2000/AP000905.html⟩. On April 24, 2002, Mbeki made his strongest statement yet that people must change their sexual behavior: "You can't be going around having hugely promiscuous sex all over the place and hope that you won't be affected." "South Africa and AIDS: Reason Prevails," *Economist* (April 27, 2002): 81.

53. *The HIV Epidemic in South Africa* (February 2001), ⟨http://www.uct.ac.za/depts/mmi/jmoodie/anco.html⟩.

54. Jimmy Volmink, Patrice Matchaba, and Merrick Zwarenstein, *Reducing Mother-to-Child Transmission of HIV Infection in South Africa* (New York: Milbank Memorial Fund, 2001).

55. Neil Soderlund, Karen Zwi, Anthony Kinghorn, and Glenda Gray, "Prevention of Vertical Transmission of HIV: Analysis of Cost-Effectiveness of Options Available in South Africa," *British Medical Journal* 318 (June 19, 1999): 1650–56.

56. "Shifting Stance, Beijing Shows Drama on AIDS," *NYT*, December 2, 2001.

57. Rachel L. Swarns, "A Bold Move on AIDS in South Africa," *NYT*, February 5, 2002.

58. *Minister of Health and Others v. Treatment Action Campaign and Others*, CCT 08/02, decided April 4, 2002, ⟨http://www.concourt.gov.za/date2002.html⟩.

59. Bernhard Schwartlander, John Stover, Neff Walker, et al., "Resource Needs for HIV/AIDS," *Science* 292 (2001): 2434–36.

60. Commission on Macroeconomics and Health, *Macroeconomics and Health: Investing in Health for Economic Development* (Geneva: WHO, 2001).

61. Editorial, "Global Fund Confronts AIDS," *NYT*, December 13, 2001.

62. Global Fund to Fight AIDS, Tuberculosis, and Malaria, ⟨http://www.globalfundatm.org/index.html⟩.

63. Sarah Boseley, "AIDS Bigger Problem Than Terrorism," *The Guardian*, December 14, 2001, ⟨http://www.guardian.co.uk/aids/story/0,7369,618493,00.html⟩.

64. Priya Alagiri, Todd Summers, and Jennifer Kates, *Global Spending on HIV/AIDS in Resource-Poor Settings* (Menlo Park, Calif.: Henry J. Kaiser Family Foundation, 2002).

65. CSIS HIV/AIDS Task Force, "The Global Fund to Fight AIDS, TB, and Malaria Progress Report," February 2003, p. 1; "Global Fund Observer Newsletter" 8, March 24, 2003, ⟨http://www.aidspan.org/AidspanGfo/archives/newsletter/issue8.htm⟩.

66. Commission on Macroeconomics and Health, *Investing in Health for Economic Development*.

67. Paul Blustein, "Bush to Announce Three-Year AIDS Spending Initiative," *Washington Post*, June 19, 2002.

68. Stanecki, *AIDS Pandemic.*

69. Paul Farmer et al., "Community-Based Treatment of Advanced HIV Disease: Introducing DOT-HAART (Directly Observed Therapy with Highly Active Antiretroviral Therapy)," *BWHO* 79 (2001): 1145–51.

70. Kenneth A. Freedberg et al., "The Cost-Effectiveness of Combination Antiretroviral Therapy for HIV Disease," *NEJM* 344 (March 15, 2001): 824–31.

71. UNAIDS/WHO Working Group on Global HIV/AIDS and STI Surveillance, *Zimbabwe: Epidemiological Fact Sheet on HIV/AIDS and Sexually Transmitted Infections* (Geneva: UNAIDS and WHO, 2000): 2–3, ⟨http://www.who.int/emc-hiv/fact_sheets/pdfs/Zimbabwe_EN.pdf⟩.

72. UNAIDS/WHO Working Group on Global HIV/AIDS and STI Surveillance, *Mozambique: Epidemiological Fact Sheet on HIV/AIDS and Sexually Transmitted Infections* (Geneva: UNAIDS and WHO, 2000): 2–3, ⟨http://www.who.int/emc-hiv/fact_sheets/pdfs/Mozambique_EN.pdf⟩.

73. UNAIDS/WHO Working Group on Global HIV/AIDS and STI Surveillance, *Germany: Epidemiological Fact Sheet on HIV/AIDS and Sexually Transmitted Infections* (Geneva: UNAIDS and WHO, 2000): 2–3, ⟨http://www.who.int/emc-hiv/fact_sheets/pdfs/Germany_EN.pdf⟩.

74. Beresford, "Nkosi Johnson."

75. UNAIDS, *Accelerating Access to HIV Care, Treatment, and Support* (Geneva: UNAIDS, October 2001).

76. Oxfam, *Patent Injustice: How World Trade Rules Threaten the Health of Poor People* (Oxford: Oxfam GB, 2001), ⟨http://www.oxfam.org.uk/cutthecost/downloads/patent.pdf⟩.

77. Bernard Peecoul, Pierre Chirac, Patrice Trouiller, and Jacques Pinel, "Access to Essential Drugs in Poor Countries: A Lost Battle?," *JAMA* 281 (January 27, 1999): 361–67.

78. UNAIDS, *Accelerating Access to HIV Care, Support, and Treatment* (Geneva: UNAIDS, 2000), ⟨http://www.unaids.org/acc_access⟩.

79. M. Gregg Bloche, "WTO Deference to National Health Policy: Toward an Interpretive Principle," 5 *Journal of International Economic Law* 821 (2002).

80. Oxfam, *Patent Injustice.*

81. Amir Attaran and Lee Gillespie-White, "Do Patents for Antiretroviral Drugs Constrain Access to AIDS Treatment in Africa?," *JAMA* 286 (October 17, 2001): 1886–92.

82. Kate H. Murashige, "Harmonization of Patent Laws," *Houston Journal of International Law* 16 (Spring 1994): 591–614.

83. Agreement on the Trade-Related Aspects of Intellectual Property Rights, April 15, 1994, WTO Agreement, Annex 1C, Legal Instruments—Results of the Uruguay Round, vol. 31; 33 I.L.M. 81 (1994); Keith E. Maskus, "Intellectual Property Challenges for Developing Countries," *University of Illinois Law Review* 2001 (2001): 457–74.

84. Christopher J. Kay, "Harmonization and Intellectual Property Human Rights in Least Developed Countries" (paper, Georgetown University Law Center, Health and Human Rights Seminar, December 21, 2001).

85. Lawrence O. Gostin and Zita Lazzarini, *Public Health and Human Rights in the*

AIDS Pandemic (New York: Oxford University Press, 1997), 197; *UDHR* (Geneva: United Nations, December 10, 1948), ⟨http://www.un.org/Overview/rights.html⟩.

86. Sarah M. Ford, "Compulsory Licensing Provisions under the TRIPS Agreement: Balancing Pills and Patents," *American University International Law Review* 15 (2000): 941–74.

87. Rosemary Sweeney, "The U.S. Push for Worldwide Patent Protection for Drugs Meets the AIDS Crisis in Thailand: A Devastating Collision," *Pacific Rim Law and Policy Journal* 9 (May 2000): 445–71.

88. Stanecki, *AIDS Pandemic*.

89. UNAIDS, UNICEF, and WHO, "Kenya: Epidemiological Fact Sheets on HIV/AIDS and Sexually Transmitted Infections," 2002, ⟨http://www.who.int/emc-hiv/fact_sheets/pdfs/Kenya_en.pdf⟩.

90. United Nations Office for the Coordination of Humanitarian Affairs, "Kenya: Poor ARV Programme Infrastructure Hampers Efforts," *IRIN Plus News*, January 8, 2003.

91. U.S. Census Bureau, *HIV/AIDS Surveillance: Trends and Patterns of HIV Infection in Selected Developing Countries, 2000*, ⟨http://www.census.gov/ipc/hiv/safrica.pdf⟩ and ⟨http://www.census.gov/ipc/hiv/zimbabwe.pdf⟩.

92. Clare Kapp, "WHO Faces Funding Squeeze as Richer Countries Make a Stand," *Lancet* 357 (May 26, 2001): 1683.

93. Boseley, "AIDS 'Bigger Threat Than Terrorism'"; Michael Specter, "India's Plague," *New Yorker*, December 17, 2001, 74–85.

94. Anece France-Presse, "Nigeria Buying Generic Drugs for an AIDS Treatment Trial," *NYT*, November 30, 2001.

95. Chris McGreal, "Defiant Nigeria to Import Cheap Copies of HIV Drugs," *The Guardian*, December 11, 2001, ⟨www.guardian.co.uk/aids/story/0,7369,616827,00.html⟩.

96. As proclaimed in the Global AIDS Manifesto, "We are united with a single purpose, to ensure that everyone with HIV and AIDS has access to fundamental rights of healthcare and access to life-sustaining medicines. AIDS has become a catastrophe that threatens the very future of this planet." *Global Manifesto, Durban South Africa* (July 9, 2000), ⟨http://www.actupny.org/reports/durban-access.html⟩.

97. "U.S. Drops Brazil AIDS Drugs Case," *BBC News*, June 25, 2001, ⟨http://news.bbc.co.uk/hi/english/business/newsid_1407000/1407472.stm⟩.

98. Joint Press Release of Médecins Sans Frontières, TAC, and Oxfam, "Drug Companies in South Africa Capitulate under Barrage of Public Pressure," April 19, 2001, ⟨http://www.lists.essential.org/popermail/pharm-policy/2001-April/000944.html⟩.

99. Michael Halewood, "Regulating Patent Holders: Local Working Requirements and Compulsory Licenses at International Law," *Osgoode Hall Law Journal* 35 (Summer 1997): 243–87.

100. Joint Press Release of Médecins Sans Frontières, TAC, and Oxfam, "Drug Companies in South Africa Capitulate."

101. UNAIDS, *UNAIDS Welcomes Outcome of South African Court Case* (Geneva: UNAIDS, April 19, 2001), ⟨http://www.unaids.org/whatsnew/press/eng/pressarc01/SAfrica_190401.htm⟩.

102. WTO, "Moore Welcomes News of Settlement in South African Drug Lawsuit," *WTO News* (Geneva: WTO, April 19, 2001), ‹http://www.wto.org/english/news_e/spmm_e/spmm58_e.htm›.

103. Editorial, "A Global Medicine Deal," *NYT*, January 5, 2003.

104. Dirk Albrecht et al., "Reappearance of HIV Multidrug-Resistance in Plasma and Circulating Lymphocytes after Reintroduction of Antiretroviral Therapy," *Journal of Clinical Virology* 24 (February 2002): 93–98.

105. Brian Conway et al., "Development of Drug Resistance in Patients Receiving Combinations of Zidovudine, Didanosine, and Nevirapine," *AIDS* 15 (July 6, 2001): 1269–74.

106. Joan Stephenson, "Cheaper HIV Drugs for Poor Nations Bring a New Challenge: Monitoring Treatment," *JAMA* 288 (July 10, 2002): 151–54; Paul J. Weidle et al., "HIV/AIDS Treatment and HIV Vaccines for Africa," *Lancet* 359 (June 29, 2002): 2261–67.

107. Paul Farmer et al., "Community-Based Treatment of Advanced HIV Disease: Introducing DOT-HAART (Directly Observed Therapy with Highly Active Antiretroviral Therapy)," *BWHO* 79 (2001): 1145–51.

108. Rajesh Gupta, Jim Y. Kim, Marcos A. Espinal, et al., "Responding to Market Failures in Tuberculosis Control," *Science* 293 (July 19, 2001): 1049–51.

109. Karen Zwi, Neil Soderlund, and Helen Schneider, "Cheaper Antiretrovirals to Treat AIDS in South Africa: They Are at Their Most Cost-Effective in Preventing Mother-to-Child Transmission," *British Medical Journal* 320 (June 10, 2000): 1551–52.

110. Carter Center, *River Blindness Program* (Atlanta: Carter Center, 2002), ‹http://www.cartercenter.org/healthprograms/showdoc.asp?programID=2&submenu=health programs›.

111. UNICEF, *Progress of Nations, 1998* (New York: UNICEF, 1998).

112. UNICEF, *Global Water Supply and Sanitation Sector Report* (New York: WHO and UNICEF, 1998).

113. WHO, *The World Health Report, 1998: Life in the Twenty-first Century: A Vision for All* (Geneva: WHO, 1998).

114. Marge Berer, "Reducing Perinatal HIV Transmission in Developing Countries through Antenatal and Delivery Care, and Breastfeeding: Supporting Infant Survival by Supporting Women's Survival," *BWHO* 77 (1999): 871–75; Chewe Luo, "Strategies for Prevention of Mother-to-Child Transmission of HIV," *Reproductive Health Matters* 8 (November 2000): 144–55.

115. Anne Winter, *AIDS in Africa* (Johannesburg: UNAIDS, November 30, 1998).

116. UNAIDS and WHO, *AIDS Epidemic Update* (December 2002).

117. Beth R. Santmyire, "Vertical Transmission of HIV from Mother-to-Child in Sub-Saharan Africa: Modes of Transmission and Methods for Prevention," *Obstetrical and Gynecological Survey* 56 (May 2001): 306–12.

118. "Working Group on Mother-to-Child Transmission of HIV: Rates of Mother-to-Child Transmission of HIV 1 in Africa, America, and Europe: Results from 13 Perinatal Studies," *JAIDS* 8 (April 15, 1995): 506–10.

119. Kevin M. DeCock, Mary Glenn Fowler, Eric Mercier, et al., "Prevention of

Mother-to-Child HIV Transmission in Resource-Poor Countries: Translating Research into Policy and Practice," *JAMA* 283 (March 1, 2000): 1175–82.

120. Edward M. Connor, Rhoda S. Sperling, Richard Gelber, et al., "Reduction of Maternal-Infant Transmission of Human Immunodeficiency Virus Type 1 with Zidovudine Treatment," *NEJM* 331 (November 3, 1994): 1173–80.

121. Mary Lou Lindegren, Robert H. Byers Jr., Pauline Thomas, et al., "Trends in Perinatal Transmission in HIV/AIDS in the United States," *JAMA* 282 (August 11, 1999): 531–38.

122. Angus Nicoll, Marie-Louise Newell, Eric Von Praag, Philippe Van de Perre, and Catherine Peckham, "Infant Feeding Policy and Practice in the Presence of HIV-1 Infection," *AIDS* 9 (October 1995): 107–19.

123. "Elective Caesarean-Section versus Vaginal Delivery in Prevention of Vertical HIV-1 Transmission: A Randomised Clinical Trial," *Lancet* 353 (March 27, 1999): 1035–39.

124. Lynne M. Mofesnson and James A McIntyre, "Advances and Research Directions in the Prevention of Mother-to-Child HIV-1 Transmission," *Lancet* 355 (June 24, 2000): 2237–44.

125. Elliot Marseille, James G. Kahn, and Francis Mmiro, "Cost-Effectiveness of Single-Dose Nevirapine Regimen for Mothers and Babies to Decrease Vertical HIV-1 Transmission in Sub-Saharan Africa," *Lancet* 354 (September 4, 1999): 803–9.

126. Francois Dabis, Philippi Msellati, Nicolas Meda, et al., "Six-Month Efficacy, Tolerance, and Acceptability of a Short Regimen of Oral Zidovudine to Reduce Vertical Transmission of HIV in Breastfed Children in Côte d'Ivoire and Burkina Faso: A Double-Blind Placebo-Controlled Multicentre Trial," *Lancet* 353 (March 6, 1999): 786–92; Stefan Z. Wiktor, Ehounou Ekpini, John M. Karon, et al., "Short-Course Oral Zidovudine for Prevention of Mother-to-Child Transmission of HIV-1 in Abidjan, Côte d'Ivoire: A Randomised Trial," *Lancet* 353 (March 6, 1999): 781–85; Nathan Shaffer, Rutt Chuachoowong, Philip A. Mock, et al., "Short-Course Zidovudine for Perinatal Transmission in Bangkok, Thailand: A Randomised Controlled Trial," *Lancet* 353 (March 6, 1999): 773–80.

127. Laura A. Guay, Phillipa Musoke, Thomas Fleming, et al., "Intrapartum and Neonatal Single-Dose Nevirapine Compared with Zidovudine for Prevention of Mother-to-Child Transmission of HIV-1 in Kampala, Uganda," *Lancet* 354 (September 4, 1999): 795–802.

128. Ibid.

129. CDC, "Administration of Zidovudine during Late Pregnancy to Prevent Perinatal HIV Transmission—Thailand, 1996–1998," *MMWR* 47 (March 6, 1998): 151–53.

130. Neil Soderlund, Karen Zwi, Anthony Kinghorn, and Glenda Gray, "Prevention of Vertical Transmission of HIV: Analysis of Cost-Effectiveness of Options Available in South Africa," *British Medical Journal* 318 (June 19, 1999): 1650–56.

131. UNICEF, UNAIDS, and WHO, *HIV and Infant Feeding: Guidelines for Decision-Makers* (Geneva: UNAIDS, June 1998), ‹http://www.unaids.org/publications/documents/mtct/infantpolicy.html›; Berer, "Reducing Perinatal HIV Transmission in Developing Countries."

132. Luo, "Strategies for Prevention of Mother-to-Child Transmission of HIV."

133. David Wilkinson, Salim S. Abdool Karim, and Hoosen M. Coovadia, "Short Course Antiretroviral Regimens to Reduce Maternal Transmission of HIV: May Be Effective but Shouldn't Be Allowed to Strangle Research That Might Help Africans," *British Medical Journal* 318 (February 20, 1999): 479–80.

134. Catherine Hankins, "Preventing Mother-to-Child Transmission of HIV in Developing Countries: Recent Developments and Ethical Implications," *Reproductive Health Matters* 8 (May 2000): 87–92.

135. Michael Grunwald, "In Echo of Apartheid Fight, Public Pushes S. Africa on AIDS," *Washington Post*, January 28, 2003; Chris McGreal, "Court Orders Mbeki to Provide AIDS Drug," *The Guardian*, December 15, 2001, ⟨http://www.guardian.co.uk/aids/story/0,7369,619153,00.html⟩; "South Africa to Provide AIDS Drug," *BBC News*, April 4, 2002.

136. Carel B. Ijsselmuiden and Ruth Faden, "Research and Informed Consent in Africa—Another Look," *NEJM* 326 (March 19, 1992): 830–34.

137. Berer, "Reducing Perinatal HIV Transmission in Developing Countries."

138. Luo, "Strategies for Prevention of Mother-to-Child Transmission of HIV"; Rachel Baggaley and Eric van Praag, "Antiretroviral Interventions to Reduce Mother-to-Child Transmission of Human Immunodeficiency Virus: Challenges for Health Systems, Communities, and Society," *BWHO* 78 (2000): 1036–44.

139. In a PCT, one group of persons is given the experimental treatment and one group (the control group) is given a placebo, such as a sugar pill. The incidence of transmission in the two groups is compared to determine whether the experimental treatment had any effect.

140. Ronald Bayer, "The Debate over Maternal-Fetal HIV Transmission Prevention Trials in Africa, Asia, and the Caribbean: Racist Exploitation or Exploitation of Racism?," *AJPH* 88 (April 1998): 567–70.

141. Ibid.

142. Harold Varmus and David Satcher, "Ethical Complexities of Conducting Research in Developing Countries," *NEJM* 337 (October 2, 1997): 1003–5.

143. Peter Lurie and Sidney M. Wolf, "Unethical Trials of Interventions to Reduce Perinatal Transmission of Human Immunodeficiency Virus in Developing Countries," *NEJM* 337 (September 18, 1997): 853–56.

144. Marcia Angell, "The Ethics of Clinical Research in the Third World," *NEJM* 337 (September 18, 1997): 847–49.

145. World Medical Association Declaration of Helsinki, *Ethical Principles for Medical Research Involving Human Subjects, Edinburgh, Scotland* (World Medical Association, October 2000), ⟨http://www.wma.net/e/policy/17-c_e.html⟩.

146. CIOMS, "International Guidelines for Ethical Review of Epidemiological Studies," *Law, Medicine, and Health Care* 19 (1991): 191–201.

147. Patricia Huston and Robert Peterson, "Withholding Proven Treatment in Clinical Research," *NEJM* 345 (September 20, 2001): 912–13.

148. Ezekiel J. Enanuel and Franklin G. Miller, "The Ethics of Placebo-Controlled Trials—A Middle Ground," *NEJM* 345 (September 20, 2001): 915–19; Benjamin Freedman, Kathleen Cranley Glass, and Charles Weijer, "Placebo Orthodoxy in Clini-

cal Research II: Ethical, Legal, and Regulatory Myths," *Journal of Law, Medicine, and Ethics* 24 (Fall 1996): 252–59; Benjamin Freedman, Charles Weijer, and Kathleen Cranley Glass, "Placebo Orthodoxy in Clinical Research I: Empirical and Methodological Myths," *Journal of Law, Medicine, and Ethics* 24 (Fall 1996): 243–51.

149. Angell, "Ethics of Clinical Research."

150. Marcia Angell, "Tuskegee Revisited," *Wall Street Journal*, October 28, 1997.

151. Varmus and Satcher, "Ethical Complexities of Conducting Research."

152. Michael H. Merson, Letter to the Editor, *NEJM* 338 (March 19, 1998): 836, and Donald Francis, Letter to the Editor, *NEJM* 338 (March 19, 1998): 837.

153. Salim S. Abdool Karim, "Placebo Controls in HIV Perinatal Transmission Trials: A South African's Viewpoint," *AJPH* 88 (April 1998): 564–66, and Edward K. Mbidde, Letter to the Editor, *NEJM* 338 (March 19, 1998): 837.

154. Bayer, "Debate over Maternal-Fetal HIV Transmission Prevention Trials."

155. "Perinatal HIV Intervention Research in Developing Countries Workshop Participants, Science, Ethics, and the Future of Research into Maternal Infant Transmission of HIV-1," *Lancet* 353 (March 6, 1999): 832–35.

156. Donald G. McNeil Jr., "Malarial Treatment for Chinese AIDS Patients Prompts Inquiry in U.S.," *NYT*, March 4, 2003 (investigating whether U.S. researchers aided experiments in China in which HIV-infected patients were deliberately infected with malaria in an effort to kill the AIDS virus); Daniel W. Fitzgerald and Frieda M-T Behets, "Women's Health and Human Rights in HIV Prevention Research," *Lancet* 361 (January 4, 2003): 68–69 (discussing the ethical duty of researchers to report violence against women).

157. "Fact Sheet: The President's Emergency Plan for AIDS Relief," January 29, 2003, ⟨http://www.whitehouse.gov/news/releases/2003/01/print/20030129-1.html⟩.

158. Sonya Ross, "Bush Pledges $15 Billion AIDS Relief Plan for Africa and Caribbean, Again Criticizes Iran, Iraq, North Korea," *Associated Press*, January 28, 2003.

159. Laurie Garrett, "$15 Billion Spent Wrong Way/Bush AIDS Plan Meets Resistance," *Newsday*, February 1, 2003.

160. Deb Riechmann, "Bush Signs Bill to Help Fight AIDS Worldwide," *Washington Post*, May 27, 2003.

161. Richard Marlink, "Taking Africa Seriously," *Hastings Center Report* 33 (March–April 2003): 49.

Chapter 17

1. Lawrence O. Gostin, Preface to "The Harvard Model AIDS Legislation Project: A Decade of a Maturing Epidemic: An Assessment and Directions for Future Public Policy," *American Journal of Law and Medicine* 16 (1990): 1–32; Gostin, "Public Health Strategies for Confronting AIDS: Legislative and Regulatory Policy in the United States," *JAMA* 261 (March 17, 1989): 1621–30.

2. Lawrence O. Gostin and William J. Curran, *Global Survey of AIDS Legislation* (Geneva: WHO, 1990).

3. Ronald Bayer and Cheryl Healton, "Controlling AIDS in Cuba: The Logic of Quarantine," *NEJM* 320 (April 13, 1989): 1022–24.

4. OHCHR and UNAIDS, *HIV/AIDS and Human Rights International Guidelines*, Second International Consultation on HIV/AIDS and Human Rights, Geneva, 23–25 September 1996 (New York: United Nations, 1998), ‹http://www.unaids.org/publications/documents/human/law/hright2e.pdf›.

5. Jonathan M. Mann, Lawrence O. Gostin, Sofia Gruskin, et al., "Health and Human Rights," *JHHR* 1 (1994): 6–23.

6. UNAIDS and OHCHR, *HIV/AIDS and Human Rights: International Guidelines* (Geneva: UNAIDS and OHCHR, 1998, updated 2002); Joint UNAIDS/OHCHR Press Release, "United Nations Entrenches Human Rights Principles in AIDS Response," Geneva, September 10, 2002.

7. General Comment 14, E/C.12/2000/4, July 4, 2000, ‹http://www.unhchr.ch/tbs/docs.ngf›.

8. United Nations Commission on Human Rights, Resolution 2002/31.

9. George J. Annas, "HIV/AIDS in Africa," *Lancet* 360 (November 30, 2002): 1787; Lawrence O. Gostin, "AIDS in Africa among Women and Infants: A Human Rights Framework," *Hastings Center Report* 32 (September–October 2001): 20–21.

10. M. Gregg Bloche, "WTO Deference to National Health Policy: Toward an Interpretive Principle," *Journal of International Economic Law* 5 (December 2002): 825.

11. Susan Sontag, *Illness as Metaphor and AIDS and Its Metaphors* (New York: Doubleday, 1990).

12. UNAIDS and WHO, *AIDS Epidemic Update* (Geneva: UNAIDS and WHO, December 2002), ‹http://www.unaids.org/worldaidsday/2002/press/Epiupdate.html›, 1–40.

13. Ibid., 26.

14. UNAIDS and World Bank, *HIV and Human Development: The Devastating Impact of AIDS* (Geneva: UNAIDS, 1999).

15. Commission on Macroeconomics and Health, *Macroeconomics and Health: Investing in Health for Economic Development* (Geneva: WHO, 2001).

16. Global Fund to Fight AIDS, Tuberculosis, and Malaria, ‹http://www.globalfundatm.org/index.html›.

17. Editorial, "The Global Fund Confronts AIDS," *NYT*, December 13, 2001.

18. Luc Montagnier, "A History of HIV Discovery," *Science* 298 (November 29, 2002): 1727–28; Stanley B. Prusiner, "Discovering the Cause of AIDS," *Science* 298 (November 29, 2002): 1726–27.

19. Mark Barnes, "Towards Ghastly Death: The Censorship of AIDS Education," *Columbia Law Review* 89 (April 1989): 698–724.

20. John F. Jewett and Frederick M. Hecht, "Preventive Health Care for Adults with HIV Infection," *JAMA* 269 (March 3, 1993): 1144–53.

21. Michael A. Stoto, Donna A. Almario, and Marie C. McCormick, eds., *Reducing the Odds: Preventing Perinatal Transmission of HIV in the United States* (Washington, D.C.: National Academy Press, 1999).

22. CDC, Panel on Clinical Practices for the Treatment of HIV, "Guidelines for Using Antiretroviral Agents among HIV-infected Adults and Adolescents: Recommendations of the Panel on Clinical Practices for Treatment of HIV," *MMWR* 51 (May 17, 2002): 1–55.

23. Susan J. Little et al., "Antiretroviral-Drug Resistance among Patients Recently Infected with HIV," *NEJM* 347 (August 8, 2002): 385–94; Joan Stephenson, "'Sobering' Levels of Drug-Resistant HIV Found," *JAMA* 287 (February 13, 2002): 704–5.

24. The results of the first large-scale human trial of an AIDS vaccine were disappointing; the trial failed to show that the vaccine effectively prevented HIV transmission. AVAC, "Understanding the Results of the AIDSVAX Trial," March 11, 2003.

25. UNAIDS and WHO, *AIDS Epidemic Update*; Lawrence K. Altman, "Women with HIV Reach Half of Global Cases," *NYT*, November 27, 2002.

26. CDC, *H/ASR* 13 (Atlanta: CDC, December 2001): 3; CDC, "The Global HIV and AIDS Epidemic, 2001," *MMWR* 50 (June 1, 2001): 434–39; World Bank, *Accelerating an AIDS Vaccine for Developing Countries: Recommendations for the World Bank* (May 2000), ⟨http://www.worldbank.org/aids-econ/vacc/accelerateb.pdf⟩, 1–29.

27. Office of AIDS Research, NIH, *Behavioral and Social Science HIV/AIDS-Related Research at NIH* (Bethesda, Md.: NIH, December 10, 2001), ⟨http://www.nih.gov/od/oar/about/research/behavioral/oarbehv.htm⟩.

Selected Bibliography

This list of books, reports, and articles on HIV/AIDS is arranged by topic in reverse chronological order. Each work appears only once even if it covers more than one topic.

Topics

I. History of an Epidemic

Prusiner, Stanley B. "Discovering the Cause of AIDS." *Science* 298 (November 29, 2002): 1726.

Montagnier, Luc. "A History of HIV Discovery." *Science* 298 (November 29, 2002): 1727–28.

Gallo, Robert C. "The Early Years of HIV/AIDS." *Science* 298 (November 29, 2002): 1728–30.

Karon, John M., Patricia L. Fleming, Richard W. Steketee, and Kevin M. DeCock. "HIV in the United States at the Turn of the Century: An Epidemic in Transition." *American Journal of Public Health* 91 (July 2001): 1060–68.

Bayer, Ronald, and Gerald M. Oppenheimer. *AIDS Doctors: Voices from the Epidemic: An Oral History.* New York: Oxford University Press, 2000.

Sontag, Susan. *Illness as Metaphor and AIDS and Its Metaphors.* Garden City, N.Y.: Doubleday, 1990.

Bayer, Ronald. *Private Acts, Social Consequences: AIDS and the Politics of Public Health.* New York: Free Press, 1989.

Brandt, Allan M. "AIDS in Historical Perspective: Four Lessons from the History of Sexually Transmitted Diseases." *American Journal of Public Health* 78 (April 1988): 367–71.

Fee, Elizabeth, and Daniel M. Fox, eds. *AIDS: The Burden of History.* Berkeley: University of California Press, 1988.

Schilts, Randy. *And the Band Played On: People, Politics, and the AIDS Epidemic.* New York: Penguin Books, 1988.

Altman, David. *AIDS in the Mind of America.* Garden City, N.Y.: Anchor Books, 1986.

II. Public Health, Science, and Medicine

Pruisiner, Stanley B. "Discovering the Causes of AIDS." *Science* 298 (November 29, 2002): 1126–31.

Little, Susan J. "Antiretroviral-Drug Resistance among Patients Recently Infected with HIV." *New England Journal of Medicine* 347 (August 8, 2002): 385–94.

Semaan, Salaam, and Ellen Sogolow, eds. "Do Behavioral HIV Interventions Work?: A Review and Meta-Analysis." *Journal of Acquired Immune Deficiency Syndromes* (July 1, 2002).

Stephenson, Joan. "'Sobering' Levels of Drug-Resistant HIV Found." *Journal of the American Medical Association* 287 (February 13, 2002): 704–5.

Farmer, Paul, et al. "Community-Based Treatment of Advanced HIV Disease: Introducing DOT-HAART (Directly Observed Therapy with Highly Active Antiretroviral Therapy)." *Bulletin of the World Health Organization* 79 (2001): 1145–51.

U.S. Public Health Service (USPHS) and Infectious Diseases Society of America (IDSA). "2001 USPHS/IDSA Guidelines for the Prevention of Opportunistic Infections in Persons Infected with Human Immunodeficiency Virus." *HIV Clinical Trials* 2 (November–December 2001): 493–554, ⟨http://www.ama-assn.org/special/hiv/treatmnt/guide/rr4810rev/rr4810a1rev.htm⟩.

Centers for Disease Control and Prevention (CDC). "Guidelines for the Use of Antiretroviral Agents in HIV-infected Adults and Adolescents." *Morbidity and Mortality Weekly Report* 47 (April 24, 1998): 42–82.

Connor, Edward M., et al. "Reduction of Maternal-Infant Transmission of Human Immunodeficiency Virus Type 1 with Zidovudine Treatment: Pediatric AIDS Clinical Trials Group Protocol 076 Study Group." *New England Journal of Medicine* 331 (November 3, 1994): 1173–80.

Isbell, Michael T. "AIDS and Public Health: The Enduring Relevance of a Communitarian Approach to Disease Prevention." *AIDS and Public Policy Journal* 8 (1993): 157–77.

Fischl, Margaret A., et al. "The Efficacy of Azidothymidine (AZT) in the Treatment of Patients with AIDS and AIDS-Related Complex: A Double-Blind Placebo-Controlled Trial." *New England Journal of Medicine* 317 (July 23, 1987): 185–91.

Gallo, Robert C. "The First Human Retrovirus." *Scientific American* 255 (December 1986): 88–98.

CDC. "Antibodies to a Retrovirus Etiologically Associated with Acquired Immunodeficiency Syndrome (AIDS) in Populations with Increased Incidences of the Syndrome." *Morbidity and Mortality Weekly Report* 33 (July 13, 1984): 377–79.

CDC. "Epidemiologic Aspects of the Current Outbreak of Kaposi's Sarcoma and Opportunistic Infections." *New England Journal of Medicine* 306 (January 28, 1982): 248–52.

CDC. "*Pneumocystis* Pneumonia—Los Angeles." *Morbidity and Mortality Weekly Report* 30 (June 5, 1981): 250–52.

III. Policy and Politics

Centers for Disease Control and Prevention (CDC): "Advancing HIV Prevention: New Strategies for a Changing Epidemic—United States, 2003." *Morbidity and Mortality Weekly Report* 52 (April 18, 2003): 329–32.

Stockdill, Brett C. *Activism against AIDS: At the Intersection of Sexuality, Race, and Class.* Boulder, Colo.: Lynne Rienner Publishers, 2003.

Kates, Jennifer, Richard Sorian, Jeffrey S. Crowley, and Todd A. Summers. "Critical Policy Challenges in the Third Decade of the HIV/AIDS Epidemic." *American Journal of Public Health* (July 2002): 1060–63.

Siplon, Patricia D. *AIDS and the Policy Struggle in the United States*. Washington, D.C.: Georgetown University Press, 2002.

"Proposal Seeks to Extend 'Legal Checkups' Nationwide." *AIDS Policy and Law* 16 (February 16, 2001): 1, 6–9.

Ruiz, Monica S., et al., eds. *No Time to Lose: Getting More from HIV Prevention*. Washington, D.C.: National Academy Press, 2001.

Presidential Advisory Council on HIV/AIDS. *Progress Report: Implementation of Advisory Council Recommendations* (Washington, D.C.: Presidential Advisory Council on HIV/AIDS, July 8, 1996).

Theodoulou, Stella Z., ed. *AIDS: The Politics and Policy of Disease*. Upper Saddle River, N.J.: Prentice Hall, 1996.

National Commission on AIDS. *America Living with AIDS: Transforming Anger, Fear, and Indifference into Action*. Washington, D.C.: National Commission on AIDS, 1991.

Bayer, Ronald. "Public Health Policy and the AIDS Epidemic: An End to HIV Exceptionalism." *New England Journal of Medicine* 324 (May 23, 1991): 1500–1504.

Miller, Heather G., Charles F. Turner, and Lincoln E. Moses, eds. *AIDS: The Second Decade*. Washington, D.C.: National Academy Press, 1990.

Presidential Commission. *Report of the Presidential Commission on the Human Immunodeficiency Virus Epidemic*. Washington, D.C.: GPO, 1988.

Institute of Medicine. *Confronting AIDS: Directions for Public Health, Health Care, and Research*. Washington, D.C.: National Academy Press, 1986, Update 1988.

Neslund, Verla S., Eugene W. Matthews, and William J. Curran. "The Role of CDC in the Development of AIDS Recommendations and Guidelines." *Law, Medicine, and Health Care* 15 (Summer 1987): 73–79.

U.S. Public Health Service, Office of Surgeon General. *Surgeon General's Report on Acquired Immune Deficiency Syndrome*. Rockville, Md.: Office of the Surgeon General, 1986.

IV. AIDS Education

Valdiserri, Ronald, ed. *Dawning Answers: How the HIV/AIDS Epidemic Has Helped to Strengthen Public Health*. North Carolina: Oxford University Press, 2003.

Samuels, Sarah E., and Mark D. Smith, eds. *Condoms in the Schools*. Menlo Park, Calif.: Henry J. Kaiser Family Foundation, 1993.

Barnes, Mark. "Towards Ghastly Death: The Censorship of AIDS Education." *Columbia Law Review* 89 (April 1989): 698–724.

Kirp, David L. *Learning by Heart: AIDS and School Children in America's Communities*. New Brunswick, N.J.: Rutgers University Press, 1989.

V. Law and Ethics

Webber, David W., ed. *AIDS and the Law*. 3d ed. New York: John Wiley and Sons, 1997, with 2002 Supp.

Frankowski, Stanislaw, ed. *Legal Responses to AIDS in Comparative Perspective*. The Hague: Kluwer Law International, 1998.

Gostin, Lawrence O., Zita Lazzarini, Kathleen Flaherty, and Robert Scherer. *The*

AIDS Litigation Project III: A Look at HIV/AIDS in the Courts in the 1990s. Menlo Park, Calif.: Henry J. Kaiser Family Foundation, 1996.

Leonard, Arthur S., et al., eds. *AIDS Law and Policy: Cases and Materials.* 2d ed. Houston: John Marshall Publishing Co., 1995.

Burris, Scott, Harlon L. Dalton, and Judith Leonie Miller, eds. *AIDS Law Today: A New Guide for the Public.* New Haven: Yale University Press, 1993.

Gostin, Lawrence O., and Lane Porter. *U.S. AIDS Litigation Project II: A National Survey of Federal, State, and Local Cases before Courts and Human Rights Commissions: Objective Description of Trends in AIDS Litigation.* Washington, D.C.: Department of Health and Human Services, 1991.

Gostin, Lawrence O., Lane Porter, and Hazel Sandomire. *U.S. AIDS Litigation Project I: A National Survey of Federal, State, and Local Cases before Courts and Human Rights Commissions.* Washington, D.C.: Department of Health and Human Services, 1990.

American Bar Association. *Policy on AIDS.* Chicago: American Bar Association, 1989.

Gostin, Lawrence O. "Public Health Strategies for Confronting AIDS: Legislative and Regulatory Policy in the United States." *Journal of the American Medical Association* 261 (March 17, 1989): 1621–30.

American Bar Association AIDS Coordinating Committee. *AIDS: The Legal Issues.* Washington, D.C.: American Bar Association, 1988.

Curran, William J., Lawrence O. Gostin, and Mary E. Clark. *Acquired Immunodeficiency Syndrome: Legal, Regulatory, and Policy Analysis.* Washington, D.C.: Department of Health and Human Services, 1986; reprint, Hagerstown, Md.: University Publishing Group, 1988.

VI. Human Rights

Hunt, Paul. *Economic, Social, and Cultural Rights: The Right of Everyone to the Enjoyment of the Highest Attainable Standard of Physical and Mental Health.* Geneva: United Nations Economic and Social Council (ECOSOC) Commission on Human Rights, 2003.

Fleishman, Jane. *Fatal Vulnerabilities: Reducing the Acute Risk of HIV/AIDS among Women and Girls.* Washington, D.C.: Center for Strategic and International Studies (CSIS), February 2003.

Gruskin, Sofia, and Bebe Loff. "Do Human Rights Have a Role in Public Health Work?" *Lancet* 360 (December 7, 2002): 1880.

Joint United Nations Programme on AIDS (UNAIDS) and Office of the High Commissioner for Human Rights. *HIV/AIDS and Human Rights: International Guidelines.* New York: United Nations, 1998, updated 2002.

World Health Organization (WHO). *25 Questions and Answers on Health and Human Rights.* Geneva: WHO, 2002, http://www.who.int/hhr/information/25_questions_hhr.pdf.

UNAIDS. *Handbook for Legislators on HIV/AIDS, Law, and Human Rights: Action to Combat HIV/AIDS in View of Its Devastating Human, Economic, and Social Impact.* Geneva: UNAIDS, 1999.

Mann, Jonathan M. "Medicine and Public Health, Ethics and Human Rights." *Hastings Center Report* 27 (May 1997): 6–13.

Gostin, Lawrence O., and Zita Lazzarini. *Human Rights and Public Health in the AIDS Pandemic*. New York: Oxford University Press, 1997.

VII. Privacy and Confidentiality

Gostin, Lawrence O., and James G. Hodge Jr. "Personal Privacy and Common Goods: A Framework for Balancing under the National Health Information Privacy Rule." *Minnesota Law Review* 86 (June 2002): 1439–79.

Gostin, Lawrence O., James G. Hodge Jr., and Ronald O. Valdiserri. "Informational Privacy and the Public's Health." *American Journal of Public Health* 91 (September 2001): 1388–92.

Burr, Chandler. "The AIDS Exception: Privacy vs. Public Health." *Atlantic Monthly*, June 1997, 57–67.

Association of State and Territorial Health Officials (ASTHO). *Guide to Public Health Practice: AIDS Confidentiality and Anti-Discrimination Principles: Interim Report*. Washington, D.C.: ASTHO, 1987.

VIII. Stigma, Social Risk, and Discrimination

Hermann, Donald H. J. "The Development of AIDS Federal Civil Rights Law: Antidiscrimination Law Protection of Persons with Human Immunodeficiency Virus." *Indiana Law Review* 33 (2000): 783–862.

Centers for Disease Control and Prevention. "HIV-Related Knowledge and Stigma—United States, 2000." *Morbidity and Mortality Weekly Report* 49 (December 1, 2000): 1062–64.

Note. "Name Brands: The Effects of Intrusive HIV Legislation on High-Risk Demographic Groups." *Harvard Law Review* 113 (June 2000): 2098–2117.

Webber, David W., and Lawrence O. Gostin. "Discrimination Based on HIV/AIDS and Other Health Conditions: 'Disability' as Defined under Federal and State Law." *Journal of Health Care Law and Policy* 3 (2000): 266–329.

Burris, Scott. "Studying the Legal Management of HIV-Related Stigma." *American Behavioral Scientist* 42 (April 1999): 1229–43.

Gostin, Lawrence O., Chai Feldblum, and David W. Webber. "Disability Discrimination in America: HIV/AIDS and Other Health Conditions." *Journal of the American Medical Association* 281 (February 24, 1999): 745–52.

Parmet, Wendy E. "The Supreme Court Confronts HIV: Reflections on Bragdon v. Abbott." *Journal of Law, Medicine, and Ethics* 26 (1998): 225–40.

Rubenstein, William B., Ruth Eisenberg, and Lawrence O. Gostin. *Rights of Persons Who Are HIV Positive: The Authoritative ACLU Guide to the Rights of People Living with HIV Disease and AIDS*. Carbondale: Southern Illinois University Press, 1996.

Swiss Institute of Comparative Law. *Comparative Study on Discrimination against Persons with HIV or AIDS*. Strasbourg, France: Council of Europe, 1993.

Jonsen, Albert R., and Jeff Stryker, eds. *The Social Impact of AIDS in the United States*. Washington, D.C.: National Academy Press, 1993.

Hunter, Nan D., and William B. Rubenstein, eds. *AIDS Agenda: Emerging Issues in Civil Rights*. New York: New Press, 1992.

White, Ryan. *Ryan White: My Own Story*. New York: Dial Books, 1991.

American Civil Liberties Union (ACLU). *Epidemic of Fear: A Survey of AIDS Discrimination in the 1980s and Policy Recommendations for the 1990s*. New York: ACLU AIDS Project, 1990.

Stoddard, Thomas B., and Walter Rieman. "AIDS and the Rights of the Individual: Toward a More Sophisticated Understanding of Discrimination." *Milbank Quarterly* 68, supp. 1 (1990): 143–74.

Dalton, Harlan. "AIDS in Blackface." *Daedelus* 118 (1989): 205–27.

Dannemeyer, William E. "Proposed 'Sex Survey.'" *Science* 244 (1989): 1530.

Richard A. Berk, ed. *The Social Impact of AIDS in the U.S.* Cambridge, Mass.: Abt Books, 1988.

IX. Counseling, Testing, and Screening

Centers for Disease Control and Prevention (CDC). "Approval of a New Rapid Test for HIV Antibody." *Morbidity and Mortality Weekly Report* 46 (November, 22, 2002): 1051–52.

Vermund, Stan H., and Craig M. Wilson. "Barriers to HIV Testing—Where Next?" *Lancet* 360 (October 19, 2002): 1186–87.

Pilcher, Christopher D., et al. "Real-time, Universal Screening for Acute HIV Infection in a Routine HIV Counseling and Testing Population." *Journal of the American Medical Association* 288 (July 10, 2002): 216–21.

CDC. "Revised Guidelines for HIV Counseling, Testing, and Referral." *Morbidity and Mortality Weekly Report* 50 (November 9, 2001): 1–58.

CDC. "Revised Recommendations for HIV Screening of Pregnant Women." *Morbidity and Mortality Weekly Report* 50 (November 9, 2001): 59–86.

UNAIDS and World Health Organization (WHO). *Guidelines for Using HIV Testing Technologies in Surveillance: Selection, Evaluation, and Implementation*. Geneva: WHO, 2001, ⟨http://www.who.int/emc-documents/order.html⟩.

Summers, Todd, Freya Spielberg, Chris Collins, and Thomas Coates. "Voluntary Counseling, Testing, and Referral for HIV: New Technologies, Research Findings Create Dynamic Opportunities." *Journal of Acquired Immune Deficiency Syndromes* 25, supp. 2 (2000): S128–S135.

CDC. "Anonymous or Confidential HIV Counseling and Voluntary Testing in Federally Funded Testing Sites—United States, 1995–1997." *Morbidity and Mortality Weekly Report* 48 (June 25, 1999): 509–13.

HIV Testing Action Coalition. *Statement of the National HIV Testing Action Coalition on the Necessity for Maintaining Anonymous HIV Testing Sites in All States*. Washington, D.C.: HIV Testing Action Coalition, 1997.

Field, Martha A. "Testing for AIDS: Uses and Abuses." *American Journal of Law and Medicine* 16 (1990): 33–106.

Cleary, Paul D., Michael Barry, Kenneth Mayer, Allan M. Brandt, Lawrence O.

Gostin, and Harvey V. Fineberg. "Compulsory Premarital Screening for the Human Immunodeficiency Virus: Technical and Public Health Considerations." *Journal of the American Medical Association* 258 (October 2, 1987): 1757–62.

Gostin, Lawrence O., William J. Curran, and Mary E. Clark. "The Case against Compulsory Casefinding in Controlling AIDS: Testing, Screening, and Reporting." *American Journal of Law and Medicine* 12 (1987): 1–47.

Bayer, Ronald, Carol Levine, and Susan M. Wolf. "HIV Antibody Screening: An Ethical Framework for Evaluating Proposed Programs." *Journal of the American Medical Association* 256 (October 3, 1986): 1768–74.

X. Reporting and Surveillance

Centers for Disease Control and Prevention (CDC). *HIV/AIDS Surveillance Report* 13. Atlanta: CDC, December 2001, ⟨http://www.cdc.gov/hiv/stats/hasr1302.pdf⟩.

CDC. "Updated Guidelines for Evaluating Public Health Surveillance Systems: Recommendations from the Guidelines Working Group." *Morbidity and Mortality Weekly Report* 50 (July 27, 2001): 1–36.

Health Policy Tracking Service. *Issue Brief: HIV Reporting in the States.* Washington, D.C.: Health Policy Tracking Service, National Conference of State Legislatures, April 30, 2001.

CDC. "Guidelines for National Human Immunodeficiency Virus Case Surveillance, Including Monitoring for Human Immunodeficiency Virus Infection and Acquired Immunodeficiency Syndrome." *Morbidity and Mortality Weekly Report* 48 (December 10, 1999): 1–28.

CDC. "Evaluation of HIV Case Surveillance through the Use of Non-Name Unique Identifiers—Maryland and Texas, 1994–1996." *Morbidity and Mortality Weekly Report* 46 (January 9, 1998): 1254–71.

Gostin, Lawrence O., and James G. Hodge Jr. "The 'Names Debate': The Case for National HIV Reporting in the United States." *Albany Law Review* 61 (1998): 679–743.

Gostin, Lawrence O., John W. Ward, and A. Cornelius Baker. "National HIV Case Reporting for the United States: A Defining Moment in the History of the Epidemic." *New England Journal of Medicine* 337 (October 16, 1997): 1162–67.

American Civil Liberties Union (ACLU). *HIV Surveillance and Name Reporting: A Public Health Case for Protecting Civil Liberties.* New York: An ACLU Report, 1997, ⟨http://www.aclu.org/issues/aids/namereport.html⟩.

AIDS Action Foundation. *Should HIV Test Results Be Reportable?: A Discussion of the Key Policy Questions.* Washington, D.C.: AIDS Action Foundation, 1993.

Fox, Daniel M. "From TB to AIDS: Value Conflicts in Reporting Disease." *Hastings Center Report* 16, supp. 1 (December 1986): 11–16.

XI. Partner Notification, the "Right to Know," and the "Duty to Warn"

Ainslie, Donald C. "Questioning Bioethics: AIDS, Sexual Ethics, and the Duty to Warn." *Hastings Center Report* 29 (September–October 1999): 26–35.

Gostin, Lawrence O., and James G. Hodge Jr. "Piercing the Veil of Secrecy in HIV/AIDS and Other Sexually Transmitted Diseases: Theories of Privacy and Disclosure in Partner Notification." *Duke Journal of Gender Law and Policy* 5 (Spring 1998): 9–88.

Bayer, Ronald. "AIDS Prevention—Sexual Ethics and Responsibility." *New England Journal of Medicine* 334 (June 6, 1996): 1540–42.

Rothenberg, Karen H., and Stephen J. Paskey. "The Risk of Domestic Violence and Women with HIV Infection: Implications for Partner Notification, Public Policy, and the Law." *American Journal of Public Health* 85 (November 1995): 1569–76.

Bayer, Ronald, and Kathleen Toomey. "HIV Prevention and the Two Faces of Partner Notification." *American Journal of Public Health* 82 (August 1992): 1158–64.

Toomey, Kathleen E., and Willard Cates Jr. "Partner Notification for the Prevention of HIV Infection." *AIDS* 3, supp. 1 (1989): S57–S62.

World Health Organization (WHO). *Consensus Statement from Consultation on Partner Notification for Preventing HIV Transmission.* Geneva: WHO, 1989.

Association of State and Territorial Health Officials. *Guide to Public Health Practice: HIV Partner Notification Strategies.* Washington, D.C.: Public Health Foundation, 1988.

XII. Compulsory State Powers and the Criminal Law

Lazzarini, Zita, Sarah Bray, and Scott Burris. "Evaluating the Impact of Criminal Laws on HIV Sexual Risk Behavior." *Journal of Law, Medicine, and Ethics* 30 (Summer 2002): 239–53.

Joint United Nations Programme on AIDS (UNAIDS). *Criminal Law, Public Health, and HIV Transmission: A Policy Options Paper.* Geneva: UNAIDS, June 2002.

Hodge Jr., James G., and Lawrence O. Gostin. "Handling Cases of Wilful Exposure through HIV Partner Counseling and Referral Services." *Rutgers Women's Law Reporter* 22 (2001): 45–62.

Sanchez, Lee, Stephanie Wilson, Lisa Speissegger, and Amanda Watson. *HIV/AIDS: Criminal Transmission and Exposure.* Health Policy Tracking Service, July 19, 1999, ⟨www.stateserv.hpts.org/public/issueb.nsf⟩.

Bayer, Ronald, and Amy Fairchild-Carrino. "AIDS and the Limits of Control: Public Health Orders, Quarantine, and Recalcitrant Behavior." *American Journal of Public Health* 83 (October 1993): 1471–76.

Jackson, Mark H. "The Criminalization of HIV." In *AIDS Agenda: Emerging Issues in Civil Rights*, edited by Nan D. Hunter and William B. Rubenstein, 239–70. New York: New Press, 1992.

Hermann, Donald H. J. "Criminalizing Conduct Related to HIV Transmission." *St. Louis University Public Law Review* 9 (1990): 351–78.

Gostin, Lawrence O. "The Politics of AIDS: Compulsory State Powers, Public Health, and Civil Liberties." *Ohio State Law Review* 49 (1989): 1017–58.

Field, Martha, and Kathleen Sullivan. "AIDS and the Coercive Power of the State." *Harvard Civil Rights–Civil Liberties Law Review* 23 (Winter 1988): 139–97.

Merritt, Deborah. "Communicable Disease and Constitutional Law: Controlling AIDS." *New York University Law Review* 61 (November 1986): 739–99.

Musto, David F. "Quarantine and the Problem of AIDS." *Milbank Quarterly* 64, supp. 1 (1986): 97–117.

Parmet, Wendy. "AIDS and Quarantine: The Revival of an Archaic Doctrine." *Hofstra Law Review* 14 (Fall 1985): 53–90.

XIII. Sexual Assault

Wiebe, Ellen R., Susan E. Comay, Margaret McGregor, and Sylvia Ducceschi. "Offering HIV Prophylaxis to People Who Have Been Sexually Assaulted: 16 Months' Experience in a Sexual Assault Service." *Canadian Medical Association Journal* 162 (March 7, 2000): 641–45.

Bamberger, Joshua D., Craig R. Waldo, Julie Louise Gerberding, and Mitchell H. Katz. "Post-Exposure Prophylaxis for Human Immunodeficiency Virus (HIV) Infection following Sexual Assault." *American Journal of Medicine* 106 (1999): 323–26.

Gostin, Lawrence O., Zita Lazzarini, Dianne D. Alexander, Allan M. Brandt, Kenneth H. Mayer, and Daniel C. Silverman. "HIV Testing, Counseling, and Prophylaxis after Sexual Assault." *Journal of the American Medical Association* 271 (May 11, 1994): 1436–44.

XIV. The Health Care System

Gerberding, Julie Louise. "Occupational Exposure to HIV in Health Care Settings." *New England Journal of Medicine* 348 (February 27, 2003): 826–33.

Filetoth, Zsolt. *Hospital-Acquired Infection: Causes and Control.* London: Whurr Publishers/Taylor and Francis Inc., 2003.

Zopolsky, Joe. "HIV-infected Healthcare Workers and Practice Modification." *North Dakota Law Review* 78 (2002): 77–98.

Centers for Disease Control and Prevention (CDC). "Updated U.S. Public Health Service Guidelines for the Management of Occupational Exposures to HBV, HCV, and HIV and Recommendations for Postexposure Prophylaxis." *Morbidity and Mortality Weekly Report* 50 (June 29, 2001): 1–42.

Summers, Todd. "Public Policy for Health Care Workers Infected with Human Immunodeficiency Virus." *Journal of the American Medical Association* 285 (February 21, 2001).

Fost, Norman. "Patient Access to Information on Clinicians Infected with Blood-borne Pathogens." *Journal of the American Medical Association* 284 (October 18, 2000): 1975–76.

Gostin, Lawrence O. "A Proposed National Policy on Health Care Workers Living with HIV/AIDS and Other Blood-borne Pathogens." *Journal of the American Medical Association* 284 (October 18, 2000): 1965–70.

Gerberding, Julie. "Provider-to-Patient HIV Transmission: How to Keep It Exceedingly Rare." *Annals of Internal Medicine* 130 (January 5, 1999): 64–65.

Tereskerz, Patti Miller, Richard D. Pearson, and Janine Jagger. "Infected Physicians and Invasive Procedures: National Policy and Legal Reality." *Milbank Quarterly* 77 (1999): 511–29.

American College of Surgeons. "Statement on the Surgeon and HIV Infection." *Bulletin of the American College of Surgeons* 83 (1998): 27–29.

AIDS/TB Committee of the Society for Healthcare Epidemiology of America. "Management of Healthcare Workers Infected with Hepatitis B Virus, Hepatitis C Virus, Human Immunodeficiency Virus, or Other Bloodborne Pathogens." *Infection Control and Hospital Epidemiology* 18 (1997): 349–63.

Schatz, Benjamin. "Supporting and Advocating for HIV-Positive Health Care Workers." *Bulletin of the New York Academy of Medicine* 72 (1995): 263–72.

Ciesielski, Carol, et al. "The 1990 Florida Dental Investigation: The Press and the Science." *Annals of Internal Medicine* 121 (December 1, 1994): 886–88.

Daniels, Norman. "HIV-infected Professionals, Patient Rights, and the 'Switching' Dilemma." *Journal of the American Medical Association* 267 (March 11, 1992): 1368–71.

Lo, Bernard, and Robert Steinbrook. "Health Care Workers Infected with the Human Immunodeficiency Virus: The Next Steps." *Journal of the American Medical Association* 267 (February 26, 1992): 1100–1105.

CDC. "Recommendations for Preventing Transmission of Human Immunodeficiency Virus and Hepatitis B Virus to Patients during Exposure-prone Invasive Procedures." *Morbidity and Mortality Weekly Report* 40 (July 12, 1991): 1–9.

Gostin, Lawrence O., ed. *AIDS and the Health Care System.* New Haven: Yale University Press, 1990.

Gostin, Lawrence O. "Hospitals, Health Care Professionals, and AIDS: The 'Right to Know' the Health Status of Professionals and Patients." *Maryland Law Review* 48 (1989): 12–54.

Gostin, Lawrence O. "HIV-infected Physicians and the Practice of Seriously Invasive Procedures." *Hastings Center Report* 19 (January–February 1989): 32–39.

Piorkowski, Joseph D., Jr. "Between a Rock and a Hard Place: AIDS and the Conflicting Physicians' Duties of Preventing Disease Transmission." *Georgetown Law Journal* 76 (October 1987): 169–202.

XV. Blood Supply

Feldman, Eric A., and Ronald Bayer, eds. *Blood Feuds: AIDS, Blood, and the Politics of Medical Disaster.* New York: Oxford University Press, 1999.

Leveton, Lauren B., Harold C. Sox Jr., and Michael A. Stoto, eds. *HIV and the Blood Supply: An Analysis of Crisis Decisionmaking.* Washington, D.C.: National Academy Press, 1995.

Centers for Disease Control and Prevention. "Provisional Public Health Service Interagency Recommendations for Screening Donated Blood and Plasma for Antibody to the Virus Causing Acquired Immunodeficiency Syndrome." *Morbidity and Mortality Weekly Report* 34 (January 11, 1985): 1–5.

XVI. Perinatal Transmission of HIV

Centers for Disease Control and Prevention (CDC). "HIV Testing among Pregnant Women—United States and Canada, 1998–2001." *Morbidity and Mortality Weekly Report* 51 (November 15, 2002): 1013–16.

Lazzarini, Zita, and Lorilyn Rosales. "Legal Issues concerning Public Health Efforts to Reduce Perinatal Transmission." *Yale Journal of Health Policy, Law, and Ethics* 3 (2002): 299–328.

Mofenson, Lynne M. "U.S. Public Health Service Task Force Recommendations for Use of Antiretroviral Drugs in Pregnant HIV-1 Infected Women for Maternal Health and Interventions to Reduce Perinatal HIV-1 Transmission in the United States." *Morbidity and Mortality Weekly Report* 51 (November 22, 2001): 1–38.

CDC. "Revised Recommendations for HIV Screening of Pregnant Women." *Morbidity and Mortality Weekly Report* 50 (November 9, 2001): 59–86.

Stoto, Michael A., Donna A. Almario, and Marie C. McCormick, eds. *Reducing the Odds: Preventing Perinatal Transmission of HIV in the United States*. Washington, D.C.: National Academy Press, 1999.

Bayer, Ronald. "The Debate over Maternal-Fetal HIV Transmission Prevention Trials in Africa, Asia, and the Caribbean: Racist Exploitation or Exploitation of Racism?" *American Journal of Public Health* 88 (April 1998): 567–70.

Lurie, Peter, and Sidney M. Wolf. "Unethical Trials of Interventions to Reduce Perinatal Transmission of Human Immunodeficiency Virus in Developing Countries." *New England Journal of Medicine* 337 (September 18, 1997): 853–56.

McGovern, Theresa M. "Mandatory HIV Testing and Treating of Child-Bearing Women: An Unnatural, Illegal, and Unsound Approach." *Columbia Human Rights Law Review* 28 (Spring 1997): 469–99.

Bayer, Ronald. "Rethinking the Testing of Babies and Pregnant Women for HIV Infection." *Journal of Clinical Ethics* 7 (1996): 85–87.

XVII. Injection Drug Users

Day, Dawn. *Health Emergency 2003: The Spread of Drug-Related AIDS and Hepatitis C among African Americans and Latinos*. Princeton, N.J.: Dogwood Center, 2003.

Jones, T. Stephen, and Phillip O. Coffin, guest eds. "Preventing Blood-borne Infections through Pharmacy Syringe Sales and Safe Community Syringe Disposal." *Journal of the American Pharmaceutical Association* 42 (November–December 2002).

Burris, Scott, Steffanie A. Strathdee, and Jon S. Vernick. *Syringe Access Law in the United States: A State of the Art Assessment of Law and Policy*. Washington, D.C., and Baltimore: Center for Law and the Public's Health at Georgetown University Law Center and Johns Hopkins University, 2002.

Friedman, Samuel R., Theresa Perlis, and Don C. Des Jarlais. "Laws Prohibiting Over-the-Counter Syringe Sales to Injection Drug Users: Relations to Population Density, HIV Prevalence, and HIV Incidence." *American Journal of Public Health* 91 (May 2001): 791–93.

Lazzarini, Zita. "An Analysis of Ethical Issues in Prescribing and Dispensing Syringes to Injection Drug Users." *Health Matrix* 11 (Winter 2001): 85–128.

Burris, Scott, ed. *Deregulation of Hypodermic Needles and Syringes as a Public Health Measure: A Report on Emerging Policy and Law in the United States*. Washington, D.C.: American Bar Association AIDS Coordinating Committee, 2001.

Jones, T. Stephen, and David Vlahov. "Use of Sterile Syringes and Aseptic Drug Preparation Are Important Components of HIV Prevention among Injection Drug Users." *Journal of Acquired Immune Deficiency Syndromes and Human Retrovirology* 18, supp. 1 (July 1998): S1–S5.

Gostin, Lawrence O., and Zita Lazzarini. "Prevention of HIV/AIDS among Injection Drug Users: The Theory and Science of Public Health and Criminal Justice Approaches to Disease Prevention." *Emory Law Journal* 46 (Spring 1997): 587–696.

Shalala, Donna E. *Report to the Committee on Appropriations for the Departments of Labor, Health and Human Services, and Education and Related Agencies: Needle Exchange Programs in America: Review of Published Studies and Ongoing Research*. Washington, D.C.: Department of Health and Human Services, February 18, 1997.

Burris, Scott, Davis Finucane, Heather Gallagher, and Joseph Grace. "The Legal Strategies Used in Operating Syringe Exchange Programs in the United States." *American Journal of Public Health* 86 (August 1996): 1161–66.

Des Jarlais, Don C., et al. "Maintaining Low HIV Seroprevalence in Populations of Injecting Drug Users." *Journal of the American Medical Association* 274 (October 18, 1995): 1226–31.

Normand, Jacques, David Vlahov, and Lincoln E. Moses, eds. *Preventing HIV Transmission: The Role of Sterile Needles and Bleach*. Washington, D.C.: National Academy Press, 1995.

Stryker, Jeff, and Mark D. Smith, eds. *Dimensions of HIV Prevention: Needle Exchange*. Menlo Park, Calif.: Henry J. Kaiser Family Foundation, 1993.

Fernando, M. Daniel. *AIDS and Intravenous Drug Use: The Influence of Morality, Politics, Social Science, and Race in the Making of a Tragedy*. Westport, Conn.: Praeger, 1993.

Gostin, Lawrence O. "The Inter-connected Epidemics of Drug Dependency and AIDS." *Harvard Civil Rights–Civil Liberties Law Review* 26 (Winter 1991): 113–84.

Battjes, Robert J., and Roy W. Pickens, eds. *Needle Sharing among Intravenous Drug Abusers: National and International Perspectives*. National Institute on Drug Abuse Research Monograph No. 80. Rockville, Md.: National Institute on Drug Abuse, 1988.

XVIII. Interconnected Epidemics of Sexually Transmitted Diseases and Tuberculosis

Center for Strategic and International Studies (CSIS) HIV/AIDS Task Force. *The Global Fund to Fight AIDS, TB, and Malaria Progress Report*. Washington, D.C.: CSIS, 2003, http://www.csis.org/africa/0302_globalfund.pdf.

Eng, Thomas R., and William T. Butler, eds. *The Hidden Epidemic: Confronting Sexually Transmitted Diseases*. Washington, D.C.: National Academy Press, 1997.

Gostin, Lawrence O. "The Resurgent Tuberculosis Epidemic in the Era of AIDS: Reflections on Public Health, Law, and Society." *Maryland Law Review* 54 (Winter 1995): 1–131.

Dubler, Nancy Neveloff, Ronald Bayer, Sheldon Landesman, and Amanda White. "Tuberculosis in the 1990s: Ethical, Legal, and Public Policy Issues in Screening, Treatment, and the Protection of Those in Congregate Facilities." In *The Tuberculosis Revival: Individual Rights and Social Obligations in a Time of AIDS*, 1–43. New York: United Hospital Fund of New York, 1992.

XIX. Travelers and Immigrants

Bureau of Consular Affairs. "Human Immunodeficiency Virus (HIV) Testing Requirements for Entry into Foreign Countries." Department of State, February 2002, ⟨http://travel.state.gov/HIVtestingreqs.html⟩.

Tarwater, Jeremy R. "The Tuberculosis and HIV Debate in Immigration Law: Critical Flaws in United States Academic and Anti-exclusion Arguments." *Georgetown Immigration Law Journal* 15 (Winter 2001): 357–79.

Klein, Alana. *HIV and Immigration: Final Report* (Montreal: Canadian HIV/AIDS Legal Network, 2001), ⟨http://www.aidslaw.ca/Maincontent/issues/Immigration/finalreport/Immigration2001E.pdf⟩.

Joint United Nations Programme on AIDS (UNAIDS). "Migration and HIV/AIDS." Second *Ad Hoc* Thematic Meeting, New Delhi, 9–11 December 1998. UNAIDS Programme Coordinating Board, October 28, 1998.

Ratner, Michael. "How We Closed the Guantánamo HIV Camp: The Intersection of Politics and Litigation." *Harvard Human Rights Journal* 11 (Spring 1998): 187–220.

Gostin, Lawrence O., Paul D. Cleary, Kenneth H. Mayer, Allan M. Brandt, and Eva H. Chittenden. "Screening Immigrants and International Travelers for the Human Immunodeficiency Virus." *New England Journal of Medicine* 322 (June 14, 1990): 1743–46.

National Commission on AIDS. *Resolution on U.S. Visa and Immigration Policy*. Washington, D.C.: National Commission on AIDS, December 1989.

Wolchok, Carol L. "AIDS at the Frontier: United States Immigration Policy." *Journal of Legal Medicine* 10 (1989): 127–42.

XX. The Global Reach of HIV/AIDS

Stephenson, Joan. "Growing, Evolving HIV/AIDS Pandemic Is Producing Social and Economic Fallout." *Journal of the American Medical Association* 289 (January 1, 2003): 31–33.

Joint United Nations Programme on AIDS (UNAIDS) and World Health Organization (WHO). *AIDS Epidemic Update*. Geneva: UNAIDS and WHO, December 2002, ⟨http://www.unaids.org/worldaidsday/2002/press/Epiupdate.html⟩.

DeCock, Kevin M. "Shadow on the Continent: Public Health and HIV/AIDS in Africa in the Twenty-first Century." *Lancet* 359 (July 6, 2002): 67–72.

United Nations Children's Fund (UNICEF), UNAIDS, and WHO. *Young People and HIV/AIDS: Opportunity in Crisis*. Paris: UNICEF, UNAIDS, WHO, July 2002.

Summers, Todd, Jennifer Kates, and Gillian Murphy. *The Tip of the Iceburg: The Global Impact of HIV/AIDS on Youth*. Menlo Park, Calif.: Henry J. Kaiser Family Foundation, July 2002.

Alagiri, Priya, Todd Summers, and Jennifer Kates. *Global Spending on HIV/AIDS in Resource-Poor Settings*. Menlo Park, Calif.: Henry J. Kaiser Family Foundation, July 2002.

UNAIDS, UNICEF, and U.S. Agency for International Development. *Children on the Brink, 2002: A Joint Report on Orphan Estimates and Program Strategies*. Washington, D.C.: UNAIDS, UNICEF, and USAID, July 2002.

Parker, Richard. "The Global HIV/AIDS Pandemic, Structural Inequalities, and the Politics of International Health." *American Journal of Public Health* 92 (March 2002): 343–46.

International Labour Office. *HIV/AIDS and the World of Work: An ILO Code of Practice*. Geneva: International Labour Organization Publications, 2002.

Essex, Max, ed. *AIDS in Africa*. 2d ed. New York: Kluwer Academic/Plenum Publishers, 2002.

Barnett, Tony, and Alan Whiteside. *AIDS in the Twenty-first Century: Disease and Globalization*. New York: Palgrave Macmillan, 2002.

Stanecki, Karen A. *The AIDS Pandemic in the Twenty-first Century*. Washington, D.C.: U.S. Census Bureau, 2002.

UNICEF. *Young People and HIV/AIDS: Opportunity in Crisis*. New York: UNICEF, 2002.

Folkers, Gregory K., and Anthony S. Fauci. "The AIDS Research Model: Implications for Other Infectious Diseases of Global Health Importance." *Journal of the American Medical Association* 286 (July 25, 2001): 458–61.

Centers for Disease Control and Prevention. "The Global HIV and AIDS Epidemic, 2001." *Morbidity and Mortality Weekly Report* 50 (June 1, 2001): 434–39.

UNAIDS. *HIV and Human Development: The Devastating Impact of AIDS*. Geneva: UNAIDS, 1998.

World Bank. *Confronting AIDS: Evidence from the Developing World*. Brussels: European Commission, 1998.

Varmus, Harold, and David Satcher. "Ethical Complexities of Conducting Research in Developing Countries." *New England Journal of Medicine* 337 (October 2, 1997): 1003–5.

Angell, Marcia. "The Ethics of Clinical Research in the Third World." *New England Journal of Medicine* 337 (September 18, 1997): 847–49.

World Bank. *Confronting AIDS: Public Priorities in a Global Epidemic*. New York: Oxford University Press, 1997.

Curran, William J., and Lawrence O. Gostin. *A World Wide Survey of AIDS Legislation*. Geneva: WHO, 1990.

Index of Cases

This index contains the major cases discussed in the text. Additional cases may be found in the endnotes.

General Index

AIDS phobia, xxi, 8, 36
AIDS Project Los Angeles, xxi
Alabama, 33, 192, 209
Alaska, 265, 268
American Academy of Pediatrics, 235
American Civil Liberties Union (ACLU),
 9, 111
American College of Obstetrics and
 Gynecology, 235
American College of Surgeons, 222
American Convention on Human
 Rights, 82
American Foundation for AIDS Re-
 search (AmFAR), xxiii
Americans with Disabilities Act (ADA),
 xxii, xxvii, xxx, 10, 28, 49, 50, 52, 53,
 54, 57, 112, 113, 114, 116, 119, 120,
 122, 123, 124, 130, 141, 142, 143, 223,
 225
Anal intercourse, 203, 204, 208
Angell, Marcia, 315
Annan, Kofi, 27, 109, 290, 303
Anonymous testing. See Testing:
 anonymous
Antibiotic resistance, 175
Antidiscrimination legislation, 111, 112,
 141
Anti-Drug Abuse Act, 256
Antiretroviral drugs, 208, 212
Antiretroviral resistance, xxviii. See also
 Drug resistance
Antiretroviral therapy, 118, 151, 153,
 207, 231, 235. See also Highly active
 antiretroviral therapy
Asia, xxviii, 24, 67
Assault, 189; aggravated, 189; with a
 deadly weapon, 180
Asylum, 56, 283
Asymptomatic, 135; incubation period,
 175; infection, 117, 118, 130
Attempted homicide, 180, 188–89. See
 also homicide
Australia, xiii, xiv, 251
Autonomy, 15, 18, 19, 41, 43, 55, 57, 64,
 65, 70, 72, 73, 75, 99, 135, 137, 139,

143, 146, 174, 181, 212, 228, 233,
238
Azidothymidine (AZT). See Zidovudine

Baby AIDS Bill, 234
Bathhouses, 6, 29, 34, 144
Battery, 187; infected sexual, 189
Bayer, Ronald, 315
Bergalis, Kimberly, xxxi, 16, 17
Biting, 36, 45, 186, 188, 194, 196
Blood, 6, 136, 140, 186, 188, 196, 214,
 215
—autologous donation of, 31
—directed donation of, 31
—donors, 6, 31, 186, 187, 190, 192
—selling of, 194
—suppliers, 6, 28, 30, 32, 70; liability of,
 30, 31–32
—transfusion recipients: duty to dis-
 close to, 31, 46
Blood-borne pathogen: safety standard,
 222, 223; transmission of, 218, 228
Blood-to-blood contact, 222
Botswana, xxi, xxiii, 80, 290, 317
Boylan-Town Act, 257–58
Bragdon, Randon, 28
Brazil, 308
Breast feeding, 206, 213, 311, 312
Breast milk, 192
Brennan, William, 109, 111, 141, 219
British Columbia, 205
Brundtland, Gro Harlem, 217
Bubonic plague, 7
Bureau of Citizenship and Immigration
 Services (BCIS), 22, 283. See also Im-
 migration and Naturalization Service
Burkina Faso, 314
Bush, George W., xvi, xxiii, xxiv, xxviii,
 xxix, 92, 93, 96, 303, 309, 316–17, 321

California, 29, 46, 123, 155, 161, 168,
 173, 179, 218, 221, 234, 258, 267
California Prostitutes Education Project
 (CAL-PEP), 134, 168
Canada, 21, 221, 226, 280

—law, 112–19, 220; future of, in America, 130
—definition of major life activity, 11, 120–22, 129
—mitigating measures, 11, 121
—in public accommodations, 50
—requirement of reasonable accommodations, 49, 114, 116–17, 224
—"regarded as" disabled, 121–22
—state law: 49, 57, 124–27; HIV-specific statutes, 127–28; judicial interpretations of, 129; limitations on use of HIV testing or test results, 128–29; statutory definitions of disability, 127
—substantial limitation, 121
—undue hardships, 117
Disclosure: of HIV infection, 9, 37, 38, 44, 45, 94, 101, 105, 161, 198, 229, 241; judicially ordered, 45, 98, 105
Discrimination, xxiii, xxv, xxx, 10–11, 12, 28, 38, 41, 42, 48–53, 57, 61, 64, 66, 67, 72, 73, 79, 86, 101, 109–130, 135, 142, 143, 146, 147, 153, 158, 160, 161, 177, 198, 227, 229, 237–38, 245; employment, 10, 49–50, 90, 127–28, 153, 161; health care, 10, 51, 128, 161; housing, 10, 51, 90, 153, 161; insurance, 10, 52–53, 90, 161; military, 52. *See also* Antidiscrimination legislation; Disability discrimination
Divorce, 5, 29, 39, 67
Double-gloving, 223, 228
Dominican Republic, 314
Drug dependency, xxxi, 19, 247–75 passim
Drug Enforcement Administration (DEA), 254
Drug-injection equipment, 186, 192, 247–75
Drug paraphernalia, 20, 253–57; laws, 253–57, 266–67, 271–72
Drug possession laws, 252–53
Drug resistance, 182
Drugs, generic, xvi, xxiii, 308–9

Duty of care, 172
Duty to disclose, xxx, 46, 47, 169, 170, 172, 173, 176
Duty to inform, 172
Duty to protect workers, 37
Duty to provide care, 10
Duty to warn, xxx, 169, 170, 172, 173, 176

Eighth Amendment, 54, 55, 56
Eighth International Conference on AIDS, xxiv, xxv, 21; protest of U.S. immigration policy during, 280
Ejaculate, 203, 204, 208
Eleventh Amendment, 123
Elliott, Richard, 196
Emotional distress, 226
Employment, 43, 57, 66
Employment discrimination. *See* Discrimination: employment
Employment Retirement Income Security Act (ERISA), 52
Endocarditis, 249
End-stage illness, 154
Enzyme immuno-assay (EIA), 136
Equal Employment Opportunity Commission (EEOC), 52; guidelines, 116, 224
Ethics, xxx, 11, 15, 19, 27, 99; of human subject research in resource-poor countries, 311–16; of partner notification, 173–74; of screening and testing pregnant women, 18–19, 236–40; of syringe prescription statutes, 264
Ethiopia, 314, 317
Europe, xxviii, 24, 82, 168, 167, 250, 251, 289
Exigent circumstances, 214
Expanded Syringe Access Demonstration Program, 266
Expedited trial, 38
Exposure-prone procedures, 16, 17, 219, 225, 228, 229

Failure to diagnose HIV/AIDS, 5, 29, 35
"Failure to inform," 47, 192

Health Omnibus Programs Extension (HOPE) Act, xxvii

Helms, Jesse, xxv, 281

Helms Amendment (U.S. Immigration and Nationality Act), xxv, 22, 281

Helsinki Declaration, 314

Hemophilia, 6, 8, 30, 31, 32, 181

Hepatitis B Virus (HBV), 11, 12, 16, 19, 146, 152, 203, 217, 219, 221, 249

Hepatitis C Virus (HCV), 19, 249

Herpes, 193. *See also* Genital herpes

Higgenbotham, Susan L., 201

Highly active antiretroviral therapy (HAART), xxvi, xxviii, 153, 182, 197, 304

Hispanics. *See* Latinos

HIV

—antiretroviral-resistant strains, 153

—failure to diagnose, 5, 29, 35

—failure to inform, 47, 192

—false diagnosis of, 5, 29, 35

—global effect of, xxi, xxviii–xxix, xxxii, 21–24, 289–318

—specific crimes related to, 190–95

—statutes regarding: constitutionality of, 194; and penalties, 193–94; and privacy legislation, 162

Home collection test kits, 161

Homelessness, 53, 54

Homicide, 187–88. *See also* Attempted homicide

Homophobia, xxi, 8, 110

Housing, 43, 57, 66

Housing Opportunities for People with AIDS (HOPWA) Act, xxii, xxvii

Hudson, Rock, xxv

Human Rights, xiii, xxvi, xxx, 4, 8, 13, 17; burdens, 65, 75, 77, 183, 218, 223–27, 228, 229; civil and political, xxvi, xxx, 63, 78–81; economic, social, and cultural, xxvi, xxx, 63, 78, 81; of health care workers, 21; health policies and, 53, 64–65, 67–78; impact assessment, 53, 68–78; negative and posi-

tive, 8; nonderogable, 75, 77; of travelers and immigrants, 61–87; violations of, 65–66

Human Rights Guidelines for the Protection of Persons Living with HIV/AIDS (International Guidelines), 79, 80

Human subject research, 311–16

Human T-Cell Lymphotropic Virus-Type III (HTLV-III), 153

Hypodermic syringes, 257

Illinois, 14, 129, 136, 137, 155, 161–62, 258

Immigrants, 22, 29, 33, 73, 279–88; exclusion waivers and, 22, 282–83; screening of, xxiii, 13, 279–88

Immigration, xxii, xxv, xxxii, 21, 22, 56, 279–88; accuracy of HIV tests and, 285; "designated event policy" and, 282; screening program and, 21, 22, 279–88

Immigration and Nationality Act, 21, 22, 281

Immigration and Naturalization Service (INS), 283

Immuno-fluorescence assay (IFA), 136

In-camera review, 207

Incarceration, 195

Incentive: criminal law as, 195, 197

India, 25, 66, 290, 308

Indiana, xxv, 48, 192, 234, 241

Indigence, 53–54

Individuals with Disabilities Education Act, 113

Infant (newborn) screening, 18, 234

Infectivity rate, 207

Informational privacy. *See* Privacy: informational

Informed consent, xxiii, 12, 16, 17, 18, 19, 24, 33, 55, 72, 93, 105, 192, 195, 206, 226, 235–36, 239, 240–41

Infrastructure: as barrier to treatment, 309–11

Injection drug users (IDUs), 16, 19, 20,
  25, 48, 57, 66, 72, 73, 170, 173, 111,
  181, 247–75
Inmates, 29, 137
Institute of Medicine (IOM), 18, 19, 35,
  42, 139, 148, 232–33, 234–36
Institutional Review Board (IRB), 95
Insurance companies, 43, 57, 66
Intellectual property, xvi, 305–9
Intent, criminal, 188, 194
Intentional transmission, 196, 214
Intergenerational sex, 80
International Covenant on Civil and Po-
  litical Rights (ICCPR), 8, 78
International Covenant on Economic,
  Social, and Cultural Rights (ICESCR),
  8, 78, 81, 82, 84
International Health Regulations, 22,
  287–88
International law, 62, 78, 305–9
International trade, 305–9
Iowa, 234
Isolation, 41, 63, 64, 73, 183–85; behav-
  ior-based, 183, 184; status-based, 183
Ivory Coast, 314, 317

Johnson, Earvin "Magic," 46
Johnson, Nkosi, 300
Johnson, Sterling, 287
Joint United Nations Programme on
  AIDS (UNAIDS), xiv, 296, 298, 300,
  311, 312, 313, 314, 321
Journal of Health and Human Rights,
  63

Kannabiran, Kalpana, 89
Kennedy, Anthony, 118
Kentucky, 155
Kenya, 307, 314, 317
Kimberly Bergalis Act, 16
Kirby, Michael, xviii, xxxiii
Koop, C. Everett, 30
KwaZulu Natal, 302–3

Lambda Legal Defense and Education
  Fund, xxiii
Lasso, Jose Ayala, 61
Latinos, xxvi, xxviii, 64, 233, 237, 250
Lazzarini, Zita, 194, 195
"Legal checkups," 43
Legitimate medical purpose doctrine,
  271
Levine, Mel, 256
Liberty, 5, 28, 41, 64, 70, 73, 75, 77, 80,
  184
Los Angeles, Calif., 124
Louisiana, 209, 268
Lymphadenopathy-associated virus
  (LAV), 153

Mail Order Drug Paraphernalia Control
  Act (Mail Order Act), 256–57
Maine, 155, 164, 179, 258, 267
Malaria, 249
Malawi, 314
Malpractice, 45, 227
Maluwa, Miriam, 196
Mandela, Nelson, 302
Mann, Jonathan, xiii, xiv, xix, xxxiii,
  xxxiv, xxxv, 63, 64, 67, 68, 321
Market-share liability, 32
Martin, Casey, 117
Martin Amendment (Comprehensive
  Crime Control Act), 209
Maryland, 155, 162, 188, 241, 267
Massachusetts, 37, 155, 207, 209, 258,
  267
Masturbation, 6, 34
Mayersohn, Nettie, 18, 234
Mbeki, Thabo, 23, 302
"Means-ends" inquiry, 142, 146
Media, 43, 44
Medicaid, 92, 162, 286
Medicare, 91, 92
Medicine Act, 1997, 308
Meese, Edwin, xxv
Mens rea, 186, 194
Mental illness, 184

197; alternative models for, 176; CDC guidelines on, 171; efficacy of, 174; ethical analysis of, 173

Patent protection, xxiv, 23, 24, 305–9

Patient notification, 205, 226

Pediatric AIDS Foundation, 41

Penile-vaginal intercourse, 203, 204

Pennsylvania, 45, 185, 258

Per-contact risk, 204

Perinatal transmission, xxii, xxvi, xxxi, 18, 19, 24, 118, 135, 144, 148, 153, 158, 181, 208, 231–45, 311–13

Periodic testing, 206

Permanent residence, 282–83

Pharmaceutical companies, 305–9

Pharmacy regulations, 20

Pharmacy syringe sales, 266

Phelps, Fred, 110

Philadelphia, Pa., 267

Phlebotomy, 136

Phthisiophobia, 8, 181

Piot, Peter, xvii, 61, 299

Placebo-controlled trials (PCTs), 24, 313–16

Plasma, 136

Pneumocystis pneumonia, xix, 30

Police powers, 137, 180

Polio, 8

Political sphere, xxiii, xxx, 11, 301–4

Polymerase chain reaction (PCR), 206

Postassault medical examination, 205

Postassault testing, 206

Postexposure prophylaxis, 207–8, 212, 223

Post-traumatic stress disorder (PTSD), 204

Powell, Colin, xxiii, 295

Prenatal screening, 18, 19, 35, 234–40; compulsory, 239; informed consent and, 240–41; pre-test counseling and, 240; privacy safeguards and, 240–44; problems of compulsion and consent and, 238; proposals for reform, 244–45; routine, 239–40; voluntary, 238–39

Presidential Advisory Council on HIV/AIDS, xxii, xxvii, 219

Presidential Commission on AIDS, xxii, xxvii, 219

Presidential Commission on the Human Immunodeficiency Virus Epidemic, 112

Prevention, 133, 233, 235–36, 250, 295, 304

Preventive confinement, 184

Prison, 6, 7

Prisoners, 57, 141; civil rights of, 54–56; disclosure of serological status of, 54; inadequate medical treatment of, 7, 56; rights of, 7, 54–56; screening of, 13, 55; segregation of, xxiii, 7, 54, 55; state's duty to protect, 54; testing of, 7, 55

Privacy, xxiii, xxx, 6, 7, 8, 9, 11, 12, 14, 15, 18, 28, 31, 33, 34, 38, 41, 43, 44, 45, 46, 54, 55, 57, 61, 64, 70, 72, 73, 75, 77, 80, 81, 89–107, 169, 173, 178, 134, 135, 143, 144, 146, 153, 159, 160, 212, 215, 228, 229, 236, 238, 241, 245; access to one's own data and, 92, 106; claims, 174; commercial marketing and, 89, 95, 96; disclosure for purposes not related to health care, 93, 95; federal regulations on, 9, 91; of HIV registries, 161–62; HIV-specific statutes and, 9, 97; informational, 43, 89–107, 241, 245; in health care system, 91, 93; incidental disclosures and, 94; law enforcement and, 89, 95; litigation, 89; loss of, 177; minimum disclosure standard and, 94; National Privacy Rule, 92, 93, 97, 98; parents' access to minors' records and, 96; proposals for law reform and, 100–106; public health and, 95, 97, 98, 101–6; right to, 173; safeguards in individual states, 45, 97, 100, 240

Privacy Act of 1974, 91

Privacy boards, 95

Probable cause, 140, 214

Prosecutions, 197, 207, 215, 187
Prostitutes, 80, 173, 180, 187, 194, 197, 187. *See also* Sex workers
Prostitutes' Education Network, 74
Protease inhibitor, xxvi, 153
Protected health information, 102. *See also* Privacy
Public accommodations, 57
Public health powers, compulsory, 179–98
Public nuisance: bathhouses as, 34
Puerto Rico, 124, 155, 164
Punitive measures: suggested for people with HIV/AIDS, 180

Quarantine, 64, 77, 179, 183–85

Ransom, Michael, 4
Rape, 64, 66, 188, 194, 201, 202, 203, 205, 208; crisis centers, 205; shield laws, 207; survivors, 201–16 passim
Rape Trauma Syndrome, 204
Ray, Ricky, xxv, 180. *See also* Ricky Ray Hemophilia Relief Fund Act
Reagan, Ronald, xxii, xxv, xxvii, 30
Refugee status, 283
Reglementation, 168, 172
Rehabilitation Act, xxv, 112, 113, 115, 119
Reporting (of HIV cases), xxx, 14, 15, 32, 63, 64, 97, 98, 151–65
—named: 14, 97, 151–65; anonymous testing and, 160–61; privacy and security of HIV registries and, 161–62
—national HIV system and, 161–65
—numerical codes and, 155, 162
Reproduction, 117, 118, 206
Research, HIV/AIDS, 24, 64, 72; ethics in, 23, 24, 311–16
Reverse transcriptase inhibitors, 153
Rhode Island, 155, 234, 267, 268
Ricky Ray Hemophilia Relief Fund Act, xxiii, xxvii. *See also* Ray, Ricky
"Rights rhetoric," 8
Right to health, 64, 78, 81–86: core obli-

gations of, 85; implementation of, 85; normative content of, 84; violations of, 85, 86
Right to know, 9, 14–15, 43, 46, 57, 169, 172, 173, 174, 225
Risk assessment, 203–4
Robinson, Mary, 64
Routine waiver of exclusion, 282, 283
Rubber gloves, xxv, xxvii, 41, 48
Russia, 25, 290
Rwanda, 317
Ryan White Comprehensive AIDS Resources Emergency (CARE) Act, xxii, xxiv, 47, 159, 171, 209, 234

Safe syringe disposal, 273
Sanctions, criminal, 197
San Francisco, Calif., xxvii, 74, 124, 132, 160
San Francisco AIDS Foundation, xxi, xxii, xxiv, 47, 159, 171, 209
Saquinavir, xxvi
Satcher, David, 151, 315
Scientific information: withholding of, 66
Screening, HIV/AIDS, xxiii, xxx, 12, 13, 15, 29, 32–33, 57, 64, 71, 72, 73, 133–50, 231–45, 279–88
—anonymous, 145
—compulsory, 137–38, 140–43, 148, 239
—conditional, 138
—criminal defendants and, 13
—criteria for, 143–44
—employment and, 142
—government conducted or authorized, 142
—health care and, 142
—human rights burdens and, 143, 146
—least restrictive alternative and, 148–49
—paradigm for, 149–50
—premarital, 137, 145
—public acceptability of, 149
—routine, 19, 239–40; with advance

notification (opt-in), 137, 138, 139, 239; without advance notification (opt-out), 138, 139, 239
—substantial public health objective and, 144
—targeted, 236–38
—voluntary, 139–40, 146, 148, 238–39
Security, national: effect of AIDS on, xxiv, 295
Selective enforcement (of criminal law), 198
Self-determination, 75
Semen, 192, 215
Senegal, 23, 301
Seroconversion, 203, 207, 214
Serologic status, 134, 187, 192, 195, 197, 203, 208, 217, 219, 225, 227, 228. *See also* Serostatus
Serostatus, 211, 213, 216. *See also* Serologic status
Sex offenders, 33, 137, 141, 209
Sexual abuse, 80
Sexual assault, xxxi, 201–16; counseling after, 204–6, 213; postexposure prophylaxis and, 204–8; psychological burdens of, 204
Sexual taboos, 148
Sex workers, 8, 28, 48, 64, 66, 71, 72, 73, 74, 75. *See also* Prostitutes
Shalala, Donna, 21, 91
Shanti Project, xxi, 143
Shooting galleries, 20, 143
Short-course antiretroviral regimens, 312–13
"Significant risk" standard, 57
Siracusa Principles, 68
Sixth International Conference on AIDS, xxv, 282
Slavery, 75
Smallpox, 8, 11
Social hygiene movement, 172
Social Network Analysis (SNA), 169, 176, 177
Social Security Administration (SSA), 53

Soundex code, 155
South Africa, xxiii, 23, 62, 202, 300, 302, 305, 307, 308, 314, 317, 321
South African Constitutional Court, 23, 82
South America, 310
South Carolina, 160
South Dakota, 99, 194
Spain, 222
"Special needs" doctrine, 33, 140, 141, 215
Special populations, xxxi, 16
Special Rapporteur (United Nations Commission on Human Rights), 86
Spitting, 184, 188, 194, 196
Stamps, Timothy, 309
State of mind, 186, 187, 196, 214; knowing, 186, 187, 189; purposeful, 186, 187, 189; reckless, 187, 189
Stereotypes, 73, 173
Sterile syringe equipment, 247–75
Stigma, xxv, 9, 41, 57, 67, 79, 86, 94, 101, 109, 130, 135, 164, 169, 170, 173, 196, 218, 229, 237, 279
Subpoenas, 98
Sub-Saharan Africa, xxi, xxviii, 23, 25, 311–12
Sullivan, Louis, 281
Supreme Court, 30, 33, 49, 50, 51, 57, 109, 115, 116, 117, 119, 120, 121, 122, 123, 129, 130, 140, 141, 142, 143, 162, 182, 184, 207, 214, 215, 224, 256
Surgeon-to-patient transmission, 221
Surveillance, xxx, 12, 14, 29, 32, 64, 77, 89, 97, 98, 104, 151–65; confidential, 155; current status of, 154–55; history of, 152–53; future of, 164–65; of intimate behaviors, 189, 197; methods, 155; national HIV, 155–59, 198
Syphilis, 8, 11, 12, 114, 168, 170, 175, 177, 193, 203, 249, 281
Syringe, 20, 247–75; pharmacy regulations, 264–65; pharmacy sales of, 266; prescription laws, 257–64, 272; sterile, 247–75 passim

Vaccines, xxiii, xxvi, xxviii, 75
Vagueness: HIV statutes and, 194
Varmus, Harold, 315
Venereal insontium, 8, 181
Vermont, 155, 209, 267
Vertical transmission, 311
Veterans, 53
Veterans Administration, 91, 92
Viral load, xxvi, 134, 204, 221
Virginia, 258
Virulence, 204
Visa Waiver Pilot Program, 285
Voluntaristic consensus, 137
Voluntary screening. *See* Screening, voluntary

Waiver of exclusion, routine, 282, 283
Warrant, 140, 214
Washington, 155, 164, 209, 267, 269–70
Washington, D.C., 209
Western blot, 136
West Virginia, 47, 184, 209
White House, 219
White House Office of National AIDS Policy (ONAP), xxii, xxvii
Whitman Walker Clinic, xxi

"Window period," 206
Wisconsin, 36, 268
Wolfensohn, James, xvii, 3
Women, xxii, xxiv, xxvi, xxviii, 8, 19, 42, 53, 57, 64, 67, 79, 80, 177, 301; pregnant, xxix, 16, 18, 19, 23, 33, 35, 139, 144, 148, 150, 180, 231; perinatal transmission and, 231–45, 311–13
Working Group on HIV Testing, Counseling, and Prophylaxis after Sexual Assault, 202
World AIDS Day, xxvii
World Bank, 296
World Health Organization (WHO), 22, 64, 82, 288, 296, 298, 303, 311, 312, 313, 321
World Trade Organization (WTO), 24, 306, 307, 308, 309
World War II, 62
World Whores' Summit, 74

Yellow fever, 22

Zambia, 317
Zidovudine (AZT), xxii, xxvi, 207, 311
Zimbabwe, 305, 307, 314

Studies in Social Medicine

Nancy M. P. King, Gail E. Henderson, and Jane Stein, eds., *Beyond Regulations: Ethics in Human Subjects Research* (1999).

Laurie Zoloth, *Health Care and the Ethics of Encounter: A Jewish Discussion of Social Justice* (1999).

Susan M. Reverby, ed. *Tuskegee's Truths: Rethinking the Tuskegee Syphilis Study* (2000).

Beatrix Hoffman, *Wages of Sickness: The Politics of Health Insurance in Progressive America* (2000).

Margarete Sandelowski, *Devices and Desires: Gender, Technology, and American Nursing* (2000).

Keith Wailoo, *Dying in the City of the Blues: Sickle Cell Anemia and the Politics of Race and Health* (2001).

Judith Andre, *Bioethics as Practice* (2002).

Chris Feudtner, *Bittersweet: Diabetes, Insulin, and the Transformation of Illness* (2003).

Ann Folwell Stanford, *Bodies in a Broken World: Women Novelists of Color and the Politics of Medicine* (2003).

Lawrence O. Gostin, *The AIDS Pandemic: Complacency, Injustice, and Unfulfilled Expectations* (2003).

About the Author

Lawrence Gostin is an internationally recognized scholar in public health law and ethics. He is professor of law at Georgetown University; professor of public health at Johns Hopkins University; research fellow at the Centre for Socio-Legal Studies, Oxford University; and the director of the Center for Law and the Public's Health at Johns Hopkins and Georgetown Universities (CDC Collaborating Center, "Promoting Public Health through Law," ⟨http://www.publichealthlaw.net⟩). Professor Gostin is an elected lifetime member of the Institute of Medicine/National Academy of Sciences (IOM/NAS) and serves on the IOM Board on Health Promotion and Disease Prevention. He works closely with national and international public health agencies, including the World Health Organization, UNAIDS, National Institutes of Health, and the Centers for Disease Control and Prevention. He is the health law and ethics editor of the *Journal of the American Medical Association* (JAMA).

In the United Kingdom, Professor Gostin was the chief executive of the National Council for Civil Liberties and legal director of the National Association of Mental Health, where he brought landmark cases before the European Court of Human Rights. He received the Rosemary Delbridge Memorial Award from the National Consumer Council (U.K.) for the person "who has most influenced Parliament and government to act for the welfare of society." His latest books are *Public Health Law: Power, Duty, Restraint* (2000) and *Public Health Law and Ethics: A Reader* (2002).